Cynthia Maxwell, Dan Farine (Eds.)

Pregnancy and Obesity

Hot Topics in Perinatal Medicine

Edited by
Joachim W. Dudenhausen

Volume 5

Cynthia Maxwell, Dan Farine (Eds.)

Pregnancy and Obesity

DE GRUYTER

Editors
Dr. Cynthia Maxwell
Associate Professor, Department of Obstetrics and Gynaecology
University of Toronto
Toronto, Canada
cmaxwell@mtsinai.on.ca

Prof. Dan Farine
Department of Obstetrics and Gynaecology
University of Toronto
Toronto, Canada
dfarine@sympatico.ca

ISSN 2195-5573
ISBN 978-3-11-048624-7
e-ISBN (PDF) 978-3-11-048781-7
e-ISBN (EPUB) 978-3-11-048635-3

Library of Congress Cataloging-in-Publication data
A CIP catalog record for this book has been applied for at the Library of Congress.

Bibliographic information published by the Deutsche Nationalbibliothek
The Deutsche Nationalbibliothek lists this publication in the Deutsche Nationalbibliografie; detailed bibliographic data are available in the Internet at http://dnb.dnb.de.

Cover image: Comstock/Getty Images
Typesetting: Compuscript Ltd., Shannon
Printing and binding: CPI books GmbH, Leck
∞ Printed on acid-free paper
Printed in Germany

www.degruyter.com

This book is dedicated to my children Tali and Jonathan Farine. —Dan Farine

I would like to dedicate this project to the memory of my father, Dr. Samuel Briar Maxwell, who continually inspires me to stay the course and to his granddaughters, Lily and Rose Keunen; my husband, Dr. Han Keunen, for supporting me always and contributing to this work. I would like to acknowledge the efforts of Ms. Dina Maxwell JD, who kindly assisted with editing. Finally, gratitude to my wonderful mentors, Dr. Mathew Sermer, Dr. John Kingdom, and last but not least, Dr. Dan Farine, my co-editor in this project. — Cindy Maxwell

Introduction

Obesity has become the new epidemic. In the developed world, its incidence is consistently increasing to the extent that in some countries and regions, it is more common to be overweight or obese than to have a normal weight. In the developing world, there are several countries with the perplexing reality of obesity coexisting with severe malnourishment. Aside from the increasing incidence of obesity, we find that its burden in terms of individual complications as well as population impact is increasing not only in numbers but also in scope.

Pregnancy presents a unique maternal and fetal environment. Maternal complications coexist with fetal ones and both may affect the course of pregnancy as well as labor and delivery. In addition, pregnancy offers a unique opportunity in transferring obesity and its comorbidities from one generation to the next. We need to explore the issues related to this transfer in order to reduce obesity, diabetes, and metabolic syndrome in the next and future generations.There have been several textbooks on obesity and pregnancy in the last decade. This book is unique in several different ways. It looks at obesity longitudinally from preconception to puerperium. It is a clinical textbook looking at a variety of the aspects of clinical management of women with obesity. At the same time, it deals with basic concepts that do not have a direct impact on clinical management but are crucial for the understanding of the underlying mechanisms for the effects of obesity in pregnancy.

We are thankful to the authors of this book who represent a wide range of expertise. Special thanks to the editor of the series, Prof. Joachim Dudenhausen, for his ongoing support and the publisher, De Gruyter.

Cindy Maxwell and Dan Farine

https://doi.org/10.1515/9783110487817-203

Contents

Section III: **Intrapartum management**

Contributing authors

Chapter 1
Miha Lučovnik, Natasa Tul, Isaac Blickstein
mihalucovnik@yahoo.com;
natasa.tul@kclj.si;
issac_b@clalit.org.il

Chapter 2
Natasa Tul, Isaac Blickstein
natasa.tul@kclj.si;
issac_b@clalit.org.il

Chapter 3
Sarah Crimmins, Julie Rosen, E. Albert Reece,
Menachem Miodovnik
scrimmins@FPI.umaryland.edu;
jwu@som.umaryland.edu;
areece@som.umaryland.edu;
menachem.miodovnik@nih.gov

Chapter 4
Shali Mazaki Tovi, Edi Vaisbuch
shalimazaki@gmail.com;
evaisbuch@gmail.com

Chapter 5
Aubrey R Raimondi, Eyal Sheiner
aubrey.raimondi@gmail.com;
sheiner@bgu.ac.il

Chapter 6
Ellen Greeblatt, Marta Wais
Ellen.Greenblatt@sinaihealthsystem.ca
marta.wais@sinaihealthsystem.ca

Chapter 7
Claire Jones, and Crystal Chan
crystalchan@mtsinai.on.ca;
Claire.Jones@sinaihealthsystem.ca

Chapter 8
Dana Vitner, Kristen Harris, Dan Farine,
Cynthia Maxwell
vitnerdana@gmail.com;
kristin.harris@mail.utoronto.ca
cmaxwell@mtsinai.on.ca;
dfarine@mtsinai.on.ca

Chapter 9
Irene Cetin, Francesca Parisi,
Martina I. Mazzocco
Irene.cetin@unimi.it;
francesca.parisi288@gmail.com;
martina.mazzocco@libero.it

Chapter 10
Sean Wharton
wharton.sean@gmail.com;
ragc.wmc@gmail.com

Chapter 11
Shital Gandhi
SGandhi@mtsinai.on.ca

Chapter 12
Karim Kalache
karim.kalache@charite.de;
kamil.bremen@googlemail.com;
dkamil@sidra.org

Chapter 13
Tim Van Mieghem, Johannes Keunen,
Rory Windrim, Greg Ryan
tim.vanmieghem@sinaihealthsystem.ca;
jkeunen@mtsinai.on.ca;
rwindrim@mtsinai.on.ca;
gryan@mtsinai.on.ca

Chapter 14
Frank Chervenak, Laurence B. McCullough
fac2001@mail.med.cornell.edu;
mccullou@bcm.edu

Chapter 15
Amir Aviram, Yariv Yogev
yarivyogev@hotmail.com;
amiraviram@yahoo.com

Chapter 16
Rohan D'Souza
RD'Souza@mtsinai.on.ca

Chapter 17
Ann Kinga Malinowski, Jacqueline Parrish
amalinowski@mtsinai.on.ca;
jparrish@mtsinai.on.ca

Chapter 18
Kristin Connor
connor@lunenfeld.ca;
kristin.connor@carleton.ca

Chapter 19
Shimrit Yaniv-Salem; Gustaaf Dekker
Shimrit.Yaniv-Salem@sinaihealthsystem.ca;
gustaaf.dekker@adelaide.edu.au

Chapter 20
Stefania Ronzoni, Gian Carlo Di Renzo
stefaniaronzoni@gmail.com;
giancarlo.direnzo@unipg.it

Chapter 21
Aidan Sharkey, Mrinalini Balki
Aidan.Sharkey@sinaihealthsystem.ca;
mrinalini.balki@uhn.ca

Chapter 22
Susan Guest, Cynthia Maxwell
sguest@mtsinai.on.ca;
cmaxwell@mtsinai.on.ca

Chapter 23
Yair Sagi, Cynthia Maxwell
yair.sagi@sinaihealthsystem.ca;
cmaxwell@mtsinai.on.ca

Chapter 24
Christina Nowik, Greg Davies
daviesg@KGH.KARI.NET;
christinanowik@gmail.com

Section I: **Planning for pregnancy**

Miha Lučovnik, Nataša Tul and Isaac Blickstein

1 Epidemiology of obesity

1.1 Introduction

Obesity is a medical condition in which an excessive amount of adipose tissue has accumulated to the extent that it may impair health [1]. Excess body fat is deleterious to multiple organ systems through thrombogenic, atherogenic, oncogenic, hemodynamic, and neurohumoral mechanisms [2,3]. Numerous epidemiological studies have demonstrated associations between obesity and various diseases, such as diabetes mellitus, heart disease, and several types of cancer [2–7]. Obesity has also been shown to have a negative effect on psychosocial as well as economic aspects of life [8].

In 1997, the World Health Organization (WHO) formally recognized obesity as a global epidemic [1]. Despite multiple efforts to address this public health issue, the prevalence of obesity continues to increase [1]. As the prevalence of obesity is increasing, so is the number of obese women of reproductive age. Consequently, obesity complicates a significant proportion of pregnancies [9]. These pregnancies are at increased risk of several maternal as well as fetal adverse outcomes, which are described in more detail elsewhere in this book.

In this chapter, we will discuss different methods to diagnose excess adipose tissue (obesity). We will also review current epidemiological data on the prevalence of obesity in the general population as well as specific data on the prevalence of obesity in pregnant women.

1.2 Definitions of obesity – advantages and disadvantages of using body mass index

Obesity is defined by the WHO as excessive fat accumulation [1]. However, the amount of body fat can be assessed by many different measures. The body mass index (BMI) is the most commonly used anthropometric method to define obesity. BMI is calculated as an individual's weight in kilograms divided by the height in meters squared. This measurement was first described by a Belgian mathematician Adolphus Quetelet in the mid-19th century based on the observation that body weight was proportional to the square of the height in adults with "normal body frames" [10]. Commonly used definitions of underweight, normal weight, overweight, and obesity based on BMI were established by the WHO and are presented in Tab. 1.1 [11]. As Asian populations develop negative health consequences of obesity at a lower BMI, some nations redefined different BMI cutoffs for obesity. The Japanese defined obesity as any BMI greater than 25, whereas China uses a BMI of greater than 28 [12, 13].

https://doi.org/10.1515/9783110487817-001

Tab. 1.1: Classification of adult underweight, overweight, and obesity according to BMI [11].

Category	BMI
Underweight	<18.5
Normal weight	18.5–24.9
Overweight	25.0–29.9
Class I obesity	30.0–34.9
Class II obesity	35.0–39.9
Class III obesity	≥40.0

There are several advantages of using BMI as a diagnostic method for obesity. It is easily applicable in epidemiological studies because it only depends on two commonly measured quantities, i.e., height and weight. BMI has also been widely incorporated into clinical practice due to its noninvasiveness and simplicity. Moreover, numerous studies have shown associations between BMI-defined obesity and mortality [14–16]. BMI also correlates reasonably well with more accurate measurements of percent body fat including densitometry and dual energy X-ray absorptiometry, which are the reference methods for assessment of body composition [17–19]. This is especially true in individuals with high BMIs, indicating that BMI has good specificity and positive predictive value to diagnose obesity.

On the other hand, measuring BMI also presents some disadvantages with regard to pregnancy. The overwhelming majority of studies published on this subject used a BMI cutoff of $\geq 30\ kg/m^2$ to estimate risks of adverse perinatal outcomes associated with obesity. The main limitation of BMI is that it does not distinguish between the mass associated with bones, muscles and organs (lean body mass), and that associated with fat tissue (body fat mass). BMI, therefore, contains two factors (lean body mass and adipose tissue) that have opposite biological effects. Although adipose tissue has been associated with deleterious health outcomes, preserved lean mass is positively associated with physical fitness, higher caloric expenditure, exercise capacity, and survival [20–22]. Therefore, whereas the specificity of BMI to diagnose excess body fat is high, the sensitivity is relatively low, and as many as 50% of individuals with high body fat percentage are missed by using BMI alone [19]. This issue is even more important in pregnant women because fetal, placental, and amniotic fluid mass represent more or less an unknown part of the total body mass. Moreover, BMI provides no information on the distribution of body fat. This is an important weakness of the method because abdominal obesity has been shown to be associated with significantly greater health risks [23].

Several alternatives to BMI for determining body composition and percentage of body fat have been described and are currently being studied. They are, however, expensive, cumbersome, and/or not insufficiently accurate. Precise determination of body fat content in pregnancy is particularly challenging for several reasons. Some techniques, such as dual energy X-ray absorptiometry or computed tomography, are only rarely applied during pregnancy because of radiation exposure [24]. Methods such as magnetic resonance imaging or underwater weighing use sophisticated equipment that is not available for routine use [25]. Anthropometric measures, other than BMI, for body composition assessment rely on measurements of skinfolds in different locations (e.g., triceps, subscapular, abdominal, and mid-calf) and measurements of different circumferences (e.g., waist, arm, and thigh). Measurements are used in equations that more or less accurately estimate the body fat content [26]. Physiological changes in pregnancy affect skin tension and make measurement of skinfolds challenging, especially in the abdominal region. Consequently, only few anthropometric measurements can realistically be performed during pregnancy. Moreover, the existing anthropometric methods have often been developed for use in nonpregnant women and only rarely specifically for pregnancy [26–28]. Even pregnancy-specific anthropometric methods, however, showed large discrepancies in body composition [29]. Current knowledge, therefore, does not allow selecting a more appropriate method than BMI for reliable routine determination of body fat percentage before and during pregnancy.

In conclusion, obesity is currently most often defined by BMI. This is certainly a useful measure for basic epidemiological evaluation of obesity prevalence. However, BMI can provide misleading information on the actual content of body fat. This is especially true when BMI is measured during pregnancy.

1.3 Prevalence of obesity

Obesity has become the most prevalent preventable cause of death worldwide [5]. According to WHO data, the global prevalence of obesity in 2014 was 15% in women and 11% in men. This means that more than 600 million adults were obese in 2014 [1]. Figure 1.1 displays the WHO data on the prevalence of obesity for each country.

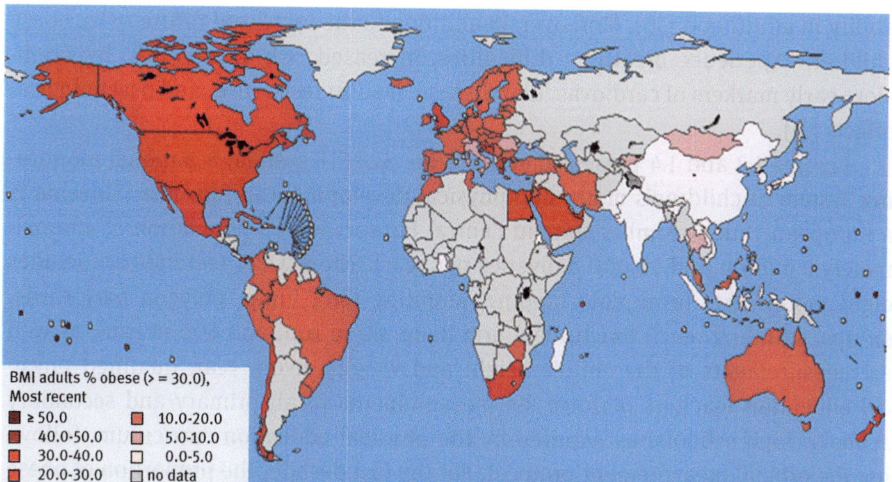

Fig. 1.1: World map displaying national data on prevalence of obesity [Source: World Health Organization; available at: http://apps.who.int/bmi/index.jsp].

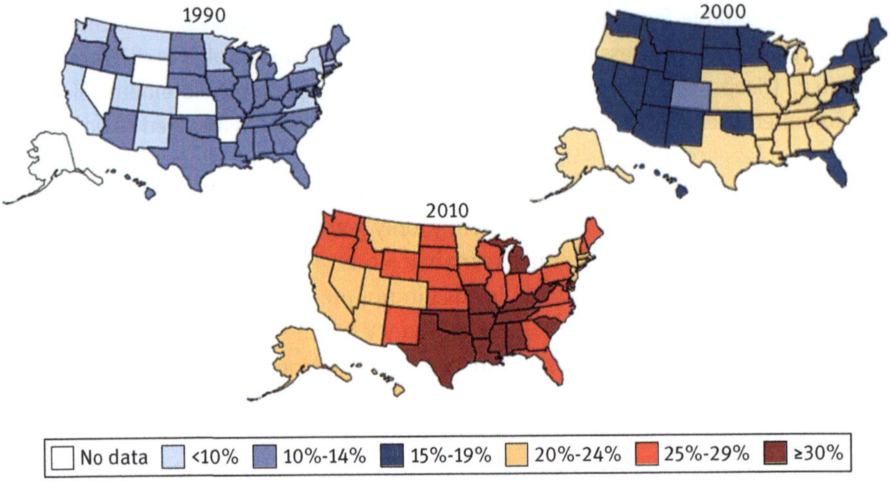

Fig. 1.2: Obesity trends among US adults. 1990, 2000, and 2010 (Source: Behavioral Risk Factor Surveillance System, CDC; available at: https://www.cdc.gov/obesity/downloads/data/obesity-trends-map_1985-2010.pdf).

Obesity trends are even more worrying than its current high prevalence. The prevalence of obesity more than doubled between 1980 and 2014 and continues to increase worldwide [1]. Figure 1.2 shows the increase in obesity rates among US adults during the period 1990 to 2000. What was once considered a problem of high-income countries is now on the rise in low- and middle-income countries as well [1]. Of special concern is the increase in obesity among children and adolescents. Childhood obesity is associated with a higher risk of obesity, premature death, and disability in adulthood [30]. Moreover, in addition to the increased future risks, obese children experience breathing difficulties, increased risk of fractures, hypertension, early markers of cardiovascular disease, insulin resistance, and psychological effects [31].

Figures 1.3 and 1.4 present data from the SLOFIT system, a national monitoring system of children's motor and physical development in Slovenia (Slovenia is a European Union member state in Central Europe, with a population of approximately 2 million and 20,000 deliveries per year). The SLOFIT test battery includes eight motor tests (arm-plate tapping, standing long jump, polygon backwards, sit-ups, standing reach touch, bent arm hang, 60 m run, and 600 m run), as well as measurements of the child's height and weight. Every year, qualified physical education teachers perform the measurements in all primary and secondary schools (high schools) as required by the physical education curriculum, following the official measurement protocol. For the last decade, the proportion of obese high school girls has been increasing (Fig. 1.3). Interestingly, we also found a high

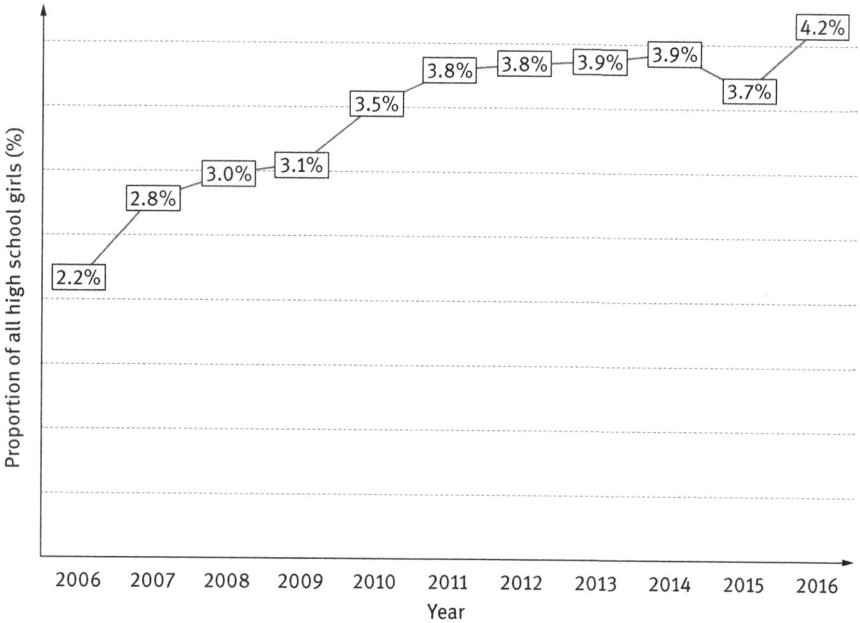

Fig. 1.3: Increase in prevalence of obesity (defined as BMI ≥30 kg/m²) among high school girls in Slovenia (unpublished data, courtesy of Gregor Starc, PhD, Faculty of Sport, University of Ljubljana, Slovenia).

proportion (44%–56%) of 18- to 19-year-old girls with normal BMI (18.5–24.9 kg/m²) but reduced exercise capacity (defined as low physical fitness index derived from the eight motor tests used in the SLOFIT system) (Fig. 1.4). These are physically unfit girls, who are most probably maintaining their normal BMI with unhealthy dietary habits and without regular physical activity. Their unhealthy lifestyle makes them at risk of health complications later in life and also during pregnancies. This emphasizes the above-mentioned shortcomings of the BMI to accurately assess body composition and risks for future health.

Given the increasing number of obese girls and short-term as well as long-term adverse health consequences of obesity, strategies to prevent obesity by healthier choices of food and regular physical activity should become a high priority in our societies. The first and the ideal goal in managing obesity-associated pregnancy complications is prevention. Clinicians should encourage changes in dietary and physical activity patterns that will lead to weight loss in obese children and adolescents. Realistically, however, the achievement of this goal is very difficult. The lifestyle that leads to obesity is often perpetuated by lack of supportive policies in many sectors: agriculture, food processing, transport, marketing, urban planning, education, and also health services.

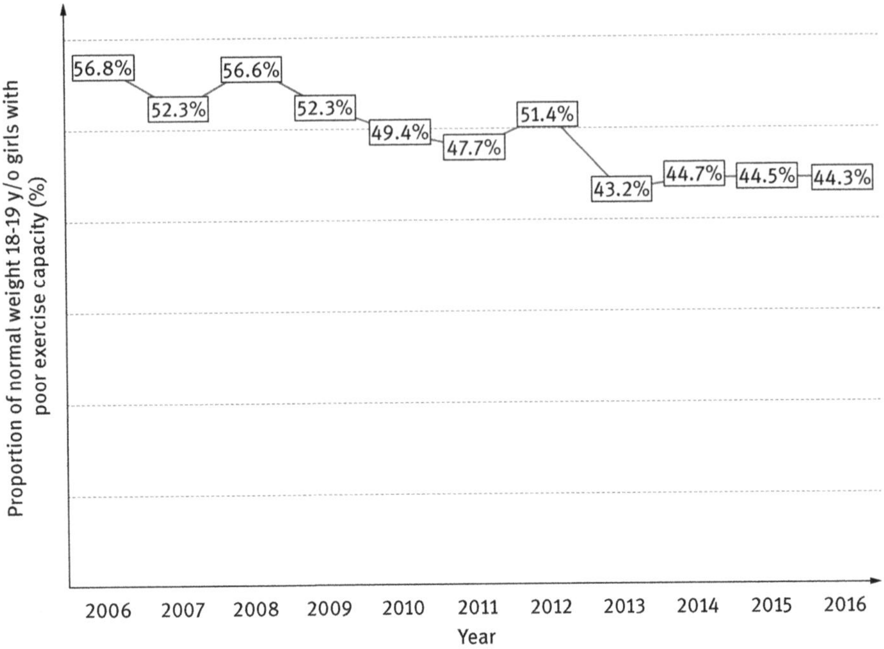

Fig. 1.4: Proportion of 18- to 19-year-old girls with normal BMI (18.5–24.9 kg/m^2) but reduced exercise capacity (unpublished data, courtesy of Gregor Starc, PhD, Faculty of Sport, University of Ljubljana, Slovenia).

1.4 Epidemiology of obesity in pregnancy

As obesity became one of the most important threats to human health in general, it also became one of the most common medical conditions complicating pregnancy [32]. At least 10% of women in industrialized counties are obese before conception, with significant variations in prevalence from country to county [9,32].

Figure 1.5 shows changes in the prevalence of prepregnancy BMI categories in Slovenia from 2002 to 2014 (data from the Slovenian National Perinatal Information System). Slovenian National Perinatal Information System registers all deliveries in Slovenia at ≥22 weeks of pregnancy or when the birth weight is ≥500 g. Registration is mandatory by law in the country's 14 maternity units and more than 140 variables are entered into a computerized database by the attending midwife and physician. These include women's height and weight. The method of registering maternal prepregnancy weight is particularly accurate and presumably without recall bias because prepregnancy data are registered very early during pregnancy. To assure quality of data collection, controls are built into the computerized system, data is audited periodically, and comparisons are made with international databases in which Slovenia

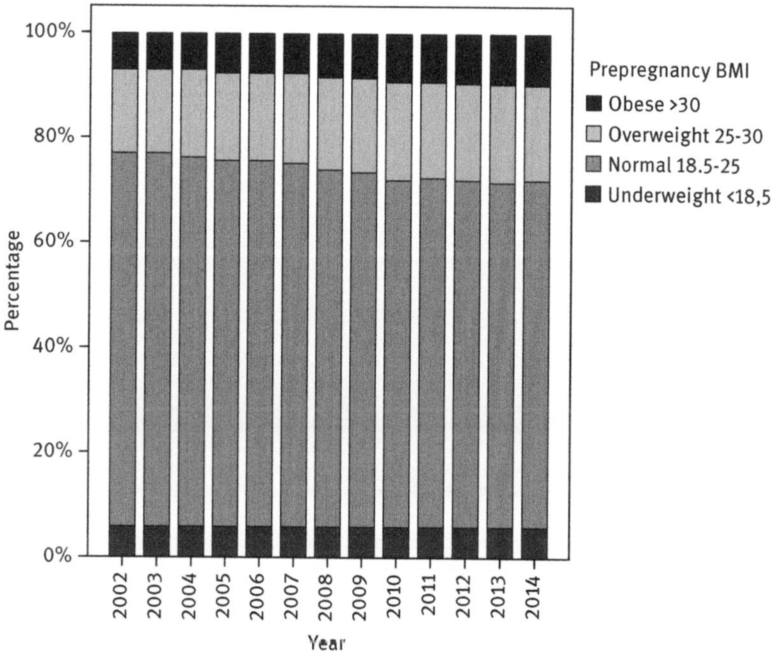

Fig. 1.5: Changes in prevalence of prepregnancy BMI categories (Slovenian National Perinatal System data).

participates. Our data on prepregnancy BMI show that the prevalence of underweight and normal weight women is decreasing, whereas the prevalence of prepregnancy overweight and obesity is increasing (Fig. 1.5). This is in accordance with data on the increasing prevalence of obesity in high school girls, as shown in Fig. 1.4. The increase in prepregnancy obesity rate is seen in all three classes of obesity, i.e., class I, II, and III as defined in Tab. 1.1 (Fig. 1.6).

Figure 1.7 shows the importance of discussing the optimal weight gain during pregnancy with obese pregnant patients. Women who were overweight or obese before pregnancy were more likely to gain more weight than recommended by the 2009 Institute of Medicine guidelines on optimal gestational weight gain shown in Tab. 1.2 [33]. Excessive gestational weight gain increases the risks of pregnancy complications beyond those related to prepregnancy overweight and obesity *per se* [33, 34]. Moreover, excessive gestational weight gain is the strongest factor for weight retention after birth and it further increases the risks of prepregnancy obesity in the next pregnancy [35]. There is evidence that receiving appropriate dietary consultation about weight gain correlates with actual weight gain within the guidelines [36]. Unfortunately, according to the literature, up to one-third of women are not counseled at all by their prenatal care providers on the appropriate and advisable weight gain during pregnancy [36].

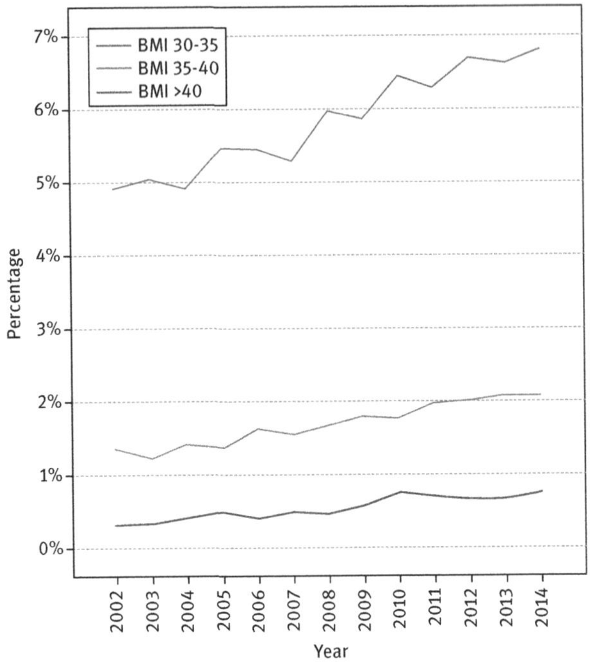

Fig. 1.6: Changes in prevalence of prepregnancy obesity class I, II, and III (Slovenian National Perinatal Information System data).

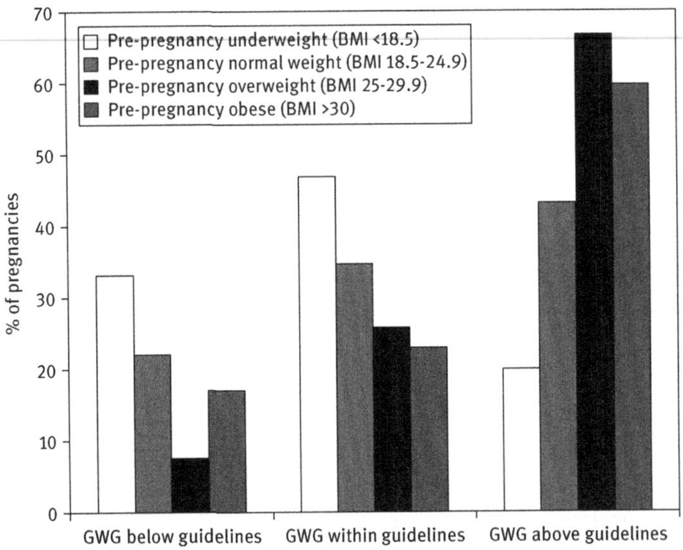

Fig. 1.7: Gestational weight gain (GWG) according to the Institute of Medicine guidelines for each prepregnancy BMI categories (Slovenian National Perinatal Information System data).

Tab. 1.2: Recommendations of gestational weight gain by prepregnancy BMI according to the 2009 Institute of Medicine guidelines [33].

Prepregnancy BMI	Singleton pregnancy	Twin pregnancy
Underweight <18.5	12.5–18 kg	Insufficient data
Normal weight 18.5–24.9	11.5–16 kg	17–25 kg
Overweight 25.0–29.9	7–11.5 kg	14–23 kg
Obesity ≥30.0	5–9 kg	11–19 kg

Bibliography

[1] WHO (World Health Organization). Obesity and overweight. Fact sheet. 2016. Available at: http://www.who.int/mediacentre/factsheets/fs311/en/index.html. Accessed: December 1, 2016.

[2] Pi-Sunyer FX. The obesity epidemic: pathophysiology and consequences of obesity. Obes Res 2002;10 [Suppl 2]:97S–104S.

[3] Poirier P, Giles TD, Bray GA, Hong Y, Stern JS, Pi-Sunyer FX, et al. Obesity and cardiovascular disease: pathophysiology, evaluation, and effect of weight loss. Arterioscler Thromb Vasc Biol 2006;26:968–76.

[4] Fontaine KR, Redden DT, Wang C, Allison DB. Years of life lost due to obesity. JAMA 2003:289, 187–93.

[5] Haslam DW, James WPT. Obesity. Lancet 2005;366:1197–1209.

[6] National Institutes of Health Consensus Development Panel. Health implications of obesity: National Institutes of Health Consensus Conference Statement. Ann Intern Med 1985;103:1073–7.

[7] Poirier P, Giles TD, Bray GA, Hong Y, Stern JS, Pi-Sunyer FX, et al. Obesity and cardiovascular disease: pathophysiology, evaluation, and effect of weight loss: an update of the 1997 American Heart Association scientific statement on obesity and heart disease from the Obesity Committee of the Council on Nutrition, Physical Activity, and Metabolism. Circulation 2006;113:898–918.

[8] Colditz GA. Economic costs of obesity. Am J Clin Nutr 1992;55:503S–507S.

[9] Yogev Y, Catalano PM. Pregnancy and obesity. Obstet Gynecol Clin N Am 2009;36:185–300.

[10] Quetelet, A. A treatise on man and the development of his faculties. Burt Franklin; New York: Originally published in 1842. Reprinted in 1968.

[11] WHO (World Health Organization). BMI classification. 2016. Available at: http://apps.who.int/bmi/index.jsp?introPage=intro_3.html Accessed: December 1, 2016.

[12] Kanazawa M, Yoshiike N, Osaka T, Numba Y, Zimmet P, Inoue S. Criteria and classification of obesity in Japan and Asia-Oceania. Asia Pac J Clin Nutr 2002;11 (Suppl) 8:S732–S737.

[13] Bei-Fan Z. Cooperative meta-analysis group of working group on obesity in China. Predictive values of body mass index and waist circumference for risk factors of certain related diseases in Chinese adults: study on optimal cut-off points of body mass index and waist circumference in Chinese adults. Asia Pac J Clin Nutr 2002;11 (Suppl) 8:S685–93.

[14] Romero-Corral A, Montori VM, Somers VK, Korinek J, Thomas RJ, Allison TG, et al. Association of bodyweight with total mortality and with cardiovascular events in coronary artery disease: a systematic review of cohort studies. Lancet 2006;368:666–78.

[15] McGee DL. Body mass index and mortality: a meta-analysis based on person-level data from twenty-six observational studies. Ann Epidemiol 2005;15:87–97.
[16] Flegal KM, Graubard BI, Williamson DF, Gail MH. Cause-specific excess deaths associated with underweight, overweight, and obesity. JAMA 2007;298:2028–37.
[17] Gallagher D, Visser M, Sepulveda D, Pierson RN, Harris T, Heymsfield SB. How useful is body mass index for comparison of body fatness across age, sex, and ethnic groups? Am J Epidemiol 1996;143:228–39.
[18] Morabia A, Ross A, Curtin F, Pichard C, Slosman DO. Relation of BMI to a dual-energy X-ray absorptiometry measure of fatness. Br J Nutr 1999;82:49–55.
[19] Romero-Corral A, Somers VK, Sierra-Johnson J, Thomas RJ, Collazo-Clavell ML, Korinek J, Allison TG, Batsis JA, Sert-Kuniyoshi FH, Lopez-Jimenez F. Accuracy of body mass index in diagnosing obesity in the adult general population. Int J Obes (Lond) 2008;32:959–66.
[20] Adams KF, Schatzkin A, Harris TB, Kipnis V, Mouw T, Ballard-Barbash R, et al. Overweight, obesity, and mortality in a large prospective cohort of persons 50–71 years old. N Engl J Med 2006;355:763–78.
[21] O'Donovan G, Owen A, Kearney EM, Jones DW, Nevill AM, Woolf-May K, et al. Cardiovascular disease risk factors in habitual exercisers, lean sedentary men and abdominally obese sedentary men. Int J Obes (Lond) 2005;29:1063–9.
[22] Goldberg AP, Busby-Whitehead MJ, Katzel LI, Krauss RM, Lumpkin M, Hagberg JM. Cardiovascular fitness, body composition, and lipoprotein lipid metabolism in older men. J Gerontol A Biol Sci Med Sci 2000;55:342–9.
[23] Fox KAA, Despres JP, Richard AJ, Brette S, Deanfield JE. Does abdominal obesity have a similar impact on cardiovascular disease and diabetes? A study of 91246 ambulant patients in 27 European countries. Eur Heart J 2009;30:3055–63.
[24] Cunningham JL, Fordham JN, Hewitt TA, Speed CA. Ultrasound velocity and attenuation at different skeletal sites compared with bone mineral density measured using dual energy X-ray absorptiometry. Br J Radiol 1996;69:25–32.
[25] Paxton A, Lederman SA, Heymsfield SB, Wang J, Thornton JC, Pierson RN Jr. Anthropometric equations for studying body fat in pregnant women. Am J Clin Nutr 1998;67:104–10.
[26] van Raaij JM, Peek ME, Vermaat-Miedema SH, Schonk CM, Hautvast JG. New equations for estimating body fat mass in pregnancy from body density or total body water. Am J Clin Nutr 1988;48:24–9.
[27] Catalano PM, Wong WW, Drago NM, Amini SB. Estimating body composition in late gestation: a new hydration constant for body density and total body water. Am J Physiol 1995;268:153–8.
[28] Paxton A, Lederman SA, Heymsfield SB, Wang J, Thornton JC, Pierson RN Jr. Anthropometric equations for studying body fat in pregnant women. Am J Clin Nutr 1998;67:104–10.
[29] Robič T, Benedik E, Fidler Mis N, Bratanič B, Rogelj I, Golja P. Challenges in determining body fat in pregnant women. Ann Nutr Metab 2013;63:341–9.
[30] Yang X, Telama R, Leskinen E, Mansikkaniemi K, Viikari JSA, Raitakari OT. Testing a model of physical activity and obesity tracking from youth to adulthood: the cardiovascular risk in young Finns study. Int J Obes (Lond) 2007;31:521–7.
[31] Centers for Disease Control (CDC). Childhood obesity facts. Available at: http://www.cdc.gov/healthyschools/obesity/facts.htm. Accessed: December 3, 2016.
[32] Lu GC, Rouse DJ, Dubard M, Cliver S, Kimberlin D, Hauth JC. The effect of increasing prevalence of maternal obesity on perinatal morbidity. Am J Obstet Gynecol 2001;185:845–9.
[33] Institute of Medicine. Weight gain during pregnancy: reexamining the guidelines. 2009. Available at: http://www.iom.edu/Reports/2009/Weight-Gain-During-Pregnancy-Reexamining-the-Guidelines.aspx. Accessed: December 1, 2012.

[34] Lucovnik M, Blickstein I, Verdenik I, Steblovnik L, Trojner Bregar A, Tul N. Impact of pre-gravid body mass index and body mass index change on preeclampsia and gestational diabetes in singleton and twin pregnancies. J Matern Fetal Neonatal Med 2014;27:1901–4.
[35] Greene GW, Smiciklas-Wright H, Scholl TO, Karp RJ. Postpartum weight change: how much of the weight gained in pregnancy will be lost after delivery? Obstet Gynecol 1988;71:701–7.
[36] Stotland NE, Haas JS, Brawarsky P, Jackson RA, Fuentes-Afflick E, Escobar RJ. Body mass index, provider advice, and target gestational weight gain. Obstet Gynecol 2005;105:663–8.

Isaac Blickstein and Nataša Tul

2 How useful are the guidelines for weight gain in pregnancy?

2.1 Introduction

Controlling maternal nutrition was often an essential part of pregnancy care. In older times, the association of obesity and both preeclampsia (PET) and large babies was already known. Thus, restricting weight gain during pregnancy to reduce PET and dystocia was generally advised. Because excessive weight gain was considered a sign of PET-associated edema, the recommended weight gain in the 1930s was up to 15 lbs. (6.8 kg) [1]. It is believed that the modern approach to maternal weight gain started with the seminal work of Hytten and Leitch [2], who in 1971, established the physiologic range of total pregnancy weight gain, the rate of gain in the second half of pregnancy, and the rate of gain associated with the best outcomes. They used data collected by other researchers of more than 3,800 women and reached three main conclusions [3]. First, that physiologic average total weight gain of the so-called "healthy primigravid women eating without restriction" is 12.5 kg – comprising 1 kg in the first trimester and the rest during the second and third trimesters. No estimates were provided for multigravid women. Second, the authors used weight gain data from a Scottish maternity hospital for 486 healthy women without weight gain control (aged 20 to 29 years, >160 cm tall, birth at 39 to 41 weeks' gestation). They found a wide range of the rate of gain during the last half of pregnancy (<0.1 to 0.9 kg/week). Third, the lowest incidence of adverse outcomes in terms of PET, low birth weight, and perinatal deaths was associated with gaining 0.45 kg/week during the second half of pregnancy [3]. Approximately two decades later, the Institute of Medicine (IOM) issued the first set of weight gain recommendations for singleton pregnancies [4]. These recommendations were subjected to numerous studies, systematically reviewed by Siega-Riz and her coworkers [5]. On the one hand, they found a strong association between excessive maternal gestational weight gain and increased fetal growth and large-for-gestational age (LGA) neonates. On the other hand, an association exists between inadequate gestational weight gain and small-for-gestational age (SGA) infants.

Almost two decades later, in 2009, the IOM issued the second set of recommendations for weight gain during pregnancy [6]. The second edition was issued because of the apparent change in the incidence of overweight and obese American women during reproductive age. Indeed, a recent survey of US adults found an age-adjusted prevalence of obesity as high as 40.4% among women, including as many as 9.9% of class 3 obesity (BMI ≥40.0 kg/m^2) [7]. Importantly, the prevalence of overall obesity and of class 3 obesity in American women showed significant linear trends for increase between 2005 and 2014 [7].

https://doi.org/10.1515/9783110487817-002

Despite these robust observations from the Institute of Medicine [4], it was not entirely clear to what extent the IOM recommended weight gain was implemented during pregnancy and which proportion of pregnant women achieved or did not achieve the recommended weight gain. Despite these shortcomings, a recent Committee Opinion released by the American College of Obstetricians and Gynecologists (ACOG) addressed maternal weight gain during pregnancy [8]. This chapter examines the limitations related to how useful the guidelines are for weight gain in pregnancy.

2.2 Accuracy and limits of weight gain estimations

Ideally, weight gain should be measured at every fixed, exact, and pre-established interval of gestation. Then, it would be possible to know exactly how much weight was gained, say, by 13 weeks, 20 weeks, and so on. Regrettably, this is impossible even in prospective studies. For example, even if the pregravid weight is known, there can be much difference in the gestational age at birth (i.e., duration of gestation varies from one case to another).

In many studies, weight gain for a given week is extrapolated by multiplying the average weekly weight gain by the number of weeks in question. For example, if a patient gained 20 kg during 40 weeks, the extrapolated weight gain at 28 weeks gestation would be 14 kg (20 kg/40 weeks = 0.5 kg/week; 0.5 kg/week × 28 weeks = 14 kg), although weight is almost never evenly gained during pregnancy.

Whereas weight during pregnancy should be measured in a relatively accurate way, the pregravid weight may suffer from recall bias, depending on the maternal recollection of when and how much she weighed before pregnancy. Quite often, this is at best an educated guess. To overcome this problem, researchers use the maternal weight at the first pregnancy check-up, at a time when the pregnant woman might suffer from nausea and vomiting or from an uncontrolled appetite, which may cause inaccurate pregravid weight recording.

Even if it is expected that all scales are regularly calibrated, there is a well-known variation across scales. Overall, the higher the weight, the less precise was the measurement, to the extent that at higher weights, more than 15% of scales were off by more than 2.3 kg [9]. This study showed that many scales are imprecise and that scales in health care settings are no more precise than those in other facilities such as primary care clinics, endocrinology clinics, weight loss facilities, and fitness centers [9].

Dietary intervention during pregnancy may also change the overall weight gain. The best example is the management of gestational diabetes mellitus (GDM) with changes of lifestyle and dietary intervention [10].

Additionally, the IOM recommendations did not specify the week of gestation to achieve the recommended weight gain, thus "term" usually lumps all gestational ages above 38 + 0 weeks. Moreover, weight gain at the end of pregnancy frequently reflects water retention, and thus, might not reflect calories-induced weight gain. At present, there is no way to establish the origin of weight gain. Finally, because not all pregnancies end at the same gestational age, some studies "round up" all pregnancies at term, ignoring differences in maternal weight in every week from 38 weeks onwards.

2.3 The recommended weight gain during pregnancy

The 2009 IOM recommended weight gain during pregnancy is supposed to balance the benefits and risks of weight gain for both mother and child's health. The first element tailors weight gain to different pregravid weight categories (BMI standards). Logically, underweight women need more weight gain than normal weight women, normal weight women need less than overweight women, and overweight women should gain less than obese women. Second, it details, within each weight category, how much should be gained during each week in the second and third trimesters. Finally, separate recommendations for twin gestations were issued. These IOM guidelines were adopted in 2013 and reaffirmed in 2015 by the ACOG Committee Opinion [8].

It seems that the guidelines issued for Americans may not be universally suitable. Fujiwara and coworkers [11] compared the weight gain of pregnant Japanese women to the IOM recommendations and reached the conclusion that the guidelines for gestational weight gain may lack external validity in Japanese women, especially for lean and normal weight women. Additionally, the ACOG Committee Opinion [8] itself voiced some reservations regarding the IOM guidelines. First, that weight gain targets, especially for overweight and obese women, seem to be too high. Second, the recommendations did not differentiate between the three degrees of obesity [12], namely, pregravid BMI 30.0 to 34.9 (Class I), BMI 35.0 to 39.9 (Class II), and BMI 40 or more (Class III or morbid obesity). Finally, the IOM recommendations failed to mention any risk related to postpartum weight retention in those who did or did not gain weight as recommended.

2.4 Weight gain in "real life" as compared with the IOM recommendations

A recent examination of a particularly accurate Slovenian database [13] examined "real life" weight gain in 173,715 patients that were, by and large, unexposed to the IOM recommendations. This cohort was composed of 5.0% (95% CI 4.9–5.1) underweight, 69.4% (95% CI, 69.1–69.6) normal weight, 17.7% (95% CI 17.5–17.9) overweight, and 7.9% (95% CI 7.7–7.9) obese patients. All in all, the recommended weight gain was achieved by roughly one-third (32.7%, 95% CI 32.5–32.9), almost half (47.6%, 95% CI 47.3–47.8) gained more than recommended, and roughly one-fifth (19.7%, 95% CI 19.5–19.5) gained less than recommended. These frequencies were remarkably similar to other studies. For example, in hospital-based data from Central Massachusetts [14], it was observed that 16.7%, 30.8%, and 52.6% were undergainers, appropriate gainers, and overgainers, respectively. A Chinese multicenter study also revealed that only 36.8% of the women gained weight within the recommended range, and 25% and 38.2% were undergainers and overgainers, respectively [15]. A US study found that 45.1% gained appropriately, whereas 31.4% and 23.5% were undergainers and overgainers, respectively [16]. Bearing in mind the difference between hospital- and population-based data, it is believed that the latter more accurately described the true frequency of mothers that gained weight as recommended. Thus, it seems that roughly two-thirds of the population needed dietary intervention to meet the IOM guidelines.

2.5 BMI category and weight gain according to the IOM recommendations

A related question to the above-mentioned observation is which BMI category is more or less likely related to weight gain according to the IOM recommendations. The Slovenian study [13] was able to reply to this question: as shown in Fig. 2.1, gaining more than recommended was much more frequent among overweight and obese mothers whereas gaining less than recommended was much more frequent among normal weight and underweight mothers. Figure 2.1 also shows that the higher the pregravid BMI, the lower the frequency of optimal weight gain. The frequency of less than optimal weight gain also decreased with increasing pregravid BMI but increased again in obese patients. In contrast, weight gain that was higher than the recommended range increased gradually from the underweight group to the overweight and obese groups.

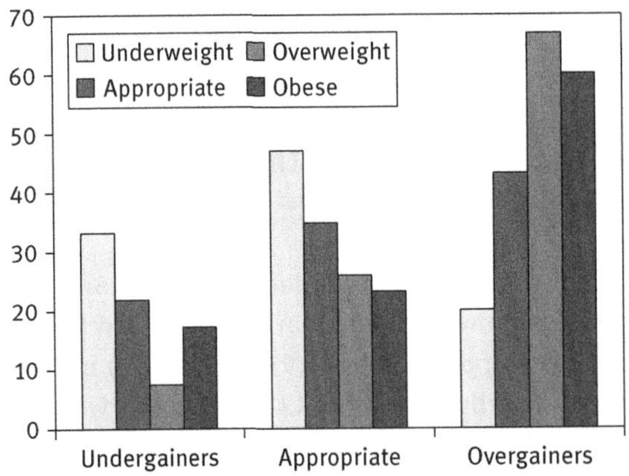

Fig. 2.1: Incidence (%) of the recommended weight gain by BMI category according to the 2009 Institute of Medicine recommendations. Adapted from Tul et al. [13].

These observations might prove clinically important for identifying the BMI subgroup that is more likely to benefit from dietary intervention. Plausibly, to meet the IOM recommendations, women with pregravid low BMIs should be encouraged to gain more weight whereas those with pregravid high BMIs should be advised to gain less weight.

2.6 Appropriate weight gain and maternal outcomes

Weight gain during pregnancy may influence maternal outcomes. Usually, studies focused on the incidence of preeclampsia, gestational diabetes, and cesarean section. Figure 2.2 shows the trend of the incidence of PET with increasing weight gain in each BMI category. The robust influence of weight gain is mainly apparent among the overweight and obese mothers, pointing to the fundamental risk of PET in pregravid overweight and obesity [10]. Because pregnant women diagnosed with GDM are more likely to keep a diet (and hence, to alter the weight gain pattern), the data related to

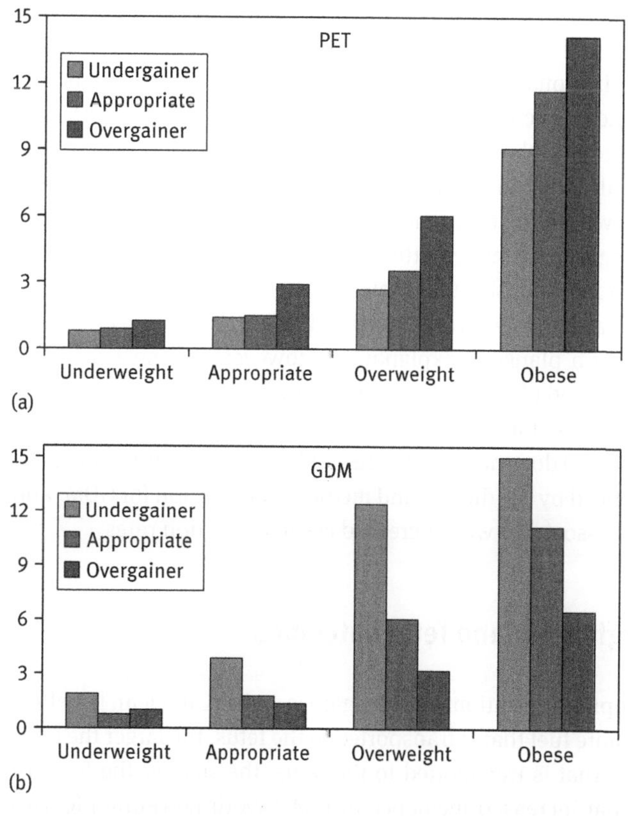

Fig. 2.2: Incidence (%) of PET and GDM by pregravid BMI category and weight gain according to the 2009 Institute of Medicine recommendations. Adapted from Tul et al. [13].

GDM (Fig. 2.2) show the effect of dietary intervention following the diagnosis of GDM, with the expected increased frequency of undergainers with each BMI category [10].

These observations are supported by the systemic review of randomized trials on the ability to reduce PET by antepartum weight management strategies. For instance, Ho et al. [17] found no evidence to suggest that antenatal weight management interventions were effective in reducing the incidence of PET in overweight and obese women. Similarly, a Dutch study [18] showed that a reduction in weight gain due to lifestyle and dietary interventions in pregnancy failed to lower the incidence of PET and GDM. Finally, the effect of treatment on patterns of weight gain in GDM pregnancies was also demonstrated by the different patterns associated with different treatment modality (diet alone, insulin, or glyburide) [19].

Another concern is the effect of weight gain on cesarean birth rates. In the analysis of 24,327 women who underwent cesarean section, Trojner-Bregar and her associates [20] found that the overall frequency of cesarean birth increases as BMI increases irrespective of weight gain pattern. However, different patterns were noted for the frequencies of urgent versus elective cesarean birth. Cedergren [21] used a prospective population-based cohort of 245,526 singleton term pregnancies to group women into five categories of BMI and three gestational weight gain categories. Despite the somewhat different categorizations of BMI and weight gain, obese women with low gestational weight gain had a decreased risk for cesarean section, whereas high gestational weight gain increased the risk for cesarean delivery in all maternal BMI classes. Similarly, Crane et al. [22] found that the rate of cesarean section was lower in women who gained weight within the recommended weight gain range than in those with excess weight gain. Regrettably, none of these studies eliminated potential confounders [20 22] and thus none were able to establish a cause-and-effect relationship between excessive gestational weight gain and increased risk of cesarean section – by itself an association without a plausible explanation. However, the most probable culprit is the increased likelihood of a large fetus (see below).

In summary, it seems that keeping women within the IOM recommended weight gain range during pregnancy (a) does not alter the risk of PET; (b) the pattern of gestational weight gain is influenced by the dietary and medical intervention for GDM; and (c) excessive weight gain is associated with increased cesarean section rates.

2.7 Appropriate weight gain and fetal outcomes

Whereas the effect of appropriate gestational weight gain is, at best, unclear, the effect on the fetus is robust: the more fuel that is transported to the fetus, the larger the fetus is. Conversely, the less fuel that is transported to the fetus, the smaller the fetus is. Figure 2.3 shows the gradual increased incidence of LGA (>90th percentile) fetuses in overgainers of all BMI categories, and the almost "mirror image" of increased incidence of SGA (<10th percentile) fetuses in undergainers of all BMI categories [13].

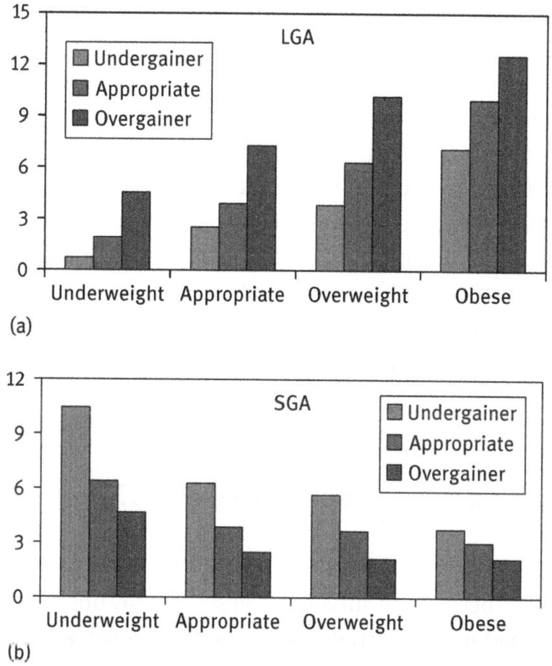

Fig. 2.3: Incidence (%) of LGA (a) and SGA (b) by pregravid BMI category and weight gain according to the 2009 Institute of Medicine recommendations. Adapted from Tul et al. [13].

As described in the Introduction, heavily restricted weight gain during pregnancy was used in older times to decrease the risk of dystocia (difficult birth). It was known that in terms of LGA and macrosomic neonates, it is better to undergain than to gain weight appropriately or to overgain weight during pregnancy. Indeed, the trend shown in Fig. 2.3 for LGA babies is the same for the trend of macrosomic (>4,000 g) babies, but needless to say that it is the fetal weight and not the maternal weight gain that may cause dystocia.

The other side of the coin is the ill effect of gaining too little on the development of SGA infants and as Fig. 2.3 shows, in terms of SGA, it is much better to overgain than to gain weight appropriately or to undergain weight during pregnancy. This statement, however, seems true for all BMI categories except for the obese mothers in whom even undergaining results in the same frequency of SGA neonates. The data shown in Fig. 2.3 relates to births at ≥38 + 0 weeks [13]. It is thus unknown if weight gain patterns are associated with SGA or growth-restricted fetuses delivered at less than 38 weeks. In contrast, a recent Irish study reviewed the current evidence on gestational weight gain [23] and called into question the advice that pregnant women are given regarding gestational weight gain and their lifestyle before, during, and after pregnancy. This conclusion was based on the weak epidemiological associations between excessive weight gain and aberrant fetal growth, mainly in obese women [23]. It seems that the truth, as always, is somewhere in the middle. Thus, undergaining and overgaining are better than appropriately gaining in terms of LGA and SGA births, respectively. Put differently, gaining weight during pregnancy as recommended by the IOM was significantly associated with an increased likelihood of SGA infants compared with overgainers and of LGA and macrosomia compared with undergainers. This information suggests that a tailored approach rather than strict adherence to the IOM recommendations may be more useful. For example, pregnant women at risk of SGA might benefit from dietary intervention that would cause overgaining whereas those at risk of LGA might from undergaining. Thus, the recommended weight gains might prove useful in the subgroups of pregnant patients who are at risk to have SGA or LGA babies.

2.8 How useful is weight gain management in pregnancy?

Based on the various considerations discussed above, one might conclude that the IOM recommendations are unrealistic because all surveys suggest that only one-third of the expecting mothers actually had an appropriate weight gain. In other words, two-thirds of the pregnant population should undergo strict or stricter dietary control to comply with the optimal weight gain range.

To explore this statement further, it is advisable to look at another practical point, namely, the evidence that interventions that might affect weight gain are useful. A recent study by the International Weight Management in Pregnancy Collaborative Group evaluated the adequacy and effectiveness of the methodological designs implemented in dietary intervention trials for overweight and obesity during pregnancy [24]. Large methodological variability existed in dietary interventions aimed to control weight gain and improve outcomes suggesting a lack of consensus that restricts the ability to convert evidence into clinical guidelines [24]. This conclusion probably explains why some authors from this Collaborative Group were unable to find in earlier studies the effect of gestational weight gain on lowering the incidence of adverse outcomes [18, 25].

Although most studies related to candidates for weight gain management focus on pregravid obese women, lean mothers have other concerns mainly related to a higher incidence of preterm and very preterm births and, consequently, a higher incidence of low and very low birth weight infants [26].

2.9 The risk of weight gain management in pregnancy

Whereas adherence to guidelines for underweight and normal weight women may be straightforward and somewhat less restrictive compared with overweight and obese women, it is unknown how many women at the upper limit of the normal range will turn overweight or obese as a result of implementing the recommended weight gain.

At the other end, Kapadia et al. [27,28] questioned whether it is safe to recommend gestational weight gain below the 2009 guidelines in obese women (i.e., weight loss rather than weight gain). Their systematic review found that undergainers had higher odds of preterm birth and SGA but, on the bright side, they enjoyed lower odds of LGA, gestational hypertension, PET, and cesarean birth rates. Despite this seemingly advantageous approach, the authors were cautious by stating that weigh gain below the guidelines cannot be routinely recommended [27,28]. The explanation for this caveat was the increased odds of SGA and a lack of information on preterm birth.

Another concern is weight retention after birth. Mannan et al. [29] evaluated the association between weight gain and long-term postpartum weight retention and BMI. They referred to the IOM recommendations and evaluated the time span for weight retention as <1 year, 1 to 9 years, and ≥15 years. The authors found that undergainers had lower weight retention than women with an adequate weight gain. Overgainers showed a U-shaped relationship over time (i.e., a decline during the early postpartum time span and then an increase in the following period). The authors concluded that undergainers or overgainers may exhibit both short-term and long-term postpartum weight imbalance. Similar conclusions were reached by Chinese researchers who apparently looked at the same studies [30].

2.10 Epilogue

The intention of the IOM weight gain recommendations was to improve maternal and fetal outcomes. However, the usefulness of these guidelines is, at best, controversial. Nonetheless, the IOM weight gain range is a powerful framework and, as the myriad publications suggest, it is a useful platform for further research to establish what is best for our pregnant patients.

Bibliography

[1] Miller D. Pregnancy weight gain guidelines in the US – a historical overview. Doctors Lounge Website. Available at: http://www.doctorslounge.com/index.php/articles/page/14732. Accessed January 03, 2017.

[2] Hytten FE, Leitch I. The physiology of human pregnancy, 2nd ed. Oxford: Blackwell Scientific Publications, 1971: 599 pp.

[3] Institute of Medicine. (US) Committee on Nutritional Status During Pregnancy and Lactation. Nutrition during pregnancy: Part I: Weight gain. Washington, DC: National Academies Press (US), 1990.

[4] Institute of Medicine. Nutrition during pregnancy. Washington, DC: National Academies Press, 1990.

[5] Siega-Riz AM, Viswanathan M, Moos MK, Deierlein A, Mumford S, Knaack J, et al. A systematic review of outcomes of maternal weight gain according to the Institute of Medicine recommendations: birthweight, fetal growth, and postpartum weight retention. Am J Obstet Gynecol 2009;20:339.e1–14.
[6] Institute of Medicine. Weight gain during pregnancy: reexamining the guidelines. Washington DC: National Academic Press, 2009.
[7] Flegal KM, Kruszon-Moran D, Carroll MD, Fryar CD, Ogden CL. Trends in obesity among adults in the United States, 2005 to 2014. JAMA 2016;315:2284–91.
[8] American College of Obstetricians and Gynecologists. Weight gain during pregnancy. Committee Opinion No. 548. Obstet Gynecol 2013;121:210–2.
[9] Stein RJ, Haddock CK, Poston WS, Catanese D, Spertus JA. Precision in weighing: a comparison of scales found in physician offices, fitness centers, and weight loss centers. Public Health Rep. 2005;120:266–70.
[10] Lucovnik M, Blickstein I, Verdenik I, Steblovnik L, Trojner Bregar A, Tul N. Impact of pre-gravid body mass index and body mass index change on preeclampsia and gestational diabetes in singleton and twin pregnancies. J Matern Fetal Neonatal Med. 2014;27:1901–4.
[11] Fujiwara K, Aoki S, Kurasawa K, Okuda M, Takahashi T, Hirahara F. Associations of maternal pre-pregnancy underweight with small-for-gestational-age and spontaneous preterm birth, and optimal gestational weight gain in Japanese women. J Obstet Gynaecol Res 2014;40:988–94.
[12] Society of Obstetricians and Gynaecologists of Canada. Clinical Practice Guidelines 239; Obesity in pregnancy. February 2010.
[13] Tul N, Bregar AT, Steblovnik L, Verdenik I, Lucovnik M, Blickstein I. A population-based comparison between actual maternal weight gain and the Institute of Medicine weight gain recommendations in singleton pregnancies. J Perinat Med. 2016;44:389–92.
[14] Simas TA, Liao X, Garrison A, Sullivan GM, Howard AE, Hardy JR. J Impact of updated Institute of Medicine guidelines on prepregnancy body mass index categorization, gestational weight gain recommendations, and needed counseling. J Womens Health (Larchmt) 2011;20:837–44.
[15] Li C, Liu Y, Zhang W. Joint and independent associations of gestational weight gain and pre-pregnancy body mass index with outcomes of pregnancy in Chinese women: a retrospective cohort study. PLoS One 2015;10:e0136850.
[16] Shamshirsaz AA, Haeri S, Ravangard SF, Sangi-Haghpeykar H, Gandhi M, Ozhand A, Spiel M, Trout S, Sadowski A, Hussain N, Campbell WA, Shamshirsaz AA. Perinatal outcomes based on the Institute of Medicine guidelines for weight gain in twin pregnancies. J Matern Fetal Neonatal Med. 2014;27:552–6.
[17] Ho LC, Saunders KA, Owen DJ, Ibrahim UN, Bhattacharya S. Are antenatal weight management interventions effective in preventing preeclampsia? Systematic review of randomised control trials. Pregnancy Hypertens 2012;2:341–9.
[18] Ruifrok AE, van Poppel MN, van Wely M, Rogozińska E, Khan KS, de Groot CJ, Thangaratinam S, Mol BW. Association between weight gain during pregnancy and pregnancy outcomes after dietary and lifestyle interventions: a meta-analysis. Am J Perinatol. 2014;31:353–64.
[19] Brustman LE, Langer O, Bimson B, Scarpelli S, El Daouk M. Weight gain in gestational diabetes: the effect of treatment modality. J Matern Fetal Neonatal Med 2016;29:1025–9.
[20] Trojner-Bregar A, Blickstein I, Lucovnik M, Steblovnik L, Verdenik I, Tul N. The relationship between cesarean section rate in term singleton pregnancies, maternal weight, and weight gain during pregnancy. J Perinat Med 2016 44:393–6.
[21] Cedergren M. Effects of gestational weight gain and body mass index on obstetric outcome in Sweden. Int J Gynecol Obstet 2006;93:269–74.
[22] Crane JM, White J, Murphy P, Burrage L, Hutchens D. The effect of gestational weight gain by body mass index on maternal and neonatal outcomes. J Obstet Gynaecol Can. 2009;31:28–35.

[23] O'Higgins AC, Doolan A, Mullaney L, Daly N, McCartney D, Turner MJ. The relationship between gestational weight gain and fetal growth: time to take stock? J Perinat Med 2013;42:409–15.
[24] Flynn AC, Dalrymple K, Barr S, Poston L, Goff LM, Rogozińska E, et al. Dietary interventions in overweight and obese pregnant women: a systematic review of the content, delivery, and outcomes of randomized controlled trials. Nutr Rev 2016;74:312–28.
[25] Thangaratinam S, Rogozińska E, Jolly K, Glinkowski S, Duda W, Borowiack E, Roseboom T, Tomlinson J, Walczak J, Kunz R, Mol BW, Coomarasamy A, Khan KS. Interventions to reduce or prevent obesity in pregnant women: a systematic review. Health Technol Assess 2012;16:1–191.
[26] Trojner Bregar A, Blickstein I, Bržan Šimenc G, Janša V, Verdenik I, Lucovnik M, Tul N. Perinatal advantages and disadvantages of being underweight before pregnancy: a population-based study. Gynecol Obstet Invest 2017;82(3):303–306. doi: 10.1159/000447557. Epub 2016 Jul 7.
[27] Kapadia MZ, Park CK, Beyene J, Giglia L, Maxwell C, McDonald SD. Can we safely recommend gestational weight gain below the 2009 guidelines in obese women? A systematic review and meta-analysis. Obes Rev 2015;16:189–206.
[28] Kapadia MZ, Park CK, Beyene J, Giglia L, Maxwell C, McDonald SD. Weight loss instead of weight gain within the guidelines in obese women during pregnancy: a systematic review and meta-analyses of maternal and infant outcomes. PLoS One 2015 10:e0132650.
[29] Mannan M, Doi SA, Mamun AA. Association between weight gain during pregnancy and postpartum weight retention and obesity: a bias-adjusted meta-analysis. Nutr Rev 2013;71:343–52.
[30] Rong K, Yu K, Han X, Szeto IM, Qin X, Wang J, Ning Y, Wang P, Ma D. Pre-pregnancy BMI, gestational weight gain and postpartum weight retention: a meta-analysis of observational studies. Public Health Nutr 2015;18:2172–82.

Sarah D. Crimmins, Julie A. Rosen, E. Albert Reece and Menachem Miodovnik

3 The endangered intrauterine milieu: the effect of diabetes, obesity, or both

3.1 Introduction

Today, a new epidemic is threatening to increase pregnancy complications rates: the rising tides of obesity and diabetes. The prevalence of diabetes – most notably type 2 diabetes – and obesity has risen together over the last 20 years, causing a condition often referred to as "diabesity." Approximately 14% of Americans older than 20 years are diagnosed with diabetes [1], and, for those who are pregnant, the rate is similar at 16.9% [2]. In addition, nearly 50% of reproductive age women are overweight or obese [3]. In this chapter, we will review some of the common complications of pregnancy, including hypertension, preterm birth, cesarean birth, stillbirth, and macrosomia, as well as the long-term sequelae of these complications, including childhood obesity and adult diseases of fetal origin, to determine if the primary contributing factor is obesity, diabetes, or both.

3.2 Pathophysiology of diabetes and obesity

Under normal conditions, pancreatic beta cells produce insulin, which acts to reduce blood glucose. Both obesity and diabetes are associated with insulin resistance [4]. In healthy weight individuals, adipose tissue plays an important role in the storage of fuel, as well as a pivotal role in the homeostasis of energy expenditure, appetite regulation, glucose regulation, and immunity. Adipose tissue modulates glucose metabolism by releasing peptides, including nonesterified fatty acids, glycerol, hormones (leptin and adiponectin), and proinflammatory cytokines [5–7]. In individuals who are overweight or obese, the accumulation of excess fat tissue causes increased production of inflammatory cytokines, excess secretion of fatty acids, and abnormal hormone signaling, resulting in insulin resistance [8]. In addition, nutrient excess can impair inflammatory signaling, increase the production of reactive oxygen species, cause mitochondrial dysfunction, and lead to triglyceride accumulation. As the efficacy of insulin action is reduced, pancreatic beta cells increase insulin release [9,10]. When beta cells can no longer compensate, or a stress such as pregnancy occurs, hyperglycemia is induced [11].

Type 1 diabetes mellitus (T1DM) is a chronic autoimmune disorder characterized by damage to the pancreatic beta cells, which leads to insulin deficiency and hyperglycemia. The primary treatment is insulin therapy. T1DM occurs in individuals with a

https://doi.org/10.1515/9783110487817-003

genetic susceptibility in concert with environmental triggers, including viral infections [12,13]. T1DM is usually diagnosed in children and young adults, and was previously called juvenile diabetes, but can occur in anyone at any age and is not related to being overweight or obese. The prevalence, however, of overweight and obesity among US adolescent females with T1DM is approximately 27% and 13.6%, respectively [14].

Type 2 diabetes mellitus (T2DM) involves a loss of balance between insulin sensitivity and insulin responsiveness, which lead to increasing levels of glucose. The development of T2DM involves systemic insulin resistance as well as beta cell failure. The major contributor to T2DM is excess weight [1], secondary to excess fat tissue; however, other predisposing factors include genetics [15], a sedentary lifestyle, and advancing age. With the rapid increase in the rates of obesity [3,16], the incidence of T2DM in the general population and in women of reproductive age has also increased [17]. For example, in the United Kingdom, the prevalence of pregnant women with T2DM has risen sharply, with an overall increase of 354% between 1995 and 2012 [18].

Gestational diabetes mellitus (GDM) is a glucose intolerance first recognized during pregnancy. Women who develop GDM share many of the metabolic characteristics of individuals with T2DM, and the overall pathophysiology is thought to be similar. The rate of GDM has increased 23-fold between 1980 and 2010 worldwide [19]. Part of this increase in GDM incidence can be attributed to the increasing prevalence of advanced maternal age, but a great majority of cases are secondary to the obesity epidemic. For every 1 kg/m^2, an individual's body mass index (BMI) increases, the risk of GDM increases by nearly 1% [20]. For individuals with a BMI greater than 40, the risk of GDM is fivefold higher than normal weight individuals [20].

3.3 Diabesity in pregnancy and maternal complications

3.3.1 Hypertension in pregnancy

Hypertension occurs in approximately 30% of people with T1DM, 50% to 80% of people with T2DM [21], and 40% of individuals who are obese [22]. The development of hypertension and diabetes share common pathways: obesity, insulin resistance, and endothelial dysfunctional play pivotal roles in the progression of both diseases [23]. Hypertensive disorders of pregnancy include chronic hypertension, gestational hypertension, preeclampsia, and eclampsia. These disorders complicate 5% to 10% of all pregnancies but pose significant risks to pregnant women with diabetes, with rates approaching 20% [22,23]. For the purposes of this discussion, we will focus on preeclampsia.

The etiology of preeclampsia has yet to be determined, but it involves a compromise of the normal adaptive vasculature of pregnancy [24]. Insulin resistance may have a critical role in the development of preeclampsia in women with diabetes, but also may play a role in the development of the disease in individuals with impaired glucose tolerance without overt diabetes. Multiple studies have demonstrated that individuals with higher fasting insulin levels, higher fasting glucose levels, and those in the highest quartile during diabetic challenge testing have an increased the risk for preeclampsia in pregnancy [25,26]. In diabetic pregnancy with preexisting microvascular complications, such as retinopathy or diabetic kidney disease, the risk of preeclampsia is greater than 56.8% higher than in pregnancies without microvascular disease [27]. In individuals with renal involvement, the odds of developing preeclampsia are eightfold higher than in individuals without diabetic kidney disease [28].

In T1DM, preeclampsia has been linked to microvascular disease as well as glycemic control. The risk of preeclampsia also increases with the severity and duration of T1DM. Utilizing the combination of White's classification and first trimester hemoglobin A1c, Klemetti and colleagues demonstrated a step-wise increase in the risk for preeclampsia [28]. In a study of women with T1DM who were 16 to 20 weeks pregnant, a strong correlation was found in individuals with elevated A1c (>8%) and the development of preeclampsia, compared with individuals with normal A1c [29]. In addition, second and third trimester blood sugar control can significantly reduce the risk of preeclampsia, demonstrated by observations that a normal A1c (<6%) carries an 8% risk of disease, as compared with an elevated A1c (>7.5%), which carries a 23% risk of disease at 26 weeks [30].

Despite the fact that T1DM and T2DM have differing mechanisms of action, T2DM has similar effects on the development of hypertensive disorders of pregnancy, demonstrated by studies that found an 8.7% risk of preeclampsia in women with T2DM, as compared with a 2.4% risk in women without diabetes [31]. The risk of preeclampsia in women with GDM is lower than in individuals with T1DM and T2DM, but remain higher than in the general population [32–34].

Obesity alone has been shown to increase the risk of preeclampsia in pregnancy. The mechanisms by which obesity causes preeclampsia seem similar to those implicated in diabetes-induced preeclampsia, wherein oxidative stress, insulin resistance, and angiogenic factors are thought to play causal roles [35–37]. Several large population studies have demonstrated that the overall risk of preeclampsia for all obesity classes is twofold to threefold higher than normal weight individuals [38], and the risk of preeclampsia doubles for each 5 to 7 kg/m^2 increase in prepregnancy BMI, with the greatest risk for preeclampsia in women with a BMI greater than 40 [39] (Fig. 3.1) [40]. Taken together, these observations translate into a 30% attributable risk, or approximately 10%, for the development of preeclampsia in women who are obese [36].

In women with T1DM, there is an increased risk of disease development as BMI category increases: 14% (BMI of 18.5–24.9), 15% (BMI of 25.0–29.9), and 18% (BMI >30) [41]. In women with T2DM, a correlation between increased risk for preeclampsia and each BMI category is not well defined [42]. In women with GDM, obese individuals have an increased risk for preeclampsia when GDM is diagnosed (Fig. 3.1) [43]. In addition, a study of 2,037 women with GDM reported that poor glycemic control (A1c > 5.9%) and prepregnancy obesity (≥30 kg/m^2) conferred a twofold and ninefold increased risk, respectively, for the development of preeclampsia [44].

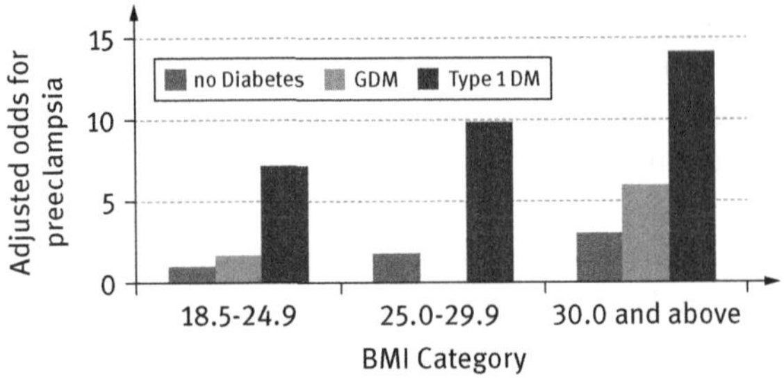

Fig. 3.1: Relationship between risk for preeclampsia, diabetes status, and BMI category. Individuals without diabetes adapted from Ovesen et al. [46]; GDM adapted from Catalano et al. [43], and T1DM adapted from Persson et al. [41].

The critical roles that insulin resistance and glycemic control play in the development of hypertensive disorders in pregnancy, in both the diabetic and obese populations, suggest that using metformin in the second trimester could reduce the risk for preeclampsia in both populations. In a double-masked, randomized control trial, obese individuals (BMI >35) without diabetes given metformin from 12 to 18 weeks' gestation had a significantly reduced rate of preeclampsia development compared with those not given the intervention [45].

3.3.2 Preterm birth

Preterm delivery complicates approximately 10% of all pregnancies. In pregnancies complicated by T1DM or T2DM that existed prior to conception (pregestational diabetes), the rate of preterm delivery was higher [47] and seemed to be related to the complications of diabetes (i.e., preeclampsia, chronic kidney disease) and to glycemic control [27]. Conflicting data exist about the incidence of spontaneous premature labor in pregnancies complicated by pregestational diabetes [48]. Studies are further confounded by the rate of iatrogenic preterm delivery. In looking at the indication for preterm delivery, Lepercq et al. [49,50] found a 9% risk of spontaneous preterm birth and a 15% risk of indicated preterm birth in women with pregestational diabetes. The risk factors identified for indicated preterm birth in women with T1DM were an elevated A1c (≥7%), the progression of diabetic kidney disease, and preeclampsia. Strict glycemic control also plays a role in reducing both spontaneous and indicated preterm birth rates in women with T2DM. A larger number of T2DM pregnancies are delivered preterm in comparison to the general population; however, the preterm birth rate decreases to 5.6% in individuals with good glycemic control (A1c <6%), versus a rate of 29.6% in those with poor glycemic control [31]. No strong associations have been observed between GDM and preterm delivery.

Conflicting results have been reported regarding preterm birth and maternal obesity, possibly due to the many confounding factors that determine the length of gestation, including hypertension, anemia, diabetes, and smoking status. For example, a Swedish population study of women with live singleton births showed increased risk of preterm delivery, especially extremely preterm delivery, with increasing BMI [51]. In contrast, Hendler et al. [52] demonstrated that obesity is inversely associated with the rate of spontaneous preterm birth. A third study found increased preterm delivery rates of 16.7% in women who were obese (BMI 30–39) and 20.3% in women who were morbidly obese (BMI ≥40), when compared with 14.5% with women who were nonobese; however, after accounting for confounders, obesity itself was not associated with prematurity [53].

When looking at the combined effects of diabetes and obesity in individuals with T1DM and obesity, the effect of obesity does not seem to change outcome. In a population study of women with T1DM in increasing BMI categories, there was no difference in the rate of preterm deliveries between the overweight and obese categories [41]. In individuals with GDM and obesity, there were higher rates of indicated preterm birth, compared with individuals with GDM and normal weight, but no difference in the in rates of spontaneous preterm birth [54]. In obese women with T2DM, the relationship with preterm birth seems independent of obesity [55]. Thus, when looking at the absolute risk of preterm birth in pregnancies complicated by diabetes and obesity, an association is not clearly defined.

3.3.3 Cesarean delivery

Cesarean delivery (CD) is associated with increased maternal morbidity [56]. The CD rate is twofold to fourfold higher in individuals with T1DM in pregnancy than in the general population [57–59]. The factors that most influence the rate of CD in T1DM are suspected macrosomia, prepregnancy BMI greater than 25, and gestational weight gain (GWG) of more than 15 kg [49]. These same factors also seem to play a role in influencing the CD rate in women with T2DM [31] and GDM [60].

The incidence of CD in the overweight and obese population is higher in comparison to the normal weight population. Exactly how BMI affects CD rate is not clearly defined; however, obesity is known to be associated with labor dysfunction (i.e., decreased uterine contractility, timing of cervical dilation, and duration and augmentation of labor) [61,62]. Compared with the nonobese patient, there is a 1:12 excess CD in moderately obese women and a 1:6 excess CD in severely obese women [63]. Brost et al. [64] found that the rate of CD increases concurrently with increasing prepregnancy BMI, and Robinson et al. [63] reported similar results.

When evaluating pregestational diabetes and obesity together, obesity seems to have a more significant role in influencing the CD rate. Ehrenberg et al. [61] observed that obesity had a dose-dependent effect on CD rates, with pregestational diabetes as a risk for CD remaining constant across BMI groups. However, for women with GDM, there seems to be an elevated risk for CD when obesity is concurrent with GDM, compared with obesity alone [43].

3.4 Diabesity in pregnancy and fetal and neonatal complications

3.4.1 Stillbirth

Stillbirth or fetal death is defined as involuntary loss after 20 weeks of gestation. The causes of stillbirth include impaired placental function (abruption, cord accidents, infection, feto-maternal hemorrhage, placental previa), fetal triggers (chromosomal anomalies, congenital malformations, infections, and hydrops), and maternal triggers (hypertension, vascular disease, advancing age, substance abuse, trauma) [65].

The prevalence of fetal deaths in women with pregestational diabetes is more than four times greater than in women without, and the risk of infant deaths is nearly double [66]. In the GDM population, the stillbirth rate is slightly higher than the general population (OR: 1.25, 95% CI: 1.11–1.41) [67]. Although the causes of stillbirth in women with GDM are unknown, congenital malformations are a common cause of stillbirth in the pregestational diabetic population, with the most common anomalies being cardiac and neural tube defects [68,69]. The higher congenital malformation rates seen in diabetic pregnancies are likely due to the altered metabolism of nutrients, especially glucose, the major teratogen of maternal diabetes in pregnancy. Hyperglycemia can lead to pathological conditions, which, in turn, can cause altered gene expression and cellular damage [70,71]. Even with strict glycemic control, transient exposure to high glucose can negatively affect the developing fetus, especially in the early stages of embryogenesis [71,72]. In addition, maternal hyperglycemia leads to overproduction of insulin by the fetal pancreas. Fetal hyperinsulinemia has been linked to hypoxia and cord blood acidemia, and acidemia has been associated with stillbirth [73].

Obesity is associated with 25% of stillbirths between 37 and 42 weeks [74], and the risk of stillbirth increases with even modest increases in BMI [75]. A BMI greater than 40 carries a relative risk of fetal death that is two to threefold higher than in individuals with a BMI of 20 [76]. Although the exact cause of fetal death in women with high BMI remains unknown, and the rate of unexplained stillbirth is high in the obese population, there is a trend between uteroplacental insufficiency, obesity, and stillbirth [77]. In addition, the etiology of abnormal metabolism found in diabetes may contribute to obesity-associated stillbirth.

The risk of stillbirth seems to be compounded by pregestational diabetes and obesity due, in large part, to an increased risk for fetal growth restriction, the single largest risk factor for stillbirth [78]. In addition, both GDM and obesity have a multiplicative effect on the risk for fetal death [79]. Thus, even stricter glycemic goals need to be applied to individuals with diabesity to reduce the risk of stillbirth.

3.4.2 Macrosomia

Macrosomia is defined as a birth weight greater than 4 kg (approximately 9 lbs.) or greater than the 90th percentile for gestational age. The primary contributors to fetal growth stem from the mother and include maternal nutrition, pregnancy weight gain, maternal age, parity, glucose intolerance, and maternal BMI. Macrosomia occurs in 15% to 45% of diabetic pregnancies [80] and is associated with increased maternal body fat and altered maternal body composition. Altered maternal body composition is also the primary reason for increased risk of birth trauma, including shoulder dystocia, hypoxic ischemic encephalopathy, and nerve palsies in infants of mothers with diabetes [81,82]. Fetuses of women with diabetes in pregnancy typically present with a significantly larger abdominal circumference in comparison to head circumference [83], and demonstrate a higher ponderal index (reflecting increased body weight relative to length) than fetuses of women without diabetes [84].

In women with euglycemia throughout pregnancy, the risk of macrosomia climbs with BMI. Owens et al. [85] found macrosomic infants were born to 15.5% of normal weight, 21.4% of overweight, and 27.8% of obese women. In a Danish population study, macrosomia increased with BMI category (Tab. 3.1) [46]. For individuals with a BMI greater than 40, the odds ratio of a large-for-gestational age (LGA) fetus is 3.82 (95% CI: 3.50–41.6), in comparison to normal weight individuals [40].

Poorly controlled blood glucose, as well as GWG, greatly influence fetal growth. To examine the contribution of each factor, Ehrenberg et al. [86] looked at the attributable risk of LGA in relationship to pregestational diabetes and obesity. They found that for every 100 LGA deliveries, 11 could be attributed to obesity, whereas 4 were attributed to pregestational diabetes, demonstrating that the growing number of LGA infants is more closely related to obesity than diabetes. In women with GDM alone, the odds for a birth weight greater than the 90th percentile increases, compared with women without GDM, and the addition of obesity to GDM increases the odds further (Tab. 3.1) [43].

Individuals with obesity adapted from Scott-Pillai et al. [75]; GDM adapted from Catalano et al. [43], and T1DM adapted from Ehrenberg et al. [86].

Tab. 3.1: Relationship between risk for macrosomia, diabetes status, and BMI category.

	BMI 25–29.9	**BMI 30 or greater**
Obesity alone [75]	aOR 1.5, 95% CI: 1.3–1.6	aOR 1.9, 95% CI: 1.6–2.2
Gestational diabetes [43]	aOR 4.52	aOR 5.35
Pregestational diabetes [86]	aOR 5.1, 95% CI: 2.9–8.9	aOR 4.4, 95% CI: 2.9–6.7

3.4.3 Childhood obesity

Maternal diabetes, BMI and GWG [87], and neonatal birth weight all influence the risk of childhood obesity [88]. Other contributing factors to childhood obesity include macrosomia and ethnicity [88]. No studies are available to determine the relative contribution of each of these factors. However, because the prevalence of obesity is much higher in comparison to the prevalence of diabetes, childhood obesity seems primarily influenced by maternal obesity in pregnancy. One reason for this is that the supply of nutrients that cross the placenta, either in deficiency or in overabundance, can permanently change fetal physiology and metabolism [89].

Lindsay et al. [90] demonstrated that the rate of overweight and obesity at age 7 is significantly higher in children of women with T1DM in pregnancy, compared with children of women without diabetes. For the offspring of women with T2DM, there is also a higher prevalence of childhood obesity (up to age 14). Offspring of mothers with GDM also have a significant risk of developing obesity in childhood (ages 9–11), compared with children of mothers without GDM. However, after adjusting for current maternal BMI, the association between GDM and childhood obesity does not remain significant, suggesting that childhood obesity and GDM are not fully independent of maternal BMI [91].

Studies have linked first trimester maternal BMI and obesity in children aged 3 years. In addition, a maternal BMI of 40 or greater is associated with a 28.8% obesity rate in children aged 4 years [92]. In addition, maternal weight gain of greater than 18.1 kg (40 lbs.) in pregnancy is associated with a 15% increased risk of childhood obesity [93,94]. Finally, for every 1 kg a newborn is above the mean birth weight for gestational age, there is a 30% increased risk of being overweight in childhood [95].

3.4.4 *In utero* programming of chronic disease

According to the *in utero* programming hypothesis (Barker hypothesis), size at birth is related to the risk of developing the disease later in life [96]. Although this hypothesis originally focused on children with low birth weight and accelerated growth in the first year, mounting evidence shows that this theory could also be linked to children who were macrosomic [97]. The presence of T1DM in pregnancy and GDM affects the offspring's risk of developing T2DM, cardiovascular disease, and stroke [98]. When comparing sibling pairs, one born prior to a diagnosis of diabetes and one born afterward, investigators have found a significantly higher risk of T2DM in the sibling whose *in utero* environment was influenced by hyperglycemia [99].

In the Helsinki Birth Cohort Study, associations were seen between maternal obesity in pregnancy and later development of cardiovascular disease, coronary heart disease, and stroke in the offspring [100]. Interestingly, an association between maternal BMI and T2DM in offspring was only seen in women [101].

3.5 Diabesity in pregnancy and modifiable factors

Because many of the major complications of diabesity in pregnancy are related to uncontrolled hyperglycemia and BMI, managing glycemic control and GWG are key to promoting a healthy pregnancy.

3.5.1 Glycemic control

Glucose values during pregnancy are best described as a continuous variable, and the risk to the fetus increases in a direct relationship to increasing levels of maternal glycemia [102]. For example, periconceptional hemoglobin A1c changes the risk of stillbirth in nonanomalous fetuses of women with pregestational diabetes [66]. In addition, well-controlled blood sugar reduces the risks of adverse pregnancy outcomes, even as BMI increases [103]. Langer et al. [104] showed that the presence of untreated GDM conferred a ninefold increased risk of stillbirth, neonatal macrosomia/LGA, neonatal hypoglycemia, erythrocytosis, and hyperbilirubinemia (the composite outcome) in women with a BMI of 30 or greater, compared with women who did not have GDM but had a BMI of 30 or greater. In addition, the use of insulin in morbidly obese GDM patients (BMI >35) decreased the rate of both fetal metabolic complications and the composite outcome [105]. This demonstrates the critical nature that glycemic control has on pregnancy outcome, and underscores that timing of treatment is critical to the success of pregnancy.

3.5.2 Gestational weight gain

Approximately 40% to 50% of all pregnant women experience excessive GWG (>20 lbs. or 9 kg) [106], and this number has been increasing [107]. In the morbidly obese (BMI ≥50), excessive weight gain is associated with increased odds of pregnancy-induced hypertension and CD, and the development of childhood obesity [87,108]. In addition, excessive GWG is associated with increased risk of abnormal fetal growth, independent of prepregnancy BMI and GDM treatment [109]. In a prospective maternal-child pairs study, Oken et al. [110] found that children of mothers with adequate or excessive weight gain in pregnancy had fourfold increased odds of being overweight by age 3 when compared with children of mothers with inadequate GWG.

For women who are overweight or obese prior to pregnancy, restricting GWG seems to have a positive effect on pregnancy outcomes. In individuals with BMI of

30 or greater who gained less than the recommended 11 lbs. (5 kg) [110], there was a reduction in the risk of delivering an infant with a birth weight greater than 4,000 g, without increasing the risk for a small-for-gestational age fetus [108].

The National Academy of Medicine (formerly the Institute of Medicine) made recommendations in 2009 for healthy weight gain pregnancy, which were stratified by prepregnancy BMI [111]. Since their publication nearly a decade ago, the prevalence of diabetes (which is mostly T2DM) and obesity has increased to current estimates of 9.3% and 36.5%, respectively. As the guidelines were developed for all women, regardless of prepregnancy diabetes and BMI status, and with the significant increase in diabesity in the intervening years, the target GWG may need to be adjusted.

3.6 Summary

Diabetes, obesity, and diabesity have profound effects on pregnancy and pregnancy outcomes (Fig. 3.2). The relative contributions of obesity and diabetes are different for each pregnancy-related complication. For the women who have diabetes and who are obese, the most important modifiable risk factor is maintaining glycemic control, and the second is managing GWG. By controlling both blood sugar levels and weight, women can significantly reduce their risks of hypertensive disorders in pregnancy, macrosomia and stillbirth, and reduce long-term sequelae for their offspring. Great care should be taken to thoroughly screen all overweight and obese patients who have not been previously diagnosed with diabetes for any evidence of impaired glycemic control, as this may significantly affect pregnancy outcomes. Continued careful management of patients with T1DM or T2DM prior to pregnancy, as well as those who are at risk of developing GDM, will also aid in reducing maternal and fetal complications.

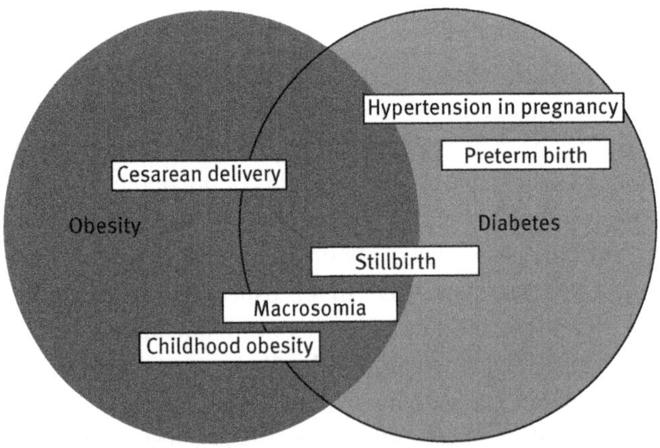

Fig. 3.2: The relative contribution between obesity and diabetes to each of the selected outcomes.

Bibliography

[1] Menke A, Casagrande S, Geiss L, Cowie CC. Prevalence of and trends in diabetes among adults in the United States, 1988–2012. JAMA 2015;314(10):1021–9.
[2] Guariguata L, Linnenkamp U, Beagley J, Whiting DR, Cho NH. Global estimates of the prevalence of hyperglycaemia in pregnancy. Diabetes Res Clin Pract 2014;103(2):176–85.
[3] Vahratian A. Prevalence of overweight and obesity among women of childbearing age: results from the 2002 National Survey of Family Growth. Matern Child Health J 2009;13(2):268–73.
[4] Reaven GM. Banting lecture 1988. Role of insulin resistance in human disease. Diabetes 1988;37(12):1595–607.
[5] Wellen KE, Hotamisligil GS. Inflammation, stress, and diabetes. J Clin Invest 2005;115(5): 1111–9.
[6] Scherer PE. Adipose tissue: from lipid storage compartment to endocrine organ. Diabetes 2006;55(6):1537–45.
[7] Shoelson SE, Lee J, Goldfine AB. Inflammation and insulin resistance. J Clin Invest 2006;116(7):1793–1801.
[8] Schuster DP. Obesity and the development of type 2 diabetes: the effects of fatty tissue inflammation. Diabetes Metab Syndr Obes 2010;3:253–62.
[9] Perley M, Kipnis DM. Plasma insulin responses to glucose and tolbutamide of normal weight and obese diabetic and nondiabetic subjects. Diabetes. 1966;15(12):867–74.
[10] Kahn SE. Clinical review 135: the importance of beta-cell failure in the development and progression of type 2 diabetes. J Clin Endocrinol and Metab 2001;86(9):4047–58.
[11] Buchanan TA, Metzger BE, Freinkel N, Bergman RN. Insulin sensitivity and B-cell responsiveness to glucose during late pregnancy in lean and moderately obese women with normal glucose tolerance or mild gestational diabetes. Am J Obst Gynecol 1990;162(4):1008–14.
[12] Knip M, Veijola R, Virtanen SM, Hyoty H, Vaarala O, Akerblom HK. Environmental triggers and determinants of type 1 diabetes. Diabetes 2005;54 Suppl 2:S125–36.
[13] Laitinen OH, Honkanen H, Pakkanen O, et al. Coxsackievirus B1 is associated with induction of beta-cell autoimmunity that portends type 1 diabetes. Diabetes 2014;63(2):446–55.
[14] Minges KE, Whittemore R, Weinzimer SA, Irwin ML, Redeker NS, Grey M. Correlates of overweight and obesity in 5529 adolescents with type 1 diabetes: the T1D Exchange Clinic Registry. Diabetes Res Clin Pract 2017;126:68–78.
[15] Robiou-du-Pont S, Bonnefond A, Yengo L, et al. Contribution of 24 obesity-associated genetic variants to insulin resistance, pancreatic beta-cell function and type 2 diabetes risk in the French population. Int J Obes (Lond) 2013;37(7):980–5.
[16] Ogden CL, Carroll MD, Kit BK, Flegal KM. Prevalence of childhood and adult obesity in the United States, 2011–2012. JAMA 2014;311(8):806–14.
[17] Lawrence JM, Contreras R, Chen W, Sacks DA. Trends in the prevalence of preexisting diabetes and gestational diabetes mellitus among a racially/ethnically diverse population of pregnant women, 1999–2005. Diabetes Care 2008;31(5):899–904.
[18] Coton SJ, Nazareth I, Petersen I. A cohort study of trends in the prevalence of pregestational diabetes in pregnancy recorded in UK general practice between 1995 and 2012. BMJ Open 2016;6(1):e009494.
[19] Lavery JA, Friedman AM, Keyes KM, Wright JD, Ananth CV. Gestational diabetes in the United States: temporal changes in prevalence rates between 1979 and 2010. BJOG 2016;124(5):804–813
[20] Torloni MR, Betran AP, Horta BL, et al. Prepregnancy BMI and the risk of gestational diabetes: a systematic review of the literature with meta-analysis. Obes Rev 2009;10(2):194–203.
[21] Landsberg L, Molitch M. Diabetes and hypertension: pathogenesis, prevention and treatment. Clin Exp Hypertens 2004;26(7–8):621–8.

[22] Mokdad AH, Ford ES, Bowman BA, et al. Prevalence of obesity, diabetes, and obesity-related health risk factors, 2001. JAMA 2003;289(1):76–9.
[23] Sowers JR. Insulin resistance and hypertension. Am J Physiol Heart Circ Physiol 2004;286(5):H1597–602.
[24] Ness RB, Sibai BM. Shared and disparate components of the pathophysiologies of fetal growth restriction and preeclampsia. Am J Obst Gynecol 2006;195(1):40–9.
[25] Joffe GM, Esterlitz JR, Levine RJ, et al. The relationship between abnormal glucose tolerance and hypertensive disorders of pregnancy in healthy nulliparous women. Calcium for Preeclampsia Prevention (CPEP) Study Group. Am J Obst Gynecol Oct 1998;179(4):1032–7.
[26] Solomon CG, Carroll JS, Okamura K, Graves SW, Seely EW. Higher cholesterol and insulin levels in pregnancy are associated with increased risk for pregnancy-induced hypertension. Am J Hypertens 1999;12(3):276–82.
[27] Reece EA, Sivan E, Francis G, Homko CJ. Pregnancy outcomes among women with and without diabetic microvascular disease (White's classes B to FR) versus non-diabetic controls. Am J Perinatol 1998;15(9):549–55.
[28] Klemetti MM, Laivuori H, Tikkanen M, Nuutila M, Hiilesmaa V, Teramo K. White's classification and pregnancy outcome in women with type 1 diabetes: a population-based cohort study. Diabetologia 2016;59(1):92–100.
[29] Hsu CD, Hong SF, Nickless NA, Copel JA. Glycosylated hemoglobin in insulin-dependent diabetes mellitus related to preeclampsia. Am J Perinatol 1998;15(3):199–202.
[30] Maresh MJ, Holmes VA, Patterson CC, et al. Glycemic targets in the second and third trimester of pregnancy for women with type 1 diabetes. Diabetes Care 2015;38(1):34–42.
[31] Abell SK, Boyle JA, de Courten B, et al. Impact of type 2 diabetes, obesity and glycaemic control on pregnancy outcomes. Aust N Z J Obstet Gynaecol 2017;57(3):308–314.
[32] Schneider S, Freerksen N, Rohrig S, Hoeft B, Maul H. Gestational diabetes and preeclampsia – similar risk factor profiles? Early Hum Dev 2012;88(3):179–84.
[33] Nerenberg KA, Johnson JA, Leung B, et al. Risks of gestational diabetes and preeclampsia over the last decade in a cohort of Alberta women. J Obstet Gynaecol Can 2013;35(11):986–94.
[34] Ostlund I, Haglund B, Hanson U. Gestational diabetes and preeclampsia. Eur J Obstet Gynecol Reprod Biol 15 2004;113(1):12–6.
[35] Bodnar LM, Ness RB, Harger GF, Roberts JM. Inflammation and triglycerides partially mediate the effect of prepregnancy body mass index on the risk of preeclampsia. Am J Epidemiol 15 2005;162(12):1198–1206.
[36] Roberts JM, Bodnar LM, Patrick TE, Powers RW. The role of obesity in preeclampsia. Pregnancy Hypertens 2011;1(1):6–16.
[37] Wolf M, Kettyle E, Sandler L, Ecker JL, Roberts J, Thadhani R. Obesity and preeclampsia: the potential role of inflammation. Obstet Gynecol 2001;98(5 Pt 1):757–62.
[38] Sebire NJ, Jolly M, Harris JP, et al. Maternal obesity and pregnancy outcome: a study of 287,213 pregnancies in London. Int J Obes Relat Metab Disord 2001;25(8):1175–82.
[39] O'Brien TE, Ray JG, Chan WS. Maternal body mass index and the risk of preeclampsia: a systematic overview. Epidemiology (Cambridge, MA) 2003;14(3):368–74.
[40] Cedergren MI. Maternal morbid obesity and the risk of adverse pregnancy outcome. Obstet Gynecol 2004;103(2):219–24.
[41] Persson M, Pasupathy D, Hanson U, Westgren M, Norman M. Pre-pregnancy body mass index and the risk of adverse outcome in type 1 diabetic pregnancies: a population-based cohort study. BMJ Open 2012;2(1):e000601.
[42] Persson M, Cnattingius S, Wikstrom AK, Johansson S. Maternal overweight and obesity and risk of pre-eclampsia in women with type 1 diabetes or type 2 diabetes. Diabetologia 2016;59(10):2099–105.

[43] Catalano PM, McIntyre HD, Cruickshank JK, et al. The hyperglycemia and adverse pregnancy outcome study: associations of GDM and obesity with pregnancy outcomes. Diabetes Care 2012;35(4):780–6.
[44] Barquiel B, Herranz L, Grande C, et al. Body weight, weight gain and hyperglycaemia are associated with hypertensive disorders of pregnancy in women with gestational diabetes. Diabetes Metab 2014;40(3):204–10.
[45] Syngelaki A, Nicolaides KH, Balani J, et al. Metformin versus placebo in obese pregnant women without diabetes mellitus. N Engl J Med 2016;374(5):434–43.
[46] Ovesen P, Rasmussen S, Kesmodel U. Effect of prepregnancy maternal overweight and obesity on pregnancy outcome. Obstet Gynecol 2011;118(2 Pt 1):305–12.
[47] Gizzo S, Patrelli TS, Rossanese M, et al. An update on diabetic women obstetrical outcomes linked to preconception and pregnancy glycemic profile: a systematic literature review. TheScientificWorldJournal 2013;2013:254901.
[48] von Kries R, Kimmerle R, Schmidt JE, Hachmeister A, Bohm O, Wolf HG. Pregnancy outcomes in mothers with pregestational diabetes: a population-based study in North Rhine (Germany) from 1988 to 1993. Eur J Paediatr 1997;156(12):963–7.
[49] Lepercq J, Le Meaux JP, Agman A, Timsit J. Factors associated with cesarean delivery in nulliparous women with type 1 diabetes. Obstet Gynecol 2010;115(5):1014–20.
[50] Lepercq J, Coste J, Theau A, Dubois-Laforgue D, Timsit J. Factors associated with preterm delivery in women with type 1 diabetes: a cohort study. Diabetes Care 2004;27(12): 2824–28.
[51] Cnattingius S, Villamor E, Johansson S, et al. Maternal obesity and risk of preterm delivery. JAMA 2013;309(22):2362–70.
[52] Hendler I, Goldenberg RL, Mercer BM, et al. The Preterm Prediction Study: association between maternal body mass index and spontaneous and indicated preterm birth. Am J Obst Gynecol. Mar 2005;192(3):882–6.
[53] Aly H, Hammad T, Nada A, Mohamed M, Bathgate S, El-Mohandes A. Maternal obesity, associated complications and risk of prematurity. J Perinatol 2010;30(7):447–51.
[54] Scifres C, Feghali M, Althouse AD, Caritis S, Catov J. Adverse outcomes and potential targets for intervention in gestational diabetes and obesity. Obstet Gynecol 2015;126(2):316–25.
[55] Knight KM, Pressman EK, Hackney DN, Thornburg LL. Perinatal outcomes in type 2 diabetic patients compared with non-diabetic patients matched by body mass index. J Matern Fetal Neonatal Med 2012;25(6):611–5.
[56] Takoudes TC, Weitzen S, Slocum J, Malee M. Risk of cesarean wound complications in diabetic gestations. Am J Obst Gynecol 2004;191(3):958–63.
[57] Evers IM, de Valk HW, Visser GH. Risk of complications of pregnancy in women with type 1 diabetes: nationwide prospective study in the Netherlands. BMJ 17 2004;328(7445):915.
[58] Jensen DM, Damm P, Moelsted-Pedersen L, et al. Outcomes in type 1 diabetic pregnancies: a nationwide, population-based study. Diabetes Care 2004;27(12):2819–23.
[59] Pregnancy outcomes in the Diabetes Control and Complications Trial. Am J Obst Gynecol 1996;174(4):1343–53.
[60] Billionnet C, Mitanchez D, Weill A, et al. Gestational diabetes and adverse perinatal outcomes from 716,152 births in France in 2012. Diabetologia 2017;60(4):636–644.
[61] Ehrenberg HM, Durnwald CP, Catalano P, Mercer BM. The influence of obesity and diabetes on the risk of cesarean delivery. Am J Obst Gynecol 2004;191(3):969–74.
[62] Lawn JE, Blencowe H, Waiswa P, et al. Stillbirths: rates, risk factors, and acceleration towards 2030. Lancet 2016;387(10018):587–603.
[63] Robinson HE, O'Connell CM, Joseph KS, McLeod NL. Maternal outcomes in pregnancies complicated by obesity. Obstet Gynecol 2005;106(6):1357–64.

[64] Brost BC, Goldenberg RL, Mercer BM, et al. The Preterm Prediction Study: association of cesarean delivery with increases in maternal weight and body mass index. Am J Obst Gynecol 1997;177(2):333–7; discussion 337–41.
[65] McClure EM, Garces A, Saleem S, et al. Global Network for Women's and Children's Health Research: probable causes of stillbirth in low- and middle-income countries using a prospectively defined classification system. BJOG 2017;Jan 31 [epub ahead of print].
[66] Tennant PW, Glinianaia SV, Bilous RW, Rankin J, Bell R. Pre-existing diabetes, maternal glycated haemoglobin, and the risks of fetal and infant death: a population-based study. Diabetologia 2014;57(2):285–94.
[67] Hutcheon JA, Kuret V, Joseph KS, Sabr Y, Lim K. Immortal time bias in the study of stillbirth risk factors: the example of gestational diabetes. Epidemiology 2013;24(6):787–90.
[68] Reece EA, Hobbins JC. Diabetic embryopathy: pathogenesis, prenatal diagnosis and prevention. Obstet Gynecol Surv 1986;41(6):325–35.
[69] Reece EA, Pinter E, Homko C, Wu YK, Naftolin F. The yolk sac theory: closing the circle on why diabetes-associated malformations occur. J Soc Gynecol Investig 1994;1(1):3–13.
[70] Eriksson UJ, Borg LA, Forsberg H, Styrud J. Diabetic embryopathy. Studies with animal and in vitro models. Diabetes 1991;40 Suppl 2:94–8.
[71] Zhao Z, Reece EA. Experimental mechanisms of diabetic embryopathy and strategies for developing therapeutic interventions. J Soc Gynecol Investig 2005;12(8):549–57.
[72] Reece EA. Diabetes in women. Philadelphia, PA.: Lippincott Williams and Williams; 2004.
[73] Salvesen DR, Brudenell JM, Proudler AJ, Crook D, Nicolaides KH. Fetal pancreatic beta-cell function in pregnancies complicated by maternal diabetes mellitus: relationship to fetal acidemia and macrosomia. Am J Obst Gynecol, 1993;168(5):1363–9.
[74] Yao R, Ananth CV, Park BY, Pereira L, Plante LA. Obesity and the risk of stillbirth: a population-based cohort study. Am J Obst Gynecol. May 2014;210(5):457.e451–9.
[75] Scott-Pillai R, Spence D, Cardwell CR, Hunter A, Holmes VA. The impact of body mass index on maternal and neonatal outcomes: a retrospective study in a UK obstetric population, 2004–2011. BJOG 2013;120(8):932–9.
[76] Aune D, Saugstad OD, Henriksen T, Tonstad S. Maternal body mass index and the risk of fetal death, stillbirth, and infant death: a systematic review and meta-analysis. JAMA 2014;311(15):1536–46.
[77] Kristensen J, Vestergaard M, Wisborg K, Kesmodel U, Secher NJ. Pre-pregnancy weight and the risk of stillbirth and neonatal death. BJOG 2005;112(4):403–8.
[78] Gardosi J, Madurasinghe V, Williams M, Malik A, Francis A. Maternal and fetal risk factors for stillbirth: population based study. BMJ 2013;346:f108.
[79] Yao R, Park BY, Caughey AB. The effects of maternal obesity on perinatal outcomes among those born small for gestational age. J Matern Fetal Neonatal Med. 2017 Jun;30(12):1417–1422.
[80] Moore TR, Catalano P. Diabetes in Pregnancy. In: Creasy RK, Resnik R, Iams JD, Lockwood CJ, Moore T, Greene M eds. Creasy & Resnik's Maternal fetal medicine: principles and practice, 7th edition. Philadelphia: WB Saunders; 2014.
[81] Spain JE, Tuuli MG, Macones GA, Roehl KA, Odibo AO, Cahill AG. Risk factors for serious morbidity in term nonanomalous neonates. Am J Obstet Gynecol 2015;212(6):799.e791–7.
[82] Tsang RC, Ballard J, Braun C. The infant of the diabetic mother: today and tomorrow. Clin Obstet Gynecol 1981;24(1):125–47.
[83] Hammoud NM, Visser GH, Peters SA, Graatsma EM, Pistorius L, de Valk HW. Fetal growth profiles of macrosomic and non-macrosomic infants of women with pregestational or gestational diabetes. Ultrasound Obstet Gynecol 2013;41(4):390–7.
[84] Sacks DA, Black MH, Li X, Montoro MN, Lawrence JM. Adverse pregnancy outcomes using the International Association of the Diabetes and Pregnancy Study Groups criteria: glycemic thresholds and associated risks. Obstet Gynecol 2015;126(1):67–73.

[85] Owens LA, O'Sullivan EP, Kirwan B, Avalos G, Gaffney G, Dunne F. ATLANTIC DIP: the impact of obesity on pregnancy outcome in glucose-tolerant women. Diabetes Care 2010;33(3): 577–9.
[86] Ehrenberg HM, Mercer BM, Catalano PM. The influence of obesity and diabetes on the prevalence of macrosomia. Am J Obstet Gynecol 2004;191(3):964–8.
[87] Mourtakos SP, Tambalis KD, Panagiotakos DB, et al. Association between gestational weight gain and risk of obesity in preadolescence: a longitudinal study (1997–2007) of 5125 children in Greece. J Hum Nutr Diet 2017;30(1):51–58.
[88] Hammoud NM, de Valk HW, van Rossem L, Biesma DH, Wit JM, Visser GH. Growth and BMI during the first 14 y of life in offspring from women with type 1 or type 2 diabetes mellitus. Ped Res 2017;81(2):342–8.
[89] de Boo HA, Harding JE. The developmental origins of adult disease (Barker) hypothesis. Aust N Z J Obstet Gynaecol 2006;46(1):4–14.
[90] Lindsay RS, Nelson SM, Walker JD, et al. Programming of adiposity in offspring of mothers with type 1 diabetes at age 7 years. Diabetes Care 2010;33(5):1080–5.
[91] Zhao P, Liu E, Qiao Y, et al. Maternal gestational diabetes and childhood obesity at age 9–11: results of a multinational study. Diabetologia 2016;59(11):2339–48.
[92] Whitaker RC. Predicting preschooler obesity at birth: the role of maternal obesity in early pregnancy. Pediatrics 2004;114(1):e29–36.
[93] Hivert MF, Rifas-Shiman SL, Gillman MW, Oken E. Greater early and mid-pregnancy gestational weight gains are associated with excess adiposity in mid-childhood. Obesity (Silver Spring) 2016;24(7):1546–53.
[94] Hillier TA, Pedula KL, Vesco KK, Oshiro CE, Ogasawara KK. Impact of maternal glucose and gestational weight gain on child obesity over the first decade of life in normal birth weight infants. Matern Child Health J 2016;20(8):1559–68.
[95] Gillman MW, Rifas-Shiman S, Berkey CS, Field AE, Colditz GA. Maternal gestational diabetes, birth weight, and adolescent obesity. Pediatrics 2003;111(3):e221–6.
[96] Barker DJ. The fetal and infant origins of adult disease. BMJ 17 1990;301(6761):1111.
[97] Leddy MA, Power ML, Schulkin J. The impact of maternal obesity on maternal and fetal health. Rev Obstet Gynecol 2008;1(4):170–8.
[98] Clausen TD, Mathiesen ER, Hansen T, et al. High prevalence of type 2 diabetes and pre-diabetes in adult offspring of women with gestational diabetes mellitus or type 1 diabetes: the role of intrauterine hyperglycemia. Diabetes Care 2008;31(2):340–6.
[99] Dabelea D, Hanson RL, Lindsay RS, et al. Intrauterine exposure to diabetes conveys risks for type 2 diabetes and obesity: a study of discordant sibships. Diabetes 2000;49(12):2208–11.
[100] Eriksson JG, Sandboge S, Salonen M, Kajantie E, Osmond C. Maternal weight in pregnancy and offspring body composition in late adulthood: findings from the Helsinki Birth Cohort Study (HBCS). Ann Med 2015;47(2):94–9.
[101] Eriksson JG, Sandboge S, Salonen MK, Kajantie E, Osmond C. Long-term consequences of maternal overweight in pregnancy on offspring later health: findings from the Helsinki Birth Cohort Study. Ann Med 2014;46(6):434–8.
[102] Langer O. Management of obesity in GDM: old habits die hard. J Matern Fetal Neonatal Med 2008;21(3):165–71.
[103] Langer O, Yogev Y, Xenakis EM, Brustman L. Overweight and obese in gestational diabetes: the impact on pregnancy outcome. Am J Obstet Gynecol 2005;192(6):1768–76.
[104] Langer O. Obesity or diabetes: which is more hazardous to the health of the offspring? J Matern Fetal Neonatal Med 2016;29(2):186–90.
[105] Yogev Y, Langer O. Pregnancy outcome in obese and morbidly obese gestational diabetic women. Eur J Obstet Gynecol Reprod Biol 2008;137(1):21–6.

[106] Chu SY, Callaghan WM, Bish CL, D'Angelo D. Gestational weight gain by body mass index among US women delivering live births, 2004–2005: fueling future obesity. Am J Obst Gynecol 2009;200(3):271.e271–7.
[107] Johnson JL, Farr SL, Dietz PM, Sharma AJ, Barfield WD, Robbins CL. Trends in gestational weight gain: the Pregnancy Risk Assessment Monitoring System, 2000–2009. Am J Obst Gynecol 2015;212(6):806.e801–8.
[108] Swank ML, Marshall NE, Caughey AB, et al. Pregnancy outcomes in the super obese, stratified by weight gain above and below Institute of Medicine guidelines. Obstet Gynecol 2014;124(6):1105–10.
[109] Blackwell SC, Landon MB, Mele L, et al. Relationship between excessive gestational weight gain and neonatal adiposity in women with mild gestational diabetes mellitus. Obstet Gynecol 2016;128(6):1325–32.
[110] Oken E, Taveras EM, Kleinman KP, Rich-Edwards JW, Gillman MW. Gestational weight gain and child adiposity at age 3 years. Am J Obst Gynecol 2007;196(4):322.e321–8.
[111] Council IoMaNR. Weight gain during pregnancy; reexamining the guidelines. Washington, DC 2009.

Shali Mazaki-Tovi and Edi Vaisbuch

4 Adipokines and pathophysiology of pregnancy complications

4.1 Introduction

4.1.1 Leptin

Leptin, a 167 amino acid is the product of the human leptin gene and it was first described by Zhang et al. in 1994 [1]. This 16 kDa protein is a pleiotropic adipokine that has been implicated in a vast array of physiologic and pathologic conditions including: energy homeostasis, glucose metabolism, innate and adaptive immune response, appetite, neuroendocrine function, bone metabolism, insulin resistance, obesity, cardiovascular disease, and reproductive fitness [2]. Leptin is secreted mainly by white adipose tissue, although not exclusively as several tissues and cells have been demonstrated to secrete this adipokine, including the human placenta [3]. During pregnancy, the placenta contributes a substantial amount of leptin to both maternal and fetal circulations as suggested by a dramatic decrease in circulating concentrations of this adipokine within a few days after delivery in both mothers [4] and neonates [5].

4.1.2 Adiponectin

Adiponectin, which was identified independently by four groups [6–9], is the most abundant gene (*AMP1*) product of adipose tissue. It circulates at relatively high concentrations [10,11] and accounts for 0.01% of the total plasma proteins. The plasma concentrations of adiponectin are paradoxically lower in obese than in nonobese individuals [6]. Adiponectin plays an important role in the pathophysiology of insulin resistance and diabetes [12], atherosclerosis [13], hypertension [14], dislipidemia [15], and angiogenesis [16]. Adiponectin circulates in human plasma in distinct forms including: (1) low-molecular weight (LMW) trimers; (2) medium-molecular weight (MMW) hexamers; and (3) high-molecular weight (HMW) oligomers (12–18 subunits) [17]. The importance of this observation stems from the fact that these adiponectin multimers can exert distinct biological effects [17], activate different single transduction pathways [18,19], and may have different affinities to the adiponectin receptors [20].

https://doi.org/10.1515/9783110487817-004

4.2 Maternal circulating leptin and adiponectin in complications of pregnancy

4.2.1 Maternal circulating leptin and complications of pregnancy

The association between maternal circulating leptin and preeclampsia has been investigated extensively (Tab. 4.1). Williams et al. [21] have conducted a nested case-control study that included 38 women with preeclampsia and 192 normotensive pregnant women. Blood samples were obtained between 15 and 22 weeks of gestations, before any clinical signs or symptoms of preeclampsia were apparent. There was a disparity in maternal serum leptin concentrations in the second trimester between normal weight and overweight/obese women. Whereas among normal weight pregnant women, those with preeclampsia had a significantly higher leptin concentration than normotensive women (20.5 ± 10.9 ng/mL vs. 13.6 ± 6.8 ng/mL, $P = 0.005$, a 33% increase), such difference was not detected among overweight/obese pregnant women with and without preeclampsia (22.3 ± 7.5 ng/mL vs. 27.8 ± 12.1 ng/mL, respectively; $P = 0.084$). These results were adjusted for prepregnancy maternal BMI, fetal gender, parity, as well as ethnic origin.

Anim-Nyame et al. [22] have conducted a longitudinal study including seven normal pregnant women and eight patients who subsequently developed preeclampsia. The investigators reported that circulating maternal leptin in women destined to develop preeclampsia were significantly higher starting after 20 weeks of gestation. An opposite pattern in maternal plasma leptin concentrations has been observed after 32 weeks between the two groups: whereas in normal pregnant women there was a decrease, patients who were destined to develop preeclampsia had a significant increase in circulating leptin. The elevated maternal plasma leptin concentration in patients with preeclampsia were consistent with the clinical presentation of the disease [22].

Similar findings were reported by Chappell et al. [23], who conducted a prospective case-control study in which leptin, placental growth factor, and plasminogen activator inhibitor were measured repeatedly during pregnancy in 21 women who later developed preeclampsia and in 17 normal pregnant women. The serum leptin concentration was significantly higher in the preeclampsia group than in the control (74%; 95% CI, 21%–135%). Consistent with the above-mentioned observations, numerous cross-sectional studies have reported an association between increased maternal circulating leptin and preeclampsia [24–28].

It is not clear why preeclampsia is associated with increased maternal circulating leptin. One possible explanation is increased secretion by the placenta [24]. As the increase in maternal circulating leptin precedes the clinical manifestations of preeclampsia, enhanced excretion by the kidneys seems unlikely. Similarly, the effect of high leptin in maternal circulation and the potential contribution to the pathophysiology of preeclampsia remain elusive.

Tab. 4.1: Maternal circulating leptin in pregnant women with and without preeclampsia.

First author	Control (*n*)	Study (*n*)	Trimester at sampling	GA at sampling	Leptin concentrations	Comment
Sattar [82]	12	9	2nd and 3rd	26–39	No difference	
Mise [83]	93	32	3rd	29–41	Higher in PE	Higher in severe than mild PE
McCarthy [26]	24	24	3rd	38.2 ± 0.4	Higher in PE	
Williams [21]	192	38	2nd	15–22	Higher in PE	Higher in women destined to develop PE
Laivuori [84]	16	22	3rd	29–39	Higher in PE	
Teppa [85]	18	18	3rd	36.6 ± 0.4	Higher in PE	
Anim-Nyame [22]	13	19	2nd and 3rd	16–38	Higher in PE	Higher in women destined to develop PE
Martínez-Abundis [86]	32	26	3rd	36.2 ± 3.9	No difference	No difference between severe and mild PE
Vitoratos [87]	17	18	3rd	28–34	Higher in PE	
Laml [88]	36	36	3rd	40.1 ± 1.2	Lower in PE	
Bartha [89]	27	25	3rd	34.5 ± 3.6	Higher in PE	
Clausen [90]	71	71	2nd	18	Lower in PE	
Chappell [23]	17	21	2nd	18–24	Higher in PE	
Gursoy [91]	21	21	3rd	NA	Higher in PE	
Kafulafula [92]	92	68	3rd	34.9 ± 5.1	Higher in PE	Only black African parturients
Chan [93]	100	20	2nd	18.3 ± 1.8	No difference	
Salomon [94]	60	30	1st	7–13	No difference	
Atamer [95]	40	96	3rd	30.5 ± 3.4	Higher in PE	No difference between severe and mild PE
Celik [96]	23	16	3rd	36.7 ± 0.3	No difference	
Ning [97]	487	55	1st	13	Higher in PE	Higher in women destined to develop PE
Kocyigit [98]	20	53	3rd	NA	Higher in PE	
Naruse [33]	40	15	3rd	28–40	Higher in PE	
Koçyigit [99]	30	40	3rd	NA	Higher in PE	

Tab. 4.1 (continued)

First author	Control (*n*)	Study (*n*)	Trimester at sampling	GA at sampling	Leptin concentrations	Comment
Baksu [100]	30	50	3rd	NA	No difference	
Haugen [35]	23	15	3rd	33–38	Higher in PE	
Hendler [36]	22	77	3rd	36–40	No difference	No difference between severe and mild PE
Lu [39]	42	38	3rd	29–41	Higher in PE	
Masuyama [51]	30	30	3rd	37.5 ± 2.0	Higher in PE	
Ouyang [53]	20	53	3rd	37.8 ± 0.7	Higher in PE	Higher in severe than mild PE
Savvidou [58]	44	13	2nd and 3rd	23–33	Higher in PE	
Nakatsukasa [42]	34	34	3rd	38.3 ± 2.2	Higher in PE	
Herse [54]	30	32	3rd	33.7 ± 2.5	Higher in PE	
Adali [101]	22	50	3rd	NA	Higher in PE	
Masuyama [102]	38	38	3rd	37.2 ± 1.8	Higher in PE	High in late-onset and in early-onset PE
Samolis [103]	53	37	1st	13	Higher in PE	Higher in women destined to develop PE
Stepan [46]	37	37	2nd and 3rd	23.8–39.8	Higher in PE	
Dalamaga [59]	262	106	3rd	38.2 ± 2.8	No difference	
Molvarec [104]	60	60	3rd	36–39	Higher in PE	
Masuyama [47]	56	56	3rd	36.4 ± 1.0	Higher in PE	

PE-Preeclampsia
GA-Gestational age

As expected, gestational diabetes mellitus (GDM) is also associated with elevated maternal circulating leptin. Kautzky-Willer et al. [29] determined maternal plasma leptin, insulin, and glucose in 55 patients with GDM and in 25 controls at 28 weeks of gestation. Blood samples were taken at 10, 20, 30, 60, 120, 150, and 180 minutes after 75 g oral glucose tolerance test conducted after overnight fast. Additional blood samples were obtained 8 weeks postpartum. Maternal plasma leptin concentrations were higher in women with GDM than in normal controls (24.9 ± 1.6 ng/mL vs. 18.2 ± 1.5 ng/mL; $P < 0.001$). In addition, there was a positive correlation between fasting leptin concentrations and fasting glucose ($r = 0.35$, $P < 0.01$) and fasting insulin ($r = 0.38$, $P < 0.004$). Among patients with GDM, maternal plasma leptin was negatively correlated with insulin sensitivity index ($r = -0.61$, $P < 0.006$) and positively correlated with pregestational BMI, BMI at blood sampling, and at term.

The possible contribution of leptin to the pathophysiology of GDM was studied by the group of Catalano in several longitudinal studies [30,31]. Kirwan et al. [30] conducted a study in which blood samples were obtained before pregnancy, in the first (12–14 weeks) and third (34–36 weeks) trimester from 10 normal pregnant women and 5 women who subsequently developed GDM. Insulin resistance was determined by the euglycemic-hyperinsulinemic clamp procedure. Using stepwise regression analysis, the authors concluded that leptin is the second best predictor of insulin sensitivity (after TNF-α) [30]. In a subsequent study of the same group with a similar study design, Okereke et al. [31] determined maternal serum leptin in the first, second, and third trimesters in five normal pregnant women and six patients who were destined to develop GDM. Maternal serum leptin concentrations were approximately 25% higher in patients who were destined to develop GDM than in normal pregnant women (first trimester: 42.4 ± 15.7 ng/mL vs. 34.5 ± 29.3 ng/mL; third trimester: 44.1 ± 27.2 ng/mL vs. 32.2 ± 26.0 ng/mL). The difference in maternal circulating leptin concentrations was statistically significant only in the third trimester. It seems, however, that the relatively small sample size precluded significance in the first and second trimesters. Collectively, these findings suggest that alterations in circulating leptin concentrations play a role in the pathophysiology of GDM.

4.2.2 Maternal circulating adiponectin and complications of pregnancy

In contrast to the consensus in the literature concerning the association between high maternal circulating leptin concentrations and preeclampsia, the evidence regarding maternal adiponectin concentrations in the presence of preeclampsia is inconsistent: higher [32–47], lower [48–56], and similar adiponectin concentrations [57–60] have been reported in patients with preeclampsia compared with normal pregnant women (Tab. 4.2).

Tab. 4.2: Maternal circulating adiponectin in pregnant women with and without preeclampsia.

First author	Control (*n*)	Study (*n*)	Trimester at sampling	GA at sampling	Adiponectin concentrations	Comment
Ramsay [32]	30	15	3rd	35–36	Higher in PE	
Naruse [33]	40	15	3rd	28–40	Higher in PE	
Kajantie [34]	15	22	3rd	29–39	Higher in PE	
D'Anna [48]	82	48	1st	9–13	Lower in PE	Lower in patients destined to develop PE
Haugen [35]	23	15	3rd	33–38	Higher in PE	
Hendler [36]	22	77	3rd	36–40	Higher in PE	High in mild and severe PE
Suwaki [37]	27	27	3rd	37–40	Higher in PE	
Takemura [38]	14	14	3rd	35.0 ± 4.0	Higher in PE	Selective increase in HMW in PE
Lu [39]	42	38	3rd	29–41	Higher in PE	
D'Anna [49]	36	36	1st	9–13	Lower in PE	Lower in late-onset than early-onset PE
O'Sullivan [57]	10	12	3rd	36	No difference	
Cortelazzi [50]	33	9	2nd and 3rd	20–37	Lower in PE	
Masuyama [51]	30	30	3rd	37.5 ± 2.0	Lower in PE	
Ichida [52]	81	27	3rd	NA	Lower in PE	
Ouyang [53]	20	53	3rd	37.8 ± 0.7	Lower in PE	Lower in severe than mild PE
Nien [40]	150	59	3rd	32 ± 3.6	Higher in PE	All patients had severe PE
Savvidou [58]	44	13	2nd and 3rd	23–33	No difference	
Fasshauer [41]	20	16	3rd	28.5 ± 6.7	Higher in PE	High HMW in PE
Nakatsukasa [42]	34	34	3rd	38.3 ± 2.2	Higher in PE	
Herse [54]	30	32	3rd	33.7 ± 2.5	Lower in PE	
Mazaki-Tovi [55]	225	111	3rd	29.3–38.9	Lower in PE	High HMW and LMW in PE
Masuyama [105]	38	38	3rd	37.2 ± 1.8	Higher in PE	Higher in late- but not in early-onset PE
Mori [56]	17	15	3rd	NA	Lower in PE	
Liu [44]	28	20	3rd	37.5–39.9	Higher in PE	
Nanda [45]	300	90	1st	11–13	Higher in PE	Higher in patients destined to develop PE
Stepan [46]	37	37	2nd and 3rd	23.8–39.8	Higher in PE	
Dalamaga [59]	262	106	3rd	38.2 ± 2.8	No difference	
Valdés [60]	35	10	1st	11–14	No difference	
Masuyama [47]	56	56	3rd	36.4 ± 1.0	Higher in PE	

PE-Preeclampsia
GA-Gestational age

Ramsay et al. [32] were the first to report the concentrations of adiponectin in patients with preeclampsia ($n = 15$) and controls ($n = 30$). Third trimester (35–36 weeks of gestation) maternal serum adiponectin concentrations were significantly higher in patients with preeclampsia (21.6 ± 8.18 μg/mL vs. 14.7 ± 7.06 μg/mL; $P = 0.01$). The authors described this finding as "paradoxical" because obesity and insulin resistance, which are strongly associated with low circulating adiponectin, are well-established risk factors for preeclampsia. The investigators propose several explanations for this finding including exaggerated adipocyte lipolysis, a counter-response aimed at enhancing fat utilization and attenuating endothelial damage and decreased excretion by the kidney.

D'Anna et al. [48] have conducted a nested case-control study in which maternal blood samples were obtained between 9 and 13 weeks of gestation. The study included a control group ($n = 82$) and women who subsequently developed preeclampsia ($n = 34$) or gestational hypertension ($n = 48$). When patients destined to develop either preeclampsia or gestational hypertension were grouped together, the median adiponectin concentration was significantly lower in these patients than in the control group (7.6 vs. 13.0 μg/mL; $P < 0.001$). Importantly, a comparison between the two hypertensive subgroups revealed that the median maternal plasma adiponectin was significantly lower in patients destined to develop preeclampsia than in women who subsequently had gestational hypertension (6.6 vs. 9.3 μg/mL; $P = 0.01$). When the maternal plasma adiponectin cutoff of 6.4 μg/mL was used (mean value of lower quartile of distribution among control patients), 25% of patients with gestational hypertension and 47% of patients with preeclampsia had plasma adiponectin concentration below the cutoff compared with 7% in the control group ($P < 0.001$ for both comparisons) [48].

An additional line of evidence for the relationship between adiponectin and preeclampsia comes from genetic association studies. Saarela et al. [61] determined the genotype for two single nucleotide polymorphisms (SNPs), SNP45 in exon 2 and SNP276 in intron 2, in the adiponectin gene in 133 Finnish women with preeclampsia and 245 normotensive controls. In addition, the authors conducted an analysis of the pair of loci haplotype to examine the estimated haplotype frequencies of these SNPs among the two study groups. The authors reported that the TT genotype vs. the pooled G genotypes in SNP276 was associated with protection against preeclampsia (odds ratio 0.27; 95% CI, 0.09–0.80).

Our group [55] has conducted a cross-sectional study to determine whether preeclampsia is associated with changes in circulating adiponectin multimers. The study population included women with a normal pregnancy ($n = 225$) and patients with preeclampsia ($n = 111$). The median maternal serum concentration of total adiponectin was lower in patients with preeclampsia than in those with a normal pregnancy (5.0 μg/mL vs. 6.4 μg/mL; $P < 0.001$; Fig. 4.1). Patients with preeclampsia had a lower median serum concentrations of HMW (2.3 μg/mL vs. 3.6 μg/mL; $P < 0.001$; Fig. 4.1) and LMW adiponectin (1.0 μg/mL vs. 1.3 μg/mL; $P = 0.01$, Fig. 4.1) than those with a normal

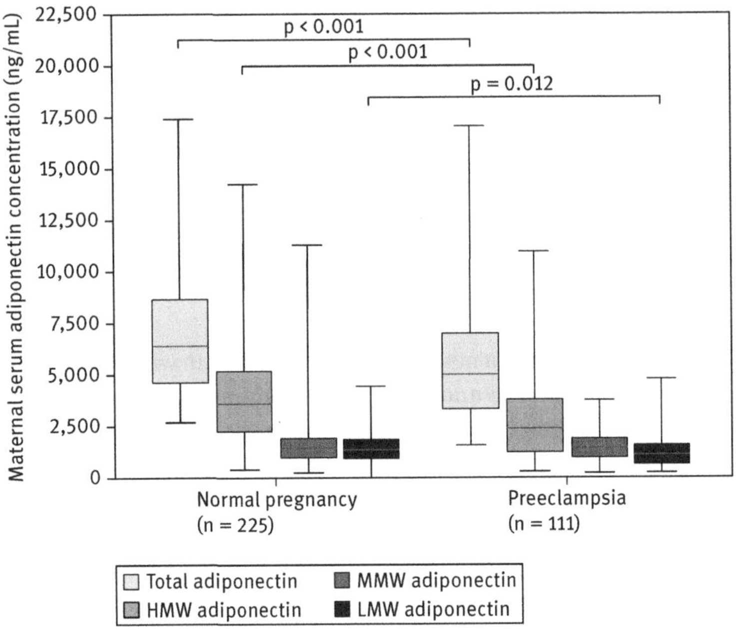

Fig. 4.1: Comparison of the median serum total, HMW, MMW, and LMW adiponectin concentrations between pregnant women with normal pregnancies and those with preeclampsia. The median maternal serum concentration of total adiponectin was lower in patients with preeclampsia than in those with a normal pregnancy. Similarly, patients with preeclampsia had lower serum concentrations of HMW and LMW adiponectin than those with a normal pregnancy. The median maternal serum concentration of MMW adiponectin did not differ between patients with preeclampsia and those with a normal pregnancy.

pregnancy. The median maternal serum concentration of MMW adiponectin did not differ between patients with preeclampsia and women with a normal pregnancy (1.3 μg/mL vs. 1.4 μg/mL; $P = 0.7$; Fig. 4.1) [55].

Differences among the two groups were not only in the absolute concentrations of adiponectin multimers but also in their relative abundance. The median maternal HMW/total adiponectin ratio was lower in patients with preeclampsia than in those with a normal pregnancy (0.46 vs. 0.55; $P < 0.001$; Fig. 4.2). In contrast, patients with preeclampsia had a higher median MMW/total adiponectin ratio (0.29 vs. 0.22; $P < 0.001$; Fig. 4.2) as well as a higher LMW/total adiponectin ratio (0.25 vs. 0.21; $P = 0.009$; Fig. 4.2) than those with a normal pregnancy [55]. Of note, the various adiponectin isoforms cannot interchange with each other after secretion [17]. Thus, the altered regulation of adiponectin multimeric complexes occurs in the adipocytes. Collectively, these results suggest that altered function of adipose tissue is a feature of preeclampsia.

In summary, several lines of evidence support the association between altered maternal circulating adiponectin concentrations and preeclampsia. Genetic

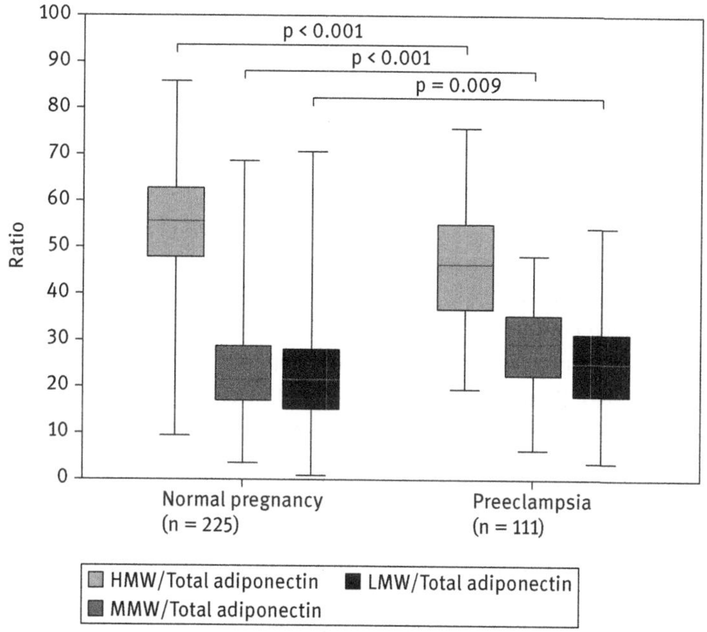

Fig. 4.2: Comparison of HMW/total adiponectin MMW/total adiponectin and LMW/total adiponectin ratio between pregnant women with normal pregnancies and those with preeclampsia. The median maternal HMW/total adiponectin ratio was lower in patients with preeclampsia than in those with a normal pregnancy. In contrast, patients with preeclampsia had a higher median MMW/total adiponectin ratio as well as a higher LMW/total adiponectin ratio than those with a normal pregnancy.

predisposition and low maternal plasma adiponectin concentration that precede the clinical stage of the disease suggest a role for adiponectin in the pathophysiology of preeclampsia. On the other hand, preeclampsia was associated with both higher and lower maternal circulating adiponectin concentrations than normal pregnant women. This inconsistency in the literature may be due to differences in the study population characteristics, definitions of preeclampsia (mild vs. severe, early- vs. late-onset), sample size or methods by which adiponectin concentrations were determined. However, although it is possible to explain some of the discrepancies by differences in study design, the inconsistency of the results may also reflect the syndromic nature of preeclampsia.

In contrast to the conflicting results concerning maternal circulating adiponectin and preeclampsia, there is an agreement that GDM is characterized by a low circulating maternal concentration of adiponectin [62–69]. This is consistent with the findings concerning the “extra-gestation” counterpart of GDM, i.e. type 2 DM. Indeed, polymorphisms of several adipokines including adiponectin [70–76] are associated with insulin resistance and type 2 DM. Moreover, compared with nondiabetic individuals, patients with type 2 DM have lower concentrations of adiponectin [77–79].

These findings laid the groundwork for the hypothesis that perturbation of adipokine homeostasis plays a role in the pathophysiology of GDM.

Retnakaran et al. [67] classified 180 pregnant women according to the results of their screening 50 g glucose challenge test and the 100 g oral glucose tolerance test into three groups: (1) GDM, (2) impaired glucose tolerance, and (3) normal glucose tolerance. The median adiponectin concentration was the lowest in the GDM group (12.3 μg/mL, interquartile range (IQR) 7.9–16.6), highest in the normal glucose tolerance group (16.2 μg/mL, IQR 12.4–19.3), and intermediate in the impaired glucose tolerance group (15.3 μg/mL, IQR 11.7–19.8; overall $P = 0.0004$).

Williams et al. [80] have conducted a prospective, nested case-control study to compare maternal plasma adiponectin concentrations between patients with GDM ($n = 41$) and controls ($n = 70$). Samples were collected at 13 weeks of gestation. The authors used a maternal plasma adiponectin cutoff of 6.4 μg/mL (lower tertile of the control group). As expected, the median maternal circulating adiponectin concentrations were significantly lower in women who subsequently developed GDM than in controls (4.4 vs. 8.1 μg/mL, $P < 0.001$). Pregnant women with adiponectin concentrations <6.4 μg/mL had a 4.6-fold increased risk of GDM than those with higher concentrations (95% CI, 1.8–11.6, adjusted for maternal BMI).

Our group [81] has conducted a cross-sectional study to determine whether GDM and pharmacological treatment (sulfonylurea vs. insulin) are associated with alterations in maternal circulating adiponectin multimers. The study included normal pregnancy ($n = 149$) and patients with GDM ($n = 72$). Thirty-three patients with GDM were managed with diet alone, 17 were treated with glyburide and 22 with insulin. The median maternal serum concentration of total adiponectin was lower in patients with GDM than in those with a normal pregnancy (3.0 ng/mL vs. 6.0 ng/mL; $P < 0.001$; Fig. 4.3). Similarly, patients with GDM had a lower median serum concentration of HMW (1.2 ng/mL vs. 3.2 ng/mL; $P < 0.001$; Fig. 4.3), MMW (8.8 ng/mL vs. 1.3 ng/mL; $P < 0.001$; Fig. 4.3), and LMW adiponectin (9.6 ng/mL vs. 1.2 ng/mL; $P < 0.001$; Fig. 4.3) than those with a normal pregnancy.

The median maternal HMW/total adiponectin ratio was lower in patients with GDM than in those with a normal pregnancy (0.37 vs. 0.54; $P < 0.001$; Fig. 4.4). In contrast, patients with GDM had a higher median MMW/total adiponectin ratio (0.30 vs. 0.23; $P < 0.001$; Fig. 4.4), and a higher LMW/total adiponectin ratio (0.32 vs. 0.21; $P < 0.001$; Fig. 4.4) than those with a normal pregnancy.

Patients with GDM who were managed with diet and those treated with a pharmacologic agent (glyburide or insulin) had comparable concentrations of total, HMW, MMW, and LMW adiponectin. The relative distribution of adiponectin isoforms was also comparable between the two groups. Similarly, there were no differences in the concentrations and relative distribution of adiponectin multimers between patients who were treated with glyburide and those treated with insulin.

Collectively, evaluation of maternal circulating total adiponectin and adiponectin isoforms in patients with GDM reveals that this condition is characterized by a pattern

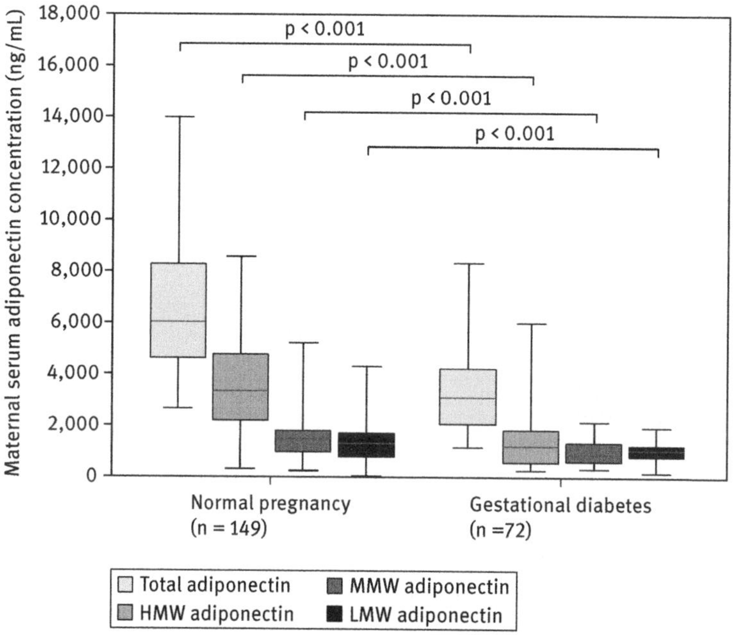

Fig. 4.3: Comparison of the median serum total, HMW, MMW, and LMW adiponectin concentrations between pregnant women with normal pregnancies and those with GDM. The median maternal serum concentration of total, HMW, MMW, and LMW were significantly lower in patients with GDM than in those with normal pregnancies.

akin to type 2 DM. In addition, the reports concerning low maternal adiponectin concentrations in patients with GDM, as well as the dysregulation of adiponectin multimers in these patients can provide a mechanistic basis for the association between adiposity and GDM. Moreover, these findings may provide a molecular mechanism to account for the association between GDM and its long-term complication, type 2 DM.

4.3 Summary

Women of reproductive age are increasingly affected by obesity. Importantly, obesity is an independent and well-established risk factor for several complications of pregnancy including preeclampsia, fetal death, GDM, congenital anomalies, and preterm labor. Although preconception weight loss is a laudable goal for overweight/obese woman, many pregnancies are not planned and recommendations for lifestyle changes aimed at reducing weight are not easily implemented. Despite the pandemic proportions of obesity in young women, the mechanism by which adipose tissue exerts its deleterious effect on gestation is not clear. The discovery of adipokines and their important role in physiological and pathological conditions provides a plausible

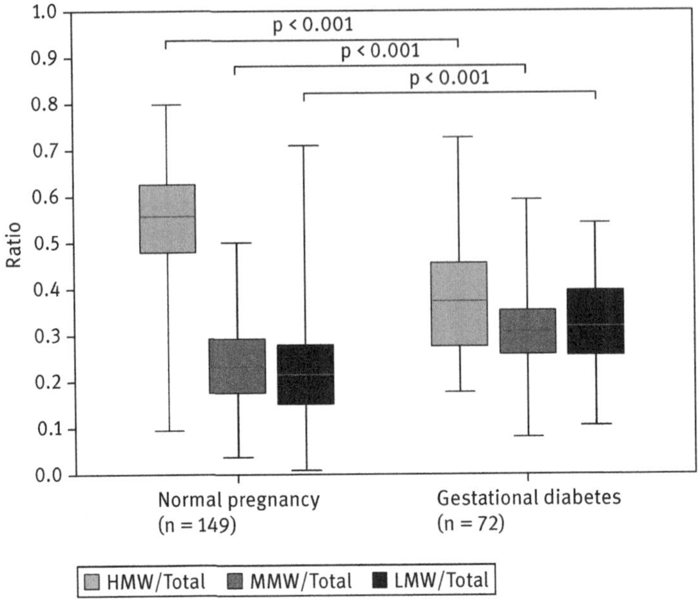

Fig. 4.4: Comparison of HMW/total adiponectin MMW/total adiponectin and LMW/total adiponectin ratios between pregnant women with normal pregnancies and those with GDM. The median maternal HMW/total adiponectin ratio was lower in patients with GDM than in those with a normal pregnancy. In contrast, patients with GDM had a higher median MMW/total adiponectin and LMW/total adiponectin ratios than those with a normal pregnancy.

molecular mechanism for the association between adiposity and metabolic- and inflammatory-related diseases. Characterization of the role played by adipokines in normal gestation and complications of pregnancy may improve the prediction and diagnosis of metabolic-related complications of pregnancy. Moreover, the implicit promise of such research is that the discovery of novel adipokines and new mechanisms of disease will identify adipokines as a target for pharmacological intervention aimed at preventing complications of pregnancy or their sequelae on the mother, fetus, and neonate.

Bibliography

[1] Zhang Y, Proenca R, Maffei M, Barone M, Leopold L, Friedman JM. Positional cloning of the mouse obese gene and its human homologue. Nature 1994;372:425–32.
[2] Kelesidis T, Kelesidis I, Chou S, Mantzoros CS. Narrative review: the role of leptin in human physiology: emerging clinical applications. Ann Intern Med 2010;152:93–100.
[3] Masuzaki H, Ogawa Y, Sagawa N, Hosoda K, Matsumoto T, Mise H, et al. Nonadipose tissue production of leptin: leptin as a novel placenta-derived hormone in humans. Nat Med 1997;3:1029–33.

[4] Sivan E, Whittaker PG, Sinha D, Homko CJ, Lin M, Reece EA, et al. Leptin in human pregnancy: the relationship with gestational hormones. Am J Obstet Gynecol 1998;179:1128–32.
[5] Sivan E, Mazaki-Tovi S, Pariente C, Efraty Y, Schiff E, Hemi R, et al. Adiponectin in human cord blood: relation to fetal birth weight and gender. J Clin Endocrinol Metab 2003;88:5656–60.
[6] Hu E, Liang P, Spiegelman BM. AdipoQ is a novel adipose-specific gene dysregulated in obesity. J Biol Chem 1996;271:10697–703.
[7] Maeda K, Okubo K, Shimomura I, Funahashi T, Matsuzawa Y, Matsubara K. cDNA cloning and expression of a novel adipose specific collagen-like factor, apM1 (AdiPose Most abundant gene transcript 1). Biochem Biophys Res Commun 1996;221:286–9.
[8] Nakano Y, Tobe T, Choi-Miura NH, Mazda T, Tomita M. Isolation and characterization of GBP28, a novel gelatin-binding protein purified from human plasma. J Biochem 1996;120:803–12.
[9] Scherer PE, Williams S, Fogliano M, Baldini G, Lodish HF. A novel serum protein similar to C1q, produced exclusively in adipocytes. J Biol Chem 1995;270:26746–9.
[10] Ahima RS, Flier JS. Adipose tissue as an endocrine organ. Trends Endocrinol Metab 2000;11:327–32.
[11] Arita Y, Kihara S, Ouchi N, Takahashi M, Maeda K, Miyagawa J, et al. Paradoxical decrease of an adipose-specific protein, adiponectin, in obesity. Biochem Biophys Res Commun 1999;257:79–83.
[12] Hotta K, Funahashi T, Arita Y, Takahashi M, Matsuda M, Okamoto Y, et al. Plasma concentrations of a novel, adipose-specific protein, adiponectin, in type 2 diabetic patients. Arterioscler Thromb Vasc Biol 2000;20:1595–9.
[13] Ouchi N, Kihara S, Arita Y, Maeda K, Kuriyama H, Okamoto Y, et al. Novel modulator for endothelial adhesion molecules: adipocyte-derived plasma protein adiponectin. Circulation 1999;100:2473–6.
[14] Ouchi N, Ohishi M, Kihara S, Funahashi T, Nakamura T, Nagaretani H, et al. Association of hypoadiponectinemia with impaired vasoreactivity. Hypertension 2003;42:231–4.
[15] Matsubara M, Maruoka S, Katayose S. Decreased plasma adiponectin concentrations in women with dyslipidemia. J Clin Endocrinol Metab 2002;87:2764–9.
[16] Shibata R, Ouchi N, Kihara S, Sato K, Funahashi T, Walsh K. Adiponectin stimulates angiogenesis in response to tissue ischemia through stimulation of amp-activated protein kinase signaling. J Biol Chem 2004;279:28670–4.
[17] Pajvani UB, Du X, Combs TP, Berg AH, Rajala MW, Schulthess T, et al. Structure-function studies of the adipocyte-secreted hormone Acrp30/adiponectin. Implications fpr metabolic regulation and bioactivity. J Biol Chem 2003;278:9073–85.
[18] Waki H, Yamauchi T, Kamon J, Ito Y, Uchida S, Kita S, et al. Impaired multimerization of human adiponectin mutants associated with diabetes. Molecular structure and multimer formation of adiponectin. J Biol Chem 2003;278:40352–63.
[19] Tsao TS, Tomas E, Murrey HE, Hug C, Lee DH, Ruderman NB, et al. Role of disulfide bonds in Acrp30/adiponectin structure and signaling specificity. Different oligomers activate different signal transduction pathways. J Biol Chem 2003;278:50810–17.
[20] Yamauchi T, Kamon J, Ito Y, Tsuchida A, Yokomizo T, Kita S, et al. Cloning of adiponectin receptors that mediate antidiabetic metabolic effects. Nature 2003;423:762–9.
[21] Williams MA, Havel PJ, Schwartz MW, Leisenring WM, King IB, Zingheim RW, et al. Pre-eclampsia disrupts the normal relationship between serum leptin concentrations and adiposity in pregnant women. Paediatr Perinat Epidemiol 1999;13:190–204.
[22] Anim-Nyame N, Sooranna SR, Steer PJ, Johnson MR. Longitudinal analysis of maternal plasma leptin concentrations during normal pregnancy and pre-eclampsia. Hum Reprod 2000;15:2033–6.

[23] Chappell LC, Seed PT, Briley A, Kelly FJ, Hunt BJ, Charnock-Jones DS, et al. A longitudinal study of biochemical variables in women at risk of preeclampsia. Am J Obstet Gynecol 2002;187:127–36.
[24] Hauguel-De MS, Lepercq J, Catalano P. The known and unknown of leptin in pregnancy. Am J Obstet Gynecol 2006;194:1537–45.
[25] Henson MC, Castracane VD. Leptin in pregnancy: an update. Biol Reprod 2006;74:218–29.
[26] McCarthy JF, Misra DN, Roberts JM. Maternal plasma leptin is increased in preeclampsia and positively correlates with fetal cord concentration. Am J Obstet Gynecol 1999;180:731–6.
[27] Poston L. Leptin and preeclampsia. Semin Reprod Med 2002;20:131–8.
[28] Laivuori H, Kaaja R, Koistinen H, Karonen SL, Andersson S, Koivisto V, et al. Leptin during and after preeclamptic or normal pregnancy: its relation to serum insulin and insulin sensitivity. Metabolism 2000;49:259–63.
[29] Kautzky-Willer A, Pacini G, Tura A, Bieglmayer C, Schneider B, Ludvik B, et al. Increased plasma leptin in gestational diabetes. Diabetologia 2001;44:164–72.
[30] Kirwan JP, Hauguel-De MS, Lepercq J, Challier JC, Huston-Presley L, Friedman JE, et al. TNF-alpha is a predictor of insulin resistance in human pregnancy. Diabetes 2002;51:2207–13.
[31] Okereke NC, Huston-Presley L, Amini SB, Kalhan S, Catalano PM. Longitudinal changes in energy expenditure and body composition in obese women with normal and impaired glucose tolerance. Am J Physiol Endocrinol Metab 2004;287:E472–9.
[32] Ramsay JE, Jamieson N, Greer IA, Sattar N. Paradoxical elevation in adiponectin concentrations in women with preeclampsia. Hypertension 2003;42:891–4.
[33] Naruse K, Yamasaki M, Umekage H, Sado T, Sakamoto Y, Morikawa H. Peripheral blood concentrations of adiponectin, an adipocyte-specific plasma protein, in normal pregnancy and preeclampsia. J Reprod Immunol 2005;65:65–75.
[34] Kajantie E, Kaaja R, Ylikorkala O, Andersson S, Laivuori H. Adiponectin concentrations in maternal serum: elevated in preeclampsia but unrelated to insulin sensitivity. J Soc Gynecol Investig 2005;12:433–9.
[35] Haugen F, Ranheim T, Harsem NK, Lips E, Staff AC, Drevon CA. Increased plasma levels of adipokines in preeclampsia: relationship to placenta and adipose tissue gene expression. Am J Physiol Endocrinol Metab 2006;290:E326–33.
[36] Hendler I, Blackwell SC, Mehta SH, Whitty JE, Russell E, Sorokin Y, et al. The levels of leptin, adiponectin, and resistin in normal weight, overweight, and obese pregnant women with and without preeclampsia. Am J Obstet Gynecol 2005;193:979–83.
[37] Suwaki N, Masuyama H, Nakatsukasa H, Masumoto A, Sumida Y, Takamoto N, et al. Hypoadiponectinemia and circulating angiogenic factors in overweight patients complicated with pre-eclampsia. Am J Obstet Gynecol 2006;1687–92.
[38] Takemura Y, Osuga Y, Koga K, Tajima T, Hirota Y, Hirata T, et al. Selective increase in high molecular weight adiponectin concentration in serum of women with preeclampsia. J Reprod Immunol 2007;73:60–5.
[39] Lu D, Yang X, Wu Y, Wang H, Huang H, Dong M. Serum adiponectin, leptin and soluble leptin receptor in pre-eclampsia. Int J Gynaecol Obstet 2006;121–6.
[40] Nien JK, Mazaki-Tovi S, Romero R, Erez O, Kusanovic JP, Gotsch F, et al. Adiponectin in severe preeclampsia. J Perinat Med 2007;35:503–12.
[41] Fasshauer M, Waldeyer T, Seeger J, Schrey S, Ebert T, Kratzsch J, et al. Circulating high-molecular-weight adiponectin is upregulated in preeclampsia and is related to insulin sensitivity and renal function. Eur J Endocrinol 2008;158:197–201.
[42] Nakatsukasa H, Masuyama H, Takamoto N, Hiramatsu Y. Circulating leptin and angiogenic factors in preeclampsia patients. Endocr J 2008;55:565–73.
[43] Masuyama H, Segawa T, Sumida Y, Masumoto A, Inoue S, Akahori Y, et al. Different profiles of circulating angiogenic factors and adipocytokines between early- and late-onset pre-eclampsia. BJOG 2010;117:314–20.

[44] Liu Y, Zhu L, Pan Y, Sun L, Chen D, Li X. Adiponectin levels in circulation and breast milk and mRNA expression in adipose tissue of preeclampsia women. Hypertens Pregnancy 2012;31:40–9.
[45] Nanda S, Yu CK, Giurcaneanu L, Akolekar R, Nicolaides KH. Maternal serum adiponectin at 11–13 weeks of gestation in preeclampsia. Fetal Diagn Ther 2011;29:208–15.
[46] Stepan H, Philipp A, Roth I, Kralisch S, Jank A, Schaarschmidt W, et al. Serum levels of the adipokine chemerin are increased in preeclampsia during and 6 months after pregnancy. Regul Pept 2011;168:69–72.
[47] Masuyama H, Nobumoto E, Inoue S, Hiramatsu Y. Potential interaction of brain natriuretic peptide with hyperadiponectinemia in preeclampsia. Am J Physiol Endocrinol Metab 2012;302:E687–93.
[48] D'Anna R, Baviera G, Corrado F, Giordano D, Di Benedetto A, Jasonni VM. Plasma adiponectin concentration in early pregnancy and subsequent risk of hypertensive disorders. Obstet Gynecol 2005;106:340–4.
[49] D'Anna R, Baviera G, Corrado F, Giordano D, De VA, Nicocia G, et al. Adiponectin and insulin resistance in early- and late-onset pre-eclampsia. BJOG 2006;113:1264–9.
[50] Cortelazzi D, Corbetta S, Ronzoni S, Pelle F, Marconi A, Cozzi V, et al. Maternal and foetal resistin and adiponectin concentrations in normal and complicated pregnancies. Clin Endocrinol (Oxf) 2007;66:447–53.
[51] Masuyama H, Nakatsukasa H, Takamoto N, Hiramatsu Y. Correlation between soluble endoglin, vascular endothelial growth factor receptor-1 and adipocytokines in preeclampsia. J Clin Endocrinol Metab 2007;2672–9.
[52] Ichida K, Moriyama T, Morita H, Kondo T, Yoshida S, Ohara N, et al. Plasma adiponectin concentrations and placental adiponectin expression in pre-eclamptic women. Gynecol Endocrinol 2007;23:238–43.
[53] Ouyang Y, Chen H, Chen H. Reduced plasma adiponectin and elevated leptin in pre-eclampsia. Int J Gynaecol Obstet 2007;98:110–14.
[54] Herse F, Bai Y, Staff AC, Yong-Meid J, Dechend R, Zhou R. Circulating and uteroplacental adipocytokine concentrations in preeclampsia. Reprod Sci 2009;16:584–90.
[55] Mazaki-Tovi S, Romero R, Vaisbuch E, Kusanovic JP, Erez O, Gotsch F, et al. Maternal serum adiponectin multimers in preeclampsia. J Perinat Med 2009;37:349–63.
[56] Mori T, Shinohara K, Wakatsuki A, Watanabe K, Fujimaki A. Adipocytokines and endothelial function in preeclamptic women. Hypertens Res 2010;33:250–4.
[57] O'Sullivan AJ, Kriketos AD, Martin A, Brown MA. Serum adiponectin levels in normal and hypertensive pregnancy. Hypertens Pregnancy 2006;25:193–203.
[58] Savvidou MD, Sotiriadis A, Kaihura C, Nicolaides KH, Sattar N. Circulating levels of adiponectin and leptin at 23–25 weeks of pregnancy in women with impaired placentation and in those with established fetal growth restriction. Clin Sci (Lond) 2008;115:219–24.
[59] Dalamaga M, Srinivas SK, Elovitz MA, Chamberland J, Mantzoros CS. Serum adiponectin and leptin in relation to risk for preeclampsia: results from a large case-control study. Metabolism 2011;60:1539–44.
[60] Valdes ER, Lattes KA, Munoz HS, Barja PY, Papapietro KV. First-trimester adiponectin and subsequent development of preeclampsia or fetal growth restriction. Gynecol Obstet Invest 2011;72:152–6.
[61] Saarela T, Hiltunen M, Helisalmi S, Heinonen S, Laakso M. Adiponectin gene haplotype is associated with preeclampsia. Genet Test 2006;10:35–9.
[62] Ategbo JM, Grissa O, Yessoufou A, Hichami A, Dramane KL, Moutairou K, et al. Modulation of adipokines and cytokines in gestational diabetes and macrosomia. J Clin Endocrinol Metab 2006;91:4137–43.
[63] Kinalski M, Telejko B, Kuzmicki M, Kretowski A, Kinalska I. Tumor necrosis factor alpha system and plasma adiponectin concentration in women with gestational diabetes. Horm Metab Res 2005;37:450–4.

[64] Ranheim T, Haugen F, Staff AC, Braekke K, Harsem NK, Drevon CA. Adiponectin is reduced in gestational diabetes mellitus in normal weight women. Acta Obstet Gynecol Scand 2004;83:341–7.
[65] Thyfault JP, Hedberg EM, Anchan RM, Thorne OP, Isler CM, Newton ER, et al. Gestational diabetes is associated with depressed adiponectin levels. J Soc Gynecol Investig 2005;12:41–5.
[66] Worda C, Leipold H, Gruber C, Kautzky-Willer A, Knofler M, Bancher-Todesca D. Decreased plasma adiponectin concentrations in women with gestational diabetes mellitus. Am J Obstet Gynecol 2004;191:2120–4.
[67] Retnakaran R, Hanley AJ, Raif N, Connelly PW, Sermer M, Zinman B. Reduced adiponectin concentration in women with gestational diabetes: a potential factor in progression to type 2 diabetes. Diabetes Care 2004;27:799–800.
[68] Retnakaran R, Hanley AJ, Raif N, Hirning CR, Connelly PW, Sermer M, et al. Adiponectin and beta cell dysfunction in gestational diabetes: pathophysiological implications. Diabetologia 2005;48:993–1001.
[69] Tsai PJ, Yu CH, Hsu SP, Lee YH, Huang IT, Ho SC, et al. Maternal plasma adiponectin concentrations at 24 to 31 weeks of gestation: negative association with gestational diabetes mellitus. Nutrition 2005;21:1095–9.
[70] Filippi E, Sentinelli F, Trischitta V, Romeo S, Arca M, Leonetti F, et al. Association of the human adiponectin gene and insulin resistance. Eur J Hum Genet 2004;12:199–205.
[71] Gonzalez-Sanchez JL, Zabena CA, Martinez-Larrad MT, Fernandez-Perez C, Perez-Barba M, Laakso M, et al. An SNP in the adiponectin gene is associated with decreased serum adiponectin levels and risk for impaired glucose tolerance. Obes Res 2005;13:807–12.
[72] Hu FB, Doria A, Li T, Meigs JB, Liu S, Memisoglu A, et al. Genetic variation at the adiponectin locus and risk of type 2 diabetes in women. Diabetes 2004;53:209–13.
[73] Lee YY, Lee NS, Cho YM, Moon MK, Jung HS, Park YJ, et al. Genetic association study of adiponectin polymorphisms with risk of type 2 diabetes mellitus in Korean population. Diabet Med 2005;22:569–75.
[74] Menzaghi C, Ercolino T, Di PR, Berg AH, Warram JH, Scherer PE, et al. A haplotype at the adiponectin locus is associated with obesity and other features of the insulin resistance syndrome. Diabetes 2002;51:2306–12.
[75] Nakatani K, Noma K, Nishioka J, Kasai Y, Morioka K, Katsuki A, et al. Adiponectin gene variation associates with the increasing risk of type 2 diabetes in non-diabetic Japanese subjects. Int J Mol Med 2005;15:173–7.
[76] Stumvoll M, Tschritter O, Fritsche A, Staiger H, Renn W, Weisser M, et al. Association of the T-G polymorphism in adiponectin (exon 2) with obesity and insulin sensitivity: interaction with family history of type 2 diabetes. Diabetes 2002;51:37–41.
[77] Kim MJ, Yoo KH, Park HS, Chung SM, Jin CJ, Lee Y, et al. Plasma adiponectin and insulin resistance in Korean type 2 diabetes mellitus. Yonsei Med J 2005;46:42–50.
[78] Putz DM, Goldner WS, Bar RS, Haynes WG, Sivitz WI. Adiponectin and C-reactive protein in obesity, type 2 diabetes, and monodrug therapy. Metabolism 2004;53:1454–61.
[79] Weyer C, Funahashi T, Tanaka S, Hotta K, Matsuzawa Y, Pratley RE, et al. Hypoadiponectinemia in obesity and type 2 diabetes: close association with insulin resistance and hyperinsulinemia. J Clin Endocrinol Metab 2001;86:1930–5.
[80] Williams MA, Qiu C, Muy-Rivera M, Vadachkoria S, Song T, Luthy DA. Plasma adiponectin concentrations in early pregnancy and subsequent risk of gestational diabetes mellitus. J Clin Endocrinol Metab 2004;89:2306–11.
[81] Mazaki-Tovi S, Romero R, Vaisbuch E, Erez O, Mittal P, Chaiwaropongsa T, et al. Maternal serum adiponectin multimers in gestational diabetes. J Perinat Med 2009;37:637–50.

[82] Sattar N, Greer IA, Pirwani I, Gibson J, Wallace AM. Leptin levels in pregnancy: marker for fat accumulation and mobilization? Acta Obstet Gynecol Scand 1998;77:278–83.
[83] Mise H, Sagawa N, Matsumoto T, Yura S, Nanno H, Itoh H, et al. Augmented placental production of leptin in preeclampsia: possible involvement of placental hypoxia. J Clin Endocrinol Metab 1998;83:3225–9.
[84] Laivuori H, Kaaja R, Koistinen H, Karonen SL, Andersson S, Koivisto V, et al. Leptin during and after preeclamptic or normal pregnancy: its relation to serum insulin and insulin sensitivity. Metabolism 2000;49:259–63.
[85] Teppa RJ, Ness RB, Crombleholme WR, Roberts JM. Free leptin is increased in normal pregnancy and further increased in preeclampsia. Metabolism 2000;49:1043–8.
[86] Martinez-Abundis E, Gonzalez-Ortiz M, Pascoe-Gonzalez S. Serum leptin levels and the severity of preeclampsia. Arch Gynecol Obstet 2000;264:71–3.
[87] Vitoratos N, Chrystodoulacos G, Kouskouni E, Salamalekis E, Creatsas G. Alterations of maternal and fetal leptin concentrations in hypertensive disorders of pregnancy. Eur J Obstet Gynecol Reprod Biol 2001;96:59–62.
[88] Laml T, Preyer O, Hartmann BW, Ruecklinger E, Soeregi G, Wagenbichler P. Decreased maternal serum leptin in pregnancies complicated by preeclampsia. J Soc Gynecol Investig 2001;8:89–93.
[89] Bartha JL, Romero-Carmona R, Escobar-Llompart M, Comino-Delgado R. The relationships between leptin and inflammatory cytokines in women with pre-eclampsia. BJOG 2001;108:1272–6.
[90] Clausen T, Djurovic S, Reseland JE, Berg K, Drevon CA, Henriksen T. Altered plasma concentrations of leptin, transforming growth factor-beta(1) and plasminogen activator inhibitor type 2 at 18 weeks of gestation in women destined to develop pre-eclampsia. Circulating markers of disturbed placentation? Placenta 2002;23:380–5.
[91] Gursoy T, Aliefendioglu D, Aslan AT, Gunduz M, Haberal A, Senes M, et al. Preeclampsia disrupts the normal physiology of leptin. Am J Perinatol 2002;19:303–10.
[92] Kafulafula GE, Moodley J, Ojwang PJ, Kagoro H. Leptin and pre-eclampsia in black African parturients. BJOG 2002;109:1256–61.
[93] Chan TF, Su JH, Chung YF, Hsu YH, Yeh YT, Jong SB, et al. Amniotic fluid and maternal serum leptin levels in pregnant women who subsequently develop preeclampsia. Eur J Obstet Gynecol Reprod Biol 2003;108:50–3.
[94] Salomon LJ, Benattar C, Audibert F, Fernandez H, Duyme M, Taieb J, et al. Severe preeclampsia is associated with high inhibin A levels and normal leptin levels at 7 to 13 weeks into pregnancy. Am J Obstet Gynecol 2003;189:1517–22.
[95] Atamer Y, Erden AC, Demir B, Kocyigit Y, Atamer A. The relationship between plasma levels of leptin and androgen in healthy and preeclamptic pregnant women. Acta Obstet Gynecol Scand 2004;83:425–30.
[96] Celik O, Hascalik S, Ozerol E, Hascalik M, Yologlu S. Cerebrospinal fluid leptin levels in preeclampsia: relation to maternal serum leptin levels. Acta Obstet Gynecol Scand 2004;83:519–23.
[97] Ning Y, Williams MA, Muy-Rivera M, Leisenring WM, Luthy DA. Relationship of maternal plasma leptin and risk of pre-eclampsia: a prospective study. J Matern Fetal Neonatal Med 2004;15:186–92.
[98] Kocyigit Y, Bayhan G, Atamer A, Atamer Y. Serum levels of leptin, insulin-like growth factor-I and insulin-like growth factor binding protein-3 in women with pre-eclampsia, and their relationship to insulin resistance. Gynecol Endocrinol 2004;18:341–8.
[99] Kocyigit Y, Atamer Y, Atamer A, Tuzcu A, Akkus Z. Changes in serum levels of leptin, cytokines and lipoprotein in pre-eclamptic and normotensive pregnant women. Gynecol Endocrinol 2004;19:267–73.

[100] Baksu A, Ozkan A, Goker N, Baksu B, Uluocak A. Serum leptin levels in preeclamptic pregnant women: relationship to thyroid-stimulating hormone, body mass index, and proteinuria. Am J Perinatol 2005;22:161–4.
[101] Adali E, Yildizhan R, Kolusari A, Kurdoglu M, Bugdayci G, Sahin HG, et al. Increased visfatin and leptin in pregnancies complicated by pre-eclampsia. J Matern Fetal Neonatal Med 2009;1–7.
[102] Masuyama H, Segawa T, Sumida Y, Masumoto A, Inoue S, Akahori Y, et al. Different profiles of circulating angiogenic factors and adipocytokines between early- and late-onset pre-eclampsia. BJOG 2010;117:314–20.
[103] Samolis S, Papastefanou I, Panagopoulos P, Galazios G, Kouskoukis A, Maroulis G. Relation between first trimester maternal serum leptin levels and body mass index in normotensive and pre-eclamptic pregnancies — role of leptin as a marker of pre-eclampsia: a prospective case-control study. Gynecol Endocrinol 2010;26:338–43.
[104] Molvarec A, Szarka A, Walentin S, Beko G, Karadi I, Prohaszka Z, et al. Serum leptin levels in relation to circulating cytokines, chemokines, adhesion molecules and angiogenic factors in normal pregnancy and preeclampsia. Reprod Biol Endocrinol 2011;9:124.
[105] Masuyama H, Segawa T, Sumida Y, Masumoto A, Inoue S, Akahori Y, et al. Different profiles of circulating angiogenic factors and adipocytokines between early- and late-onset pre-eclampsia. BJOG 2010;117:314–20.

Aubrey R. Raimondi and Eyal Sheiner

5 Perinatal outcomes following bariatric surgery

5.1 Introduction

Obesity is an issue of epidemic proportions, with as much as 20% of pregnancies affected [1–4]. Maternal obesity has implications for both maternal and fetal outcomes including increased rates of infertility, miscarriage, gestational diabetes mellitus (GDM), gestational hypertension, preeclampsia, large-for-gestational age (LGA) infants, cesarean section, and fetal morbidity and mortality [2,3]. Bariatric surgery is a method of weight loss that has been shown to be both effective and safe. Women who achieve weight loss using bariatric surgery before pregnancy are more likely to have children with outcomes comparable to those of the general population rather than those of the obese or morbidly obese cohort [4]. Despite this, each bariatric surgery carries unique risks and benefits to maternal and fetal outcomes. This chapter will review the existing evidence regarding the effect of bariatric surgery on maternal and fetal outcomes and serve as a guide for providers.

5.2 Bariatric surgery overview

Bariatric surgery is a general term used to describe various types of surgical procedures that promote weight loss. Traditionally, surgeries were classified into either malabsorptive or restrictive procedures; however, a further understanding of the pathophysiology of weight loss reveals that the mechanisms are more nuanced than previously thought. Weight loss using bariatric surgery occurs through gastric capacity restriction, decreased time to satiety, malabsorption, neuroendocrine changes (reduced levels of ghrelin, and increased GLP-1), and subsequent overall behavior modification [5,6]. The most common procedures are Roux-en-Y gastric bypass (RYGB), sleeve gastrectomy (SG), adjustable gastric banding (AGB), and biliopancreatic diversion/duodenal switch (BD). RYGB represented 45% of bariatric procedures performed as of 2013. SG has become increasingly popular and represented 37% of bariatric procedures performed as of 2013, a nearly 600% increase since 2008. Adjustable gastric bypass represented 10% of the bariatric procedures in 2013, a marked reduction as compared with 42.3% in 2008. BD represented a mere 1.5% of bariatric procedures in 2013.

5.2.1 Roux-en-Y gastric bypass

The Roux-en-Y procedure works mainly through mechanical restriction and malabsorption (Fig. 5.1). The procedure results in considerable weight loss with approximately

https://doi.org/10.1515/9783110487817-005

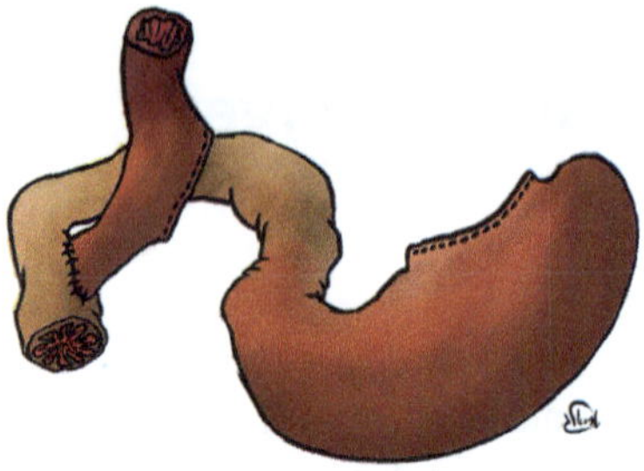

Fig. 5.1: Gastric bypass (original artwork by Dr. Michael Gluhoded).

56.2% ± 29.3% of excess body mass index (BMI) seen in the long term [7]. The procedure may result in vitamin and nutritional deficiencies including fat malabsorption, and deficits in fat-soluble vitamins, folate, iron, and zinc [8]. Of particular importance to women of child-bearing age is the potential for folate deficiency, given the role of folate in the prevention of neural tube defects. The recommendation following the Roux-en-Y procedure includes supplementation of iron, folate, calcium, vitamin B_{12}, and vitamin D [9,10]. Some studies have found no significant weight-related abnormalities following RYGB [11,12]. However, other studies have found an increased risk of low average birth weight and small-for-gestational age (SGA) babies among women following RYGB [13,14]. Therefore, although the existing evidence is inconclusive, special attention should be paid to the risk of weight-related abnormalities including SGA and intrauterine growth restriction (IUGR) [15]. Importantly, studies have documented a decreased risk of hypertensive disorders of pregnancy, GDM, and LGA babies following RYGB [16]. Furthermore, the RYGB procedure has been shown to be associated with lower postsurgical rates of diabetes mellitus type II (DMII) [17]. A shorter time-to-surgery from onset of DMII was associated with an increased rate of resolution of diabetes, indicating that earlier surgical intervention may improve overall DMII outcomes [17].

5.2.2 Sleeve gastrectomy

SG produces capacity restriction through vertical transection of the stomach [18]. The mechanism of weight loss is a combination of restriction of stomach capacity and neuroendocrine changes related to satiety signaling including ghrelin and leptin [19–21]. SG results in appreciable weight loss on par with the long- term weight loss outcomes of RYGB [7,19]. SG is an increasingly popular procedure due to the circumvention of the need for intestinal surgery, the relative simplicity and sophistication of the surgery, the decreased rates of nutritional deficiencies as compared with RYGB and BD, and the appreciable weight loss outcomes (Fig. 5.2) [22,23]. Studies examining pregnancy outcomes following SG are few and as such it is difficult to draw broad conclusions. The most comprehensive study performed to date

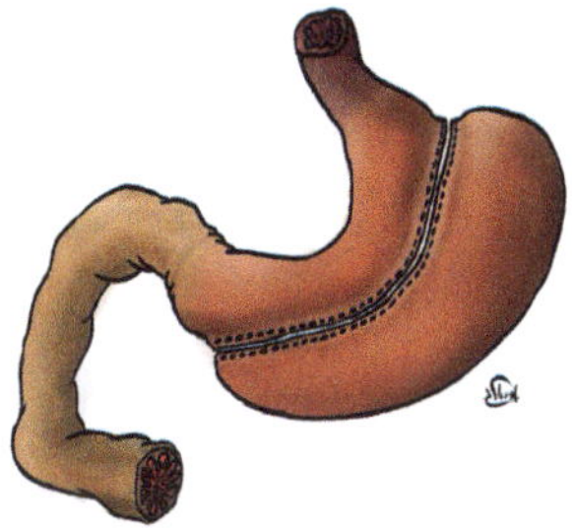

Fig. 5.2: Gastric sleeve (original artwork by Dr. Michael Gluhoded).

was by Ducarme et al. [24], which found no difference in risks of gestational vascular disorders or GDM, but increased risks of LGA births, preterm delivery, and low birth weight, specifically for women who remained obese after laparoscopic sleeve gastrectomy. However, the researchers themselves noted that the findings were limited by the lack of a comparison group. One study, which followed the outcomes of pregnancies in obese Korean patients following SG, found the SG procedure to be safe, but the study was limited by sample size as only 13 participants gave birth [25]. Another study, which looked at SG in comparison to other bariatric surgeries, found decreased levels of B_{12} postoperatively in all groups and lower average birth weights among post-BD and -RYGB but not -SG; however, only 15 of the study participants underwent SG, raising concerns that the study was underpowered to detect various outcome measures. Overall, SG is a safe and effective method of weight loss with likely similar maternal fetal outcomes as seen in RYGB or ABG; however, more studies need to be performed as the existing evidence is still preliminary.

5.2.3 Adjustable gastric banding

AGB achieves weight loss mainly through gastric capacity restriction (Fig. 5.3). The advantages of this procedure are that it is generally reversible and is not usually associated with vitamin, protein, mineral, or other nutritional issues [26,27]. The major disadvantages are that the procedure produces less impressive weight loss outcomes than that of RYGB, GS, or BD, and is not associated with some of the favorable neuroendocrine changes seen in GS [28]. As is seen in the other bariatric surgery modalities, decreased rates of GDM, LGA, and hypertensive disorders of pregnancy are found in post-AGB pregnancies as compared with an obese population [29–33]. The most common adverse effect related to AGB is gastrointestinal discomfort, including reflux, nausea, and vomiting; however, more serious, yet rare, complications include band displacement and vitamin K deficiency, both of which were related to maternal/fetal morbidity and mortality [34,35]. No guidelines have been established with regards to routine band adjustment during pregnancy, especially as the positive

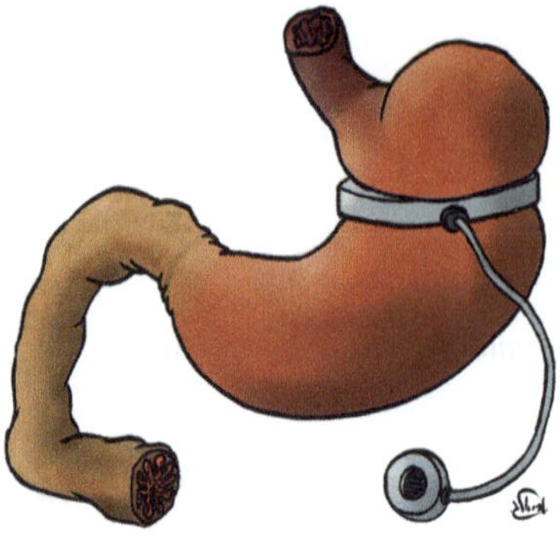

Fig. 5.3: Gastric banding (original artwork by Dr. Michael Gluhoded).

benefits of weight maintenance may outweigh the adverse side effects. Band adjustment during pregnancy is advised in cases of hyperemesis gravidarum, severe nausea, vomiting, or if there are abnormal weight fluctuations [31,32,36].

5.3 Outcomes

5.3.1 Fertility

Obesity is associated with increased rates of infertility [37,38]. Weight loss has been found to improve reproductive health outcomes [39]. As such, several researchers have tried to establish whether the weight loss associated with bariatric surgery would also improve reproductive outcomes including oligo/amenorrhea and infertility [39–42]. Few studies have found a conclusive link. Furthermore, there are multiple confounding factors including increased prevalence of infertility in the prebariatric population and increased rates of obesity in the postbariatric population as compared with average reproductive aged population. Currently there is no established link between fertility and bariatric surgery. Although it is theoretically likely that the weight loss associated with bariatric surgery would improve fertility rates, more studies must be done to examine this outcome before a conclusion can be made. At this time, it is not recommended to advise bariatric surgery solely to improve fertility [43].

5.3.2 Contraception

While the majority of contraceptives, including long acting reversible contraceptives (LARC), should in theory be unaffected by bariatric surgery status, there is concern that oral contraceptive effectiveness, including emergency contraception, may be affected by postbariatric status [44]. This concern is based on a theoretical reduction in gastrointestinal absorption of oral contraceptives due to bypass of portions of the intestines [45,46]. Several studies that examined the absorption of oral contraceptives after bariatric surgery were either inconclusive or the results were limited by comparison to normal weight controls [47]. Healthcare providers should advise patients of the paucity of clear data regarding the use of oral contraceptives after bariatric surgery. According to ACOG, if patients wish to avoid unintended pregnancy, a non-oral contraceptive is advised following bariatric surgery [48,49]. Currently, no formal studies or recommendations exist for emergency contraception. However, providers should take care to consider postsurgical BMI when advising about emergency contraceptive choice, as the efficacy of levonorgestrel decreases as BMI increases. Currently the copper IUD and ulipristal acetate still remain effective options for those women whose postsurgical BMI remains elevated, although the effect of postsurgical status on absorption of ulipristal acetate is unknown [50].

5.3.3 Time-to-conception interval

Bariatric surgery is generally associated with an increased risk for nutritional deficiencies in the postoperative period. This increased risk of nutritional deficiencies is secondary to a catabolic period of rapid weight loss. Due to the increased risk of micronutrient and macronutrient deficiencies, particularly folate and protein malabsorption, there has previously been concern about the need for an extended time-to-conception interval following bariatric surgery. Currently, the American College of Obstetrics and Gynecologists advises patients wishing to conceive following bariatric surgery to wait 12 to 24 months [51]. When examining the evidence, one study found no difference in adverse events when comparing women who conceived in the first year following bariatric surgery to women who conceived after the first year [52]. Another large, population-based study found no difference in rates of preterm delivery or SGA [53]. Additional studies have examined maternal and fetal risk factors and found no increase in adverse outcomes based on time-to-conception interval [54,55]. However, in a large population-based study published in 2016 by Parent et al. [56], which examined risks of premature birth and weight-related abnormalities among other outcomes in postbariatric surgery deliveries, a time-to-birth interval of less than 2 years was associated with increased rates of neonatal intensive care unit (NICU) admissions (12.1% vs. 17.7%; RR, 1.54; 95% CI, 1.05–2.25), preterm delivery (11.8% vs. 17.2%; RR, 1.48; 95% CI, 1.00–2.19), and SGA status (9.2% vs. 12.7%; RR, 1.51; 95% CI, 0.94–2.42). Thus, further studies will be necessary to reconcile the existing evidence in order for providers to draw definitive conclusions. The studies included here can guide the provider in advising their patients both as to the recommended time-to-conception interval and if the patient becomes pregnant before the ACOG recommended waiting period.

5.3.4 Miscarriage

There is a paucity of studies examining the effect of bariatric surgery on miscarriage rates. Thus far, those studies that have been performed have found no relationship between the two factors, but the studies are few and underpowered. Furthermore, some bariatric patients may undergo the surgery in order to address issues with infertility relating to obesity. One study found lower rates of miscarriage among the postbariatric population [57]. However, another larger and more adequately powered study found no difference in miscarriage rates [58]. Although the studies are too few and inconsistent to make a conclusive evaluation, the existing data suggests that there is little to no relationship between bariatric surgery status and miscarriage.

5.3.5 Preterm labor

Patient's with BMI >30 are at an increased risk of preterm delivery [59]. Preterm delivery complications represent a primary cause of morbidity and mortality among children under the age of five worldwide [60]. Children that are born preterm are at increased risk of developing cerebral palsy among other medical and developmental outcomes [61]. Thus far, large population based studies found no apparent increase in the risk of preterm delivery, but a shorter gestation period was noted [14,62]. Additional studies have shown an increased risk of spontaneous preterm delivery [53]. However, other studies have documented conflicting evidence and thus far a consensus has not been reached regarding the data on preterm delivery rates and bariatric surgery [32,33,58]. A recent large population based study by Stephansson et al. [63] initially noted no relationship between preterm delivery and bariatric surgery status. However, in a letter to the editor published shortly after, the same group of researchers noted that after examining an expanded cohort, a significant relationship between the risk of preterm delivery and a history of bariatric surgery was discovered. Additionally, in a large population based retrospective cohort study by Parent et al. [56], increased rates of preterm delivery were noted when comparing deliveries of nonoperative patients versus postbariatric patients, and this risk was further increased among deliveries with an operation-to-birth interval of less than 2 years. Further studies are warranted on this issue, especially considering the importance of reducing preterm deliveries as a core tenet of reducing fetal morbidity and mortality.

5.3.6 Cesarean section

Maternal obesity is associated with increased rates of cesarean section [64,65]. In one meta-analysis, researchers reported an unadjusted odds ratio of cesarean delivery of

2.89 (95%CI 2.28–3.79) among the morbidly obese population [66]. As this population is the most likely to benefit from bariatric surgery, it is useful to know whether the weight loss associated with bariatric surgery has an effect on the risk of cesarean section. Some studies have found increased crude rates of cesarean section in patients with history of bariatric surgery [40,67]. However, these rates are likely confounded by patient's personal history of cesarean section, elevated postsurgical BMI, provider bias and persistence of comorbid risk factors following bariatric surgery. In a retrospective study done by Weintraub et al. [70], significantly higher rates of prior cesarean section delivery were reported for postbariatric patients. Yet, when crude rates of postsurgical cesarean sections were controlled for presurgical cesarean section status, no statistical increase was found postoperatively. In another prospective study, rates of prior cesarean section were found to be higher in the bariatric population as compared with the general population, but the rate of emergent cesarean section was found to be lower as compared with controls [68]. Another study found no difference in cesarean section rates between the postoperative population and general community [16]. Other studies have found increased risks of cesarean section rates even after controlling for previous cesarean section and obesity among other cofounders [40]. In summary, this seems to indicate that there may be an increased risk of cesarean section among patients with a postbariatric status; however, increased crude rates of cesarean section are likely confounded by presurgical cesarean section history among other variables such as postoperative BMI. Postbariatric status is not an indication for cesarean delivery. Physicians and other mid-level providers should examine each case individually, but should not be influenced by postbariatric status when considering referral for cesarean section [48].

5.3.7 Hypertensive disorders of pregnancy

Obesity is linked to increased rates of hypertensive disorders of pregnancy. Because hypertensive disorders of pregnancy are associated with increased maternal and fetal risks [69], it is prudent to elucidate whether weight loss resulting from bariatric surgery has an effect on the risk of developing these disorders. Several studies have examined the effect of bariatric surgery status on the risk of developing hypertensive disorders of pregnancy and found a decreased risk both when compared with an obese comparison group and as compared with patients' own preoperative status [31,32,67].

One study, which examined the incidence of preeclampsia in patients after RYGB found no increased risk of preeclampsia in the postbariatric surgery group compared with the standard BMI group and a decreased risk compared with the obese cohort [70]. Similar findings of reduced risk of preeclampsia were noted in studies that examined the risk of preeclampsia and other hypertensive disorders of pregnancy following AGB and RYGB bariatric procedures [29].

Select studies have found no significant difference in rates of hypertensive disorders of pregnancy among postbariatric surgery cohorts as compared with an obese patient population [70,71]. Other studies have documented higher rates of hypertensive disorders of pregnancy among postbariatric surgery patients when compared with the general population, but decreased when compared with an elevated BMI cohort [68]. One study noted decreased rates of chronic hypertension and gestational hypertension affecting pregnancy in the postsurgical cohort [72].

In summary, the collective evidence seems to indicate that rates of hypertensive disorders of pregnancy are reduced following bariatric surgery as compared with an obese population or patient's own prebariatric surgery rates, but do not normalize to that of the general nonobese population.

5.3.8 Gestational diabetes mellitus

Obesity and GDM have been found in multiple studies to be robustly related and the risks for pregnancy complications seem to persist even if patients are able to attain euglycemia [73–75]. There are a number of issues associated with GDM during pregnancy including increased risk of shoulder dystocia, LGA infants, and hypoglycemic episodes in the postpartum period [76,77]. Preliminary studies have indicated that weight loss may reduce the risk of developing GDM [73]. Furthermore, weight loss resulting from bariatric surgery may reduce the risk of developing GDM [78]. In a large study that looked at deliveries in the Swedish Medical Birth Register, lower risks of GDM and LGA were noted in postbariatric surgery patients when compared with controls matched for BMI among other variables [14]. A population based study by Sheiner et al. [40] reported higher crude rates of GDM when patients were compared with the obese population, yet this relationship did not persist once BMI and other confounding factors were controlled. Additional studies confirm the finding that decreased rates of GDM are noted when postbariatric patients are compared with an obese population [32,67]. Yet, when rates of GDM in the postbariatric population are compared with the general population or the patient's own preoperative rates, the evidence was not conclusive [31,41,79]. Therefore, the rates of GDM in the postbariatric population are reduced when compared with an obese population; however, they are likely higher than those found in the general population.

5.3.9 Birth weight

It is well known that maternal BMI influences fetal birth weight and that the occurrence of LGA infants increases as BMI increases [80,81]. Conversely, the risk for a LGA infant decreases as maternal BMI decreases, a tenet that holds true for weight loss subsequent to bariatric surgery [67]. However, rates of LGA infants born to the postbariatric surgery population are still higher than those found in the general population [14].

Furthermore, as the risk of LGA infant decreases subsequent to maternal weight loss, the risk for SGA increases. In fact, some studies have found an elevated crude rate of weight-related abnormalities such as IUGR and SGA [82]. An additional large population-based study published recently also noted increased risks of SGA infants among the postbariatric surgery cohort [66]. This risk for SGA was increased if the operation-to-birth interval was less than 2 years. Further research is necessary to expound on the risks and nature of fetal weight-related abnormalities, including SGA, following bariatric surgery and to determine the significance of these outcomes if the relationship is confirmed.

5.3.10 Fetal malformations

Maternal obesity is associated with fetal malformations including neural tube defects, cardiac defects, and cleft lip/palate [83,84]. Bariatric surgery, in theory, may reduce risks of these malformations through a reduction in BMI, yet theoretically could be related to an increased risk due to micronutrient deficiencies [85]. After controlling for preterm delivery and maternal age, one study found no relationship between bariatric status and fetal malformations despite an increased crude rate of fetal malformations [67]. A study by Sheiner et al. [40] also showed no relationship between bariatric surgery and fetal malformations. This finding was confirmed by an additional study by Josefsson et al. [86], in which researchers noted that postbariatric status had no effect on the rates of fetal malformations when compared with the general population. The evidence thus far is reassuring for the provider when counseling patients on the risks of fetal malformation [87]. However, providers should continue to monitor patients for micronutrient deficiencies and provide appropriate treatment. Current guidelines recommend screening and treatment for deficiencies in folate, iron, calcium, vitamin B_{12}, vitamin D, and protein each trimester [48]. The risk for fetal malformations should continue to be evaluated in light of the patient's postbariatric BMI. Obesity will continue to be an independent risk factor for fetal malformations postoperatively as it would preoperatively [85].

5.3.11 Postpartum and fetal outcomes

Overall, postbariatric deliveries have similar fetal outcomes as compared with deliveries in the general population. One study, which looked at postbariatric surgery deliveries as compared with the deliveries of an obese cohort that had not undergone bariatric surgery, found no difference in complication rates [54]. Another study by Sheiner et al. [40] noted no differences in perinatal complications in postbariatric deliveries as compared with the general population. Although no differences in rates of adverse outcomes, such as perinatal mortality, postpartum hemorrhage, or Apgar scores, have been documented, more data is needed to elucidate the risk of preterm delivery and SGA infants [88].

5.4 Summary

Bariatric surgery is a safe and effective way to achieve weight loss in conjunction with nutrition and other behavior modification. Women who undergo bariatric surgery may experience an improvement in fertility, but surgery is not advised solely to improve fertility outcomes. Following bariatric surgery, ACOG recommends a time-to-conception interval of 12 to 24 months. Although the evidence is mixed, a recent study documented increased risks of preterm delivery, SGA, and NICU admissions for time-to-birth intervals of less than 2 years. There is a theoretical risk of decreased absorption of oral contraceptives and emergency contraception; however, no conclusive studies have been performed. Postsurgical BMI is an important consideration when recommending emergency contraception as levorgenestrel has been shown to have decreasing efficacy at increasing BMI. In the postsurgical cohort, the risk of developing hypertensive disorders of pregnancy, GDM, and LGA babies are lower. However, rates of weight-related abnormalities such as SGA might be higher in the postsurgical cohort. More research is necessary to establish the relationship between postsurgical status and preterm birth, although recent studies suggest that the rates may be higher. Postsurgical patients should be monitored for micronutrient deficiencies and repletion should be given as necessary. Band adjustment is advised for post-AGB patients experiencing excessive nausea, vomiting, or abnormal weight gain in pregnancy. If medical issues arise, the women's health care provider should consult with a bariatric surgeon for care management.

Bibliography

[1] Fisher SC, Kim SY, Sharma AJ, Rochat R, Morrow B. Is obesity still increasing among pregnant women? Prepregnancy obesity trends in 20 states, 2003–2009. Prev Med 2013;56(6):372–8.

[2] Catalano P, Ehrenberg H. The short- and long-term implications or maternal obesity on the mother and her offspring. BJOG 2006;113:1126–33.

[3] Liu Y, Dai W, Dai X, Li Z. Prepregnancy body mass index and gestational weight gain with the outcome of pregnancy: a 13-year study of 292,568 cases in China. Gynecol Obstet 2012;286(4):905–11.

[4] Kral JG, Biron S, Simard S, Hould FS, Lebel S, Marceau S, Marceau P. Large maternal weight loss from obesity surgery prevents transmission of obesity to children who were followed for 2 to 18 years. Pediatrics 2006;118(6):e1644–9.

[5] Nguyen NT, Blackstone RP, Morton JM, Ponce J, Rosenthal R, editors. The ASMBS textbook of bariatric surgery: Volume 1: Bariatric surgery. Springer, 2014.

[6] Nguyen NT, Blackstone RP, Morton JM, Ponce J, Rosenthal R, editors. The ASMBS textbook of bariatric surgery: Volume 2: Bariatric surgery. Springer, 2015.

[7] Himpens J, Verbrugghe A, Cadière GB, Everaerts W, Greve JW. Long-term results of laparoscopic Roux-en-Y gastric bypass: evaluation after 9 years. Obes Surg 2012;22(10):1586–93.
[8] Bloomberg R, Fleishman A, Nalle J, Herron D, Kini S. Nutritional deficiencies following bariatric surgery: what have we learned? Obes Surg 2005;15(2):145–54.
[9] Poitou BC, Ciangura C, Coupaye M, Czernichow S, Bouillot JL, Basdevant A. Nutritional deficiency after gastric bypass: diagnosis, prevention and treatment. Diabetes Metab 2007;33(1):13–24.
[10] Wax JR, Pinette MG, Cartin A, Blackstone J. Female reproductive issues following bariatric surgery. Obstet Gynecol Surv 2007;62(9):595–604.
[11] Wax JR, Cartin A, Wolff R, Lepich S, Pinette MG, Blackstone J. Pregnancy following gastric bypass surgery for morbid obesity: maternal and neonatal outcomes. Obes Surg 2008;18(5):540–4.
[12] Sheiner E, Balaban E, Dreiher J, Levi I, Levy A. Pregnancy outcome in patients following different types of bariatric surgeries. Obes Surg 2009;19(9):1286–92.
[13] Haddow JE, Hill LE, Kloza EM, Thanhauser D. Neural tube defects after gastric bypass. Lancet 1986;1(8493):1330.
[14] Johansson K, Cnattingius S, Naslund I, Roos N, Trolle L, Granath F, Stephansson O, Neovius M. Outcomes of pregnancy after bariatric surgery. Engl J Med 2015;372(9):814–24.
[15] Martin L, Chavez GF, Adams MJ, Jr., Mason EE, Hanson JW, Haddow JE, et al. Gastric bypass surgery as maternal risk factor for neural tube defects. Lancet 1988;1(8586):640–641.
[16] Wittgrove AC, Jester L, Wittgrove P, Clark GW. Pregnancy following gastric bypass for morbid obesity. Obes Surg 1998 Aug;8(4):461–4.
[17] Schauer PR, Burguera B, Ikramuddin S, Cottam D, Gourash W, Hamad G, Eid GM, Mattar S, Ramanathan R, Barinas-Mitchel E, Rao RH. Effect of laparoscopic Roux-en Y gastric bypass on type 2 diabetes mellitus. Ann Surg 2003;238(4):467–85.
[18] Alvarenga ES, Menzo EL, Szomstein S, Rosenthal RJ. Safety and efficacy of 1020 consecutive laparoscopic sleeve gastrectomies performed as a primary treatment modality for morbid obesity. A single-center experience from the metabolic and bariatric surgical accreditation quality and improvement program. Surg Endosc 2015:1–6.
[19] Bohdjalian A, Langer FB, Shakeri-Leidenmühler S, Gfrerer L, Ludvik B, Zacherl J, Prager G. Sleeve gastrectomy as sole and definitive bariatric procedure: 5-year results for weight loss and ghrelin. Obes Surg 2010;20(5):535–40.
[20] Perello M, Scott MM, Sakata I, Lee CE, Chuang JC, Osborne-Lawrence S, Rovinsky SA, Elmquist JK, Zigman JM. Functional implications of limited leptin receptor and ghrelin receptor coexpression in the brain. J Comp Neurol 2012;520(2):281–94.
[21] Meier U, Gressner AM. Endocrine regulation of energy metabolism: review of pathobiochemical and clinical chemical aspects of leptin, ghrelin, adiponectin, and resistin. Clin Chem 2004;50(9):1511–25.
[22] Gehrer S, Kern B, Peters T, Christoffel-Courtin C, Peterli R. Fewer nutrient deficiencies after laparoscopic sleeve gastrectomy (LSG) than after laparoscopic Roux-Y-gastric bypass (LRYGB)—a prospective study. Obes Surg 2010;20(4):447–53.
[23] Kehagias I, Karamanakos SN, Argentou M, Kalfarentzos F. Randomized clinical trial of laparoscopic Roux-en-Y gastric bypass versus laparoscopic sleeve gastrectomy for the management of patients with BMI <50 kg/m^2. Obes Surg 2011;21(11):1650–6.
[24] Ducarme G, Chesnoy V, Lemarié P, Koumaré S, Krawczykowski D. Pregnancy outcomes after laparoscopic sleeve gastrectomy among obese patients. Int J Gynaecol Obstet 2015;130(2):127–31.
[25] Han SM, Kim WW, Moon R, Rosenthal RJ. Pregnancy outcomes after laparoscopic sleeve gastrectomy in morbidly obese Korean patients. Obes Surg 2013;23(6):756–9.
[26] Tice J, Karliner L, Walsh J, Petersen A, Feldman M. Gastric banding or bypass? A systematic review comparing the two most popular bariatric procedures. Am J Med 2008;121(10):885–93.

[27] Buchwald H, Avidor Y, Braunwald E, et al. Bariatric surgery: a systematic review and meta-analysis. JAMA 2004;292(14):1724–37.
[28] O'Brien PE, Dixon JB, Brown W, Schachter LM, Chapman L, Burn AJ, Dixon ME, Scheinkestel C, Halket C, Sutherland LJ, Korin A. The laparoscopic adjustable gastric band (Lap-Band®): a prospective study of medium-term effects on weight, health and quality of life. Obes Surg 2002;12(5):652–60.
[29] Lapolla A, Marangon M, Dalfrà MG, Segato G, De Luca M, Fedele D, Favretti F, et al. Pregnancy outcome in morbidly obese women before and after laparoscopic gastric banding Obes Surg 2010;20:1251–7.
[30] Skull AJ, Slater GH, Duncombe JE, Fielding GA. Laparoscopic adjustable banding in pregnancy: safety, patient tolerance and effect on obesity-related pregnancy outcomes. Obes Surg 2004;14:230–5.
[31] Dixon JB, Dixon ME, O'Brien PE. Birth outcomes in obese women after laparoscopic adjustable gastric banding. Obstet Gynecol 2005;106(5 Pt 1):965–72.
[32] Ducarme G, Revaux A, Rodrigues A, Aissaoui F, Pharisien I, Uzan M. Obstetric outcome following laparoscopic adjustable gastric banding. Int J Gynaecol Obstet 2007;98:244–7.
[33] Patel JA, Patel NA, Thomas RL, Nelms JK, Colella JJ. Pregnancy outcomes after laparoscopic Roux-en-Y gastric bypass. Surg Obes Relat Dis 2008;4(1):39–45.
[34] Bar-Zohar D, Azem F, Klausner J, Abu-Abeid S. Pregnancy after laparoscopic adjustable gastric banding: perinatal outcome is favorable also for women with relatively high gestational weight gain. Surg Endosc 2006;20(10):1580–3.
[35] Eerdekens A, Debeer A, Van HG, De BC, Sachar V, Guelinckx I, et al. Maternal bariatric surgery: adverse outcomes in neonates. Eur J Pediatr 2010;169(2):191–6.
[36] Martin LF, Finigan KM, Nolan TE. Pregnancy after adjustable gastric banding. Obstet Gynecol 2000;95(6 Pt 1):927–30.
[37] Crosignani PG, Colombo M, Vegetti W, Somigliana E, Gessati A, Ragni G. Overweight and obese anovulatory patients with polycystic ovaries: parallel improvements in anthropometric indices, ovarian physiology and fertility rate induced by diet. Hum Reprod 2003;18(9):1928–32.
[38] Pasquali R, Pelusi C, Genghini S, Cacciari M, Gambineri A. Obesity and reproductive disorders in women. Hum Reprod Update 2003;9(4):359–72.
[39] Clark AM, Thornley B, Tomlinson L, Galletley C, Norman RJ. Weight loss in obese infertile women results in improvement in reproductive outcome for all forms of fertility treatment. Hum Reprod 1998;13(6):1502–5.
[40] Sheiner E, Levy A, Silverberg D, Menes TS, Levy I, Katz M, et al. Pregnancy after bariatric surgery is not associated with adverse perinatal outcome. Am J Obstet Gynecol 2004;190(5):1335–40.
[41] Sheiner E, Menes TS, Silverberg D, Abramowicz JS, Levy I, Katz M, et al. Pregnancy outcome of patients with gestational diabetes mellitus following bariatric surgery. Am J Obstet Gynecol 2006;194(2):431–5.
[42] Gosman GG, King WC, Schrope B, Steffen KJ, Strain GW, Courcoulas AP, Flum DR, Pender JR, Simhan HN. Reproductive health of women electing bariatric surgery. Fertility and sterility 2010;94(4):1426–31.
[43] Khan R. Infertility, pregnancy, and bariatric surgery. In: Obesity, bariatric and metabolic surgery 2016 (pp. 623–7). Springer International Publishing.
[44] Paulen ME, Zapata LB, Cansino C, Curtis KM, Jamieson DJ. Contraceptive use among women with a history of bariatric surgery: a systematic review. Contraception 2010;82(1):86–94.
[45] Victor A, Odlind V, Kral JG. Oral contraceptive absorption and sex hormone binding globulins in obese women: effects of jejunoileal bypass. Gastroenterol Clin North Am 1987;16(3):483–91.
[46] Gerrits EG, Ceulemans R, van HR, Hendrickx L, Totte E. Contraceptive treatment after biliopancreatic diversion needs consensus. Obes Surg 2003;13(3):378–82.

[47] Padwal R, Brocks D, Sharma AM. A systematic review of drug absorption following bariatric surgery and its theoretical implications. Obes Rev 2010;11(1):41–50.
[48] Armstrong C. ACOG guidelines on pregnancy after bariatric surgery. Am Fam Physician. 2010;81(7):905–6.
[49] Merhi ZO. Challenging oral contraception after weight loss by bariatric surgery. Gynecol Obstet Invest 2007;64(2):100–2.
[50] Fok WK, Blumenthal PD. Update on emergency contraception. Curr Opin Obstet Gynecol 2016;28(6):522–9.
[51] American College of Obstetricians and Gynecologists. ACOG practice bulletin no 105: bariatric surgery and pregnancy. Obstet Gynecol 2009;113:1405–13.
[52] Sheiner E, Edri A, Balaban E, et al. Pregnancy outcome of patients who conceive during or after the first year following bariatric surgery. Am J Obstet Gynecol 2011;204:50e1–6.
[53] Roos N, Neovius M, Cnattingius A, et al. Perinatal outcomes after bariatric surgery: nationwide population based matched cohort study. BMJ 2013;347:f6460.
[54] Ducarme G, Parisio L, Santulli P, Carbillon L, Mandelbrot L, Luton D. Neonatal outcomes in pregnancies after bariatric surgery: a retrospective multi-centric cohort study in three French referral centers. J Matern Fetal Neonatal Med 2013;26(3):275–8.
[55] Kjaer M, Nilas L. Timing of pregnancy after gastric bypass—a National Register-based cohort study. Obes Surg 2013;23(8):1281–5
[56] Parent B, Martopullo I, Weiss NS, Khandelwal S, Fay EE, Rowhani-Rahbar A. Bariatric surgery in women of childbearing age, timing between an operation and birth, and associated perinatal complications. JAMA Surg 2016;1–8.
[57] Bilenka B, Ben-Shlomo I, Cozacov C, Gold CH, Zohar S. Fertility, miscarriage and pregnancy after vertical banded gastroplasty operation for morbid obesity. Acta Obstet Gynecol Scand 1995;74(1):44.
[58] Marceau P, Kaufman D, Biron S, Hould FS, Lebel S, Marceau S, et al. Outcome of pregnancies after biliopancreatic diversion. Obes Surg 2004;14(3):318–24.
[59] McDonald SD, Han Z, Mulla S, Beyene J. Overweight and obesity in mothers and risk of preterm birth and low birth weight infants: systematic review and meta-analyses. BMJ 2010;341:c3428.
[60] Beck S, Wojdyla D, Say L, Betran AP, Merialdi M, Requejo JH, Rubens C, Menon R, Van Look PF. The worldwide incidence of preterm birth: a systematic review of maternal mortality and morbidity. Bull World Health Organ 2010;88(1):31–8.
[61] Moster D, Lie RT, Markestad T. Long-term medical and social consequences of preterm birth. N Engl J Med 2008;359(3):262–73.
[62] Kjaer MM, Lauenborg J, Breum BM, Nilas L. The risk of adverse pregnancy outcome after bariatric surgery: a nationwide register-based matched cohort study. Am J Obstet Gynecol 2013;208(6):464–e1.
[63] Stephansson O, Johansson K, Näslund I, Neovius M. Bariatric surgery and preterm birth. N Engl J Med 2016;375(8):805–6.
[64] Kulie T, Slattengren A, Redmer J, Counts H, Eglash A, Schrager S. Obesity and women's health: an evidence-based review. J Am Board Fam Med 2011;24(1):75–85.
[65] Weiss JL, Malone FD, Emig D, Ball RH, Nyberg DA, Comstock CH, Saade G, Eddleman K, Carter SM, Craigo SD, Carr SR. Obesity, obstetric complications and cesarean delivery rate—a population-based screening study. Am J Obstet Gynecol 2004;190(4):1091–7.
[66] Chu SY, Kim SY, Schmid CH, Dietz PM, Callaghan WM, Lau J, Curtis KM. Maternal obesity and risk of cesarean delivery: a meta-analysis. Obes Rev 2007;8(5):385–94.
[67] Weintraub AY, Levy A, Levi I, Mazor M, Wiznitzer A, Sheiner E. Effect of bariatric surgery on pregnancy outcome. Int J Gynaecol Obstet 2008;103(3):246–51.
[68] Berlac J, Skovlund C, Lidegaard O. Obstetrical and neonatal outcomes in women following gastric bypass: a Danish national cohort study. Acta Obstet Gynecol Scand 2014;93(5):447–53.

[69] Ananth CV, Basso O. Impact of pregnancy-induced hypertension on stillbirth and neonatal mortality in first and higher order births: a population-based study. Epidemiology 2010;21(1):118.
[70] Josefsson A, Blomberg M, Bladh M, Frederiksen SG, Sydsjö G. Bariatric surgery in a national cohort of women: sociodemographics and obstetric outcomes. Am J Obstet Gynecol 2011;205:206.e1–8.
[71] Santulli P, Mandelbrot L, Facchiano E, Dussaux C, Ceccaldi PF, Ledoux S, et al. Obstetrical and neonatal outcomes of pregnancies following gastric bypass surgery: a retrospective cohort study in a French referral centre. Obes Surg 2010;20:1501–8.
[72] Bennett WL, Gilson MM, Jamshidi R, Burke AE, Segal JB, Steele KE, et al. Impact of bariatric surgery on hypertensive disorders in pregnancy: retrospective analysis of insurance claims data. BMJ 2010;340:c1662.
[73] Artal R, Catanzaro R, Gavard J, Mostello D, Friganza J. A lifestyle intervention of weight-gain restriction: diet and exercise in obese women with gestational diabetes mellitus. Appl Physiol Nutr Metab 2007;32:596–601.
[74] Chu SY, Callaghan WM, Kim SY, Schmid CH, Lau J, England LJ, Dietz PM. Maternal obesity and risk of gestational diabetes mellitus. Diabetes Care 2007;30(8):2070–6.
[75] Yogev Y, Visser GH. Obesity, gestational diabetes and pregnancy outcome. In: Seminars in fetal and neonatal medicine 2009;14(2):77–84.
[76] Xiong X, Saunders LD, Wang FL, Demianczuk NN. Gestational diabetes mellitus: prevalence, risk factors, maternal and infant outcomes. Int J Gynaecol Obstet 2001;75(3):221–8.
[77] Langer O, Yogev Y, Xenakis EM, Brustman L. Overweight and obese in gestational diabetes: the impact on pregnancy outcome. Am J Obstet Gynecol 2005;192(6):1768–1776.
[78] Peterli R, Wolnerhanssen B, Peters T, Devaux N, Kern B, Christoffel-Courtin C, Drewe J, Von Flue M, Beglinger C. Improvement in glucose metabolism after bariatric surgery: comparison of laparoscopic Roux-en-Y gastric bypass and laparoscopic sleeve gastrectomy: a prospective randomized trial. Ann Surg 2009;250(2):234–41.
[79] Aricha-Tamir B, Weintraub AY, Levi I, Sheiner E. Downsizing pregnancy complications: a study of paired pregnancy outcomes before and after bariatric surgery. Surg Obes Relat Dis 2012;8(4):434–9.
[80] Ehrenberg HM, Mercer BM, Catalano PM. The influence of obesity and diabetes on the prevalence of macrosomia. Am J Obstet Gynecol 2004;191(3):964–8.
[81] Jensen DM, Damm P, Sorensen B, Molsted-Pedersen L, Westergaard JG, Ovesen P, et al. Pregnancy outcome and prepregnancy body mass index in 2459 glucose-tolerant Danish women. Am J Obstet Gynecol 2003;189(1):239–44.
[82] Guelinckx I, Devlieger R, Vansant G. Reproductive outcome after bariatric surgery: a critical review. Hum Reprod Update 2009;15(2):189–201.
[83] Racusin D, Stevens B, Campbell G, Aagaard KM. Obesity and the risk and detection of fetal malformations. In: Seminars in perinatology 2012;36(3):213–21.
[84] Rasmussen SA, Chu SY, Kim SY, Schmid CH, Lau J. Maternal obesity and risk of neural tube defects: a meta-analysis. Am J Obstet Gynecol 2008;198(6):611–9.
[85] Hezelgrave NL, Oteng-Ntim E. Pregnancy after bariatric surgery: a review. J Obes 2011;2011:501939.
[86] Josefsson A, Bladh M, Wirehn A, Sydsjo G. Risk for congenital malformations in offspring of women who have undergone bariatric surgery. A national cohort. BJOG 2013;120(12):1477–82.
[87] Willis K, Lieberman N, Sheiner E. Pregnancy and neonatal outcome after bariatric surgery. Best Pract Res Clin Obstet Gynaecol 2015;29(1):133–44.
[88] Willis K, Alexander C, Sheiner E. Bariatric surgery and the pregnancy complicated by gestational diabetes. Curr Diab Rep. 2016;16(4):1–1.

Ellen Greenblatt and Marta Wais

6 Conception and obesity

6.1 Introduction

The prevalence of obesity among reproductive age women is increasing, particularly in developed countries. The prevalence ranges from 14% to 20% and up to 60% in some countries [1]. As a result, there is an increasing body of literature showing the negative effects of obesity on fertility and natural conception. The effect of obesity on artificial reproductive technologies is still unclear as study data is contradictory. Weight loss, both by conservative means and bariatric surgery, has been also reviewed to look at the effects on fertility.

6.2 Natural fertility

Obesity is associated with an increased risk of menstrual irregularities and anovulation [2–4]. However, obese women with a regular ovulatory cycle still experience a lower probability of spontaneous conception [2,3,7]. Gesink Law et al. [8] studied patients trying to conceive their first pregnancy. They found that women with a body mass index (BMI) of 25 to 29.9 had an odds ratio (OR) of 0.92 (95% CI, 0.84–1.01) of conceiving each cycle whereas women with a BMI of 30 and higher had an OR of 0.82 (95% CI, 0.75–0.92). Jensen et al. [7] also looked at couples trying to conceive their first child and found that the OR of conceiving each cycle was 0.77 (95% CI, 0.70–0.84) when women had a BMI >25. van der Steeg et al. [3] looked at ovulatory women in a fertility clinic and found that women had a 4% lower pregnancy rate per kg/m^2 over a BMI of 29.

6.3 Pathophysiology

Ovulation and the menstrual cycle are controlled by a complex hormonal milieu. Although not completely understood, obesity has been demonstrated to perturb this delicate balance through several direct and indirect hormonal signals including insulin, leptin, and adipokines. Adipose tissue is an important site of steroid production and metabolism. Obese women have been shown to have a larger steroid pool than normal weight women and altered delivery of androgens and estrogens to their target organs [62]. The concentration of sex hormone-binding globulin (SHBG) is increased by estrogens and growth hormone and decreased by insulin and androgens, and the net effect leads to an overall decreased level in obese women [63]. A reduction in SHBG leads to elevated circulating free sex steroids such as testosterone,

https://doi.org/10.1515/9783110487817-006

dihydrotestosterone, and androstenedione [64]. Obesity leads to a state of relative hyperandrogenism. This may have a pathophysiological effect on ovarian function and contribute to menstrual irregularity.

One of the target organs for insulin is the ovary through the insulin receptor and the insulin-like growth factor 1 receptor. Insulin stimulates ovarian steroidogenesis in theca and granulosa cells, and enhances the stimulatory effect of luteinizing hormone through luteinizing hormone receptor upregulation [65]. Insulin also acts at the level of the pituitary, where it may enhance the sensitivity of the gonadotroph cells to the action of GnRH, further enhancing the stimulation of ovarian steroidogenesis [65]. Furthermore, insulin modulates the bioavailability of the sex steroids through inhibition of hepatic SHBG synthesis [64]. Obesity, especially central obesity, induces a state of hyperinsulinemia and insulin resistance. The most common cause of anovulatory cycles is polycystic ovarian syndrome (PCOS). Sixty-five percent of patients with PCOS are obese and this increases insulin resistance and hyperinsulinemia thereby worsening menstrual irregularities [5,6].

In response to systemic insulin resistance, there is a compensatory increase in insulin secretion. The altered insulin metabolism (insulin resistance and hyperinsulinemia) leads to reduced SHBG and hyperandrogenemia, thereby increasing the likelihood of menstrual and ovulatory disturbance in obese women. Poretsky et al. [65] demonstrated that obese women who lose weight and subsequently become ovulatory show a decrease in insulin, and an increase in SHBG.

Leptin is a hormone secreted by adipocytes and secretion increases with food intake and decreases with starvation. Leptin is a key signaling protein that relays to the magnitude of the energy stores to the hypothalamus. Leptin also has a regulatory role in reproductive function; it has stimulatory effects on the hypothalamic-pituitary-ovarian axis at normal serum concentrations but can have inhibitory effects on folliculogenesis and its control when levels are elevated, such as that seen during obesity [67].

Adipokines also participate in metabolic regulation and it has been reported that some of these substances may affect reproductive function [68]. Their exact role is unclear and more research is required to fully elucidate their role in infertility in the obese population.

6.4 Artificial reproductive technologies

In the US, one-third of adults at their peak reproductive age are considered obese [30]. Furthermore, 12% of couples will seek out infertility services at some point during their reproductive years [31]. Both conditions are multifactorial and of concern to the reproductive endocrinologist.

Koning et al. [22] published a systematic review in 2014 looking at the outcomes of assisted reproductive technology (ART) cycles in obese patients. They found 27 primarily retrospective studies and pooled the ORs. When they compared overweight and obese patients to normal weight patients, the OR of a clinical pregnancy was 0.94

(95% CI, 0.69–1.30). The OR for a live birth was 0.90 (95% CI, 0.82–1.00). The authors concluded that higher female BMIs reduce ART success rates but to a small degree and that there may be many confounding variables requiring prospective study. Although live birth rate is arguably the most important marker of success in an ART cycle, different studies have looked at different primary outcomes. Vilarino et al. [23] looked at the BMI and gonadotropin dose needed to achieve adequate ovarian follicular stimulation in an in vitro fertilization (IVF) cycle. This was a retrospective study with 752 women and 951 IVF or in vitro fertilization - intracytoplasmic sperm injection (IVF-ICSI) cycles. They found no significant difference between their BMI groups (normal weight, overweight, and obese) for total follicle stimulating hormone (FSH) dose ($p = 0.572$). They also performed a linear regression and found that being overweight ($\beta = 0.024$, $p = 0.394$) or obese ($\beta = 0.042$, $p = 0.144$) did not significantly correlate to FSH dose. After adjusting for the women's age at cycle start, the likelihood of a positive serum β-hCG result, ongoing pregnancy, or live birth was not significantly different between normal weight, overweight, and obese women. Several other studies have found similar results in regards to FSH dose [28,29]. At this time, there is no consensus in regards to the effect of increasing BMI and successful ART cycles. Several studies have shown that obesity has no effect on IVF success rates [23–25]. Many other studies have shown that increasing BMI negatively affects IVF pregnancy rates [26,27].

The largest cohort study of BMI and IVF outcomes was recently published [33]. The authors looked at 239,127 fresh IVF cycles in the US. They found that the live pregnancy rate decreased with increasing BMI from 31% in normal BMI patients to 21% in patients with a BMI of 50 and above. This was statistically significant. They also found a statistically significant progressive decline in pregnancy rate and implantation rate with increasing BMI. Due to the study size, the authors were able to perform a subgroup analysis of patients with PCOS. PCOS and obesity are often confounding variables that cannot be teased apart because of limited data points. In patients with purely PCOS-related infertility, there was a trend toward decreasing pregnancy rate and live birth rate with increasing BMI, but it was not statistically significant. This suggests that obesity is the cause for worsening outcomes.

Although many studies have looked at the effects of increasing BMI on outcomes of ART cycles, there is no clear answer. There are countless factors at play when looking at fertility, many of which we do not understand yet. Further large-scale, nationwide studies are needed to identify all the confounding variables to estimate the effect size of obesity.

6.5 Effects of obesity on conception

Planned artificial reproductive technologies represent a unique opportunity to study the different elements involved in a pregnancy such as hormone levels, oocytes, sperm, and the developing embryo and endometrium.

The negative effect of BMI of fertility is unclear. Studies have suggested that obese patients have decreased oocyte quality [27]. Many theories exist as to the molecular cause, including altered follicular fluid contents [34–36] and altered microenvironment oocyte/embryo metabolism [37]. Altered endometrial receptivity is also currently being investigated.

A study by Schliep et al. [32] included 721 couples undergoing their first fresh IVF cycle and found that the relationship between female BMI and clinical pregnancy and live birth were not statistically significant. They controlled for male and female age, parity, and partner BMI. They also noted that female BMI was not related to fertilization rate or embryo score.

Some researchers have hypothesized that the uterine environment and endometrium are significantly affected by obesity [26,58–60]. Studies looking at obese women with donor oocytes eliminate the potential effect of maternal age and lower quality of the embryo. They found significantly reduced implantation and pregnancy rates [26,59,60]. However, Luke et al. [61] demonstrated that obese women using donor oocytes had the same chance of conceiving as normal-weight women using donor oocytes, but a lower chance of live birth, suggesting that the effect of obesity on oocyte quality may be more important than the effect on endometrial receptivity.

Another frequently overlooked component in natural conception is sexual function and sexuality. Obesity has been shown to have a negative effect on sexual self-esteem and body image concerns [38,39]. Studies have shown an inverse relationship between BMI and arousal, lubrication, orgasm, and satisfaction [40]. All these factors lead to a decreased incidence of coitus with increasing BMI [41]. In regards to natural conception, it is important to consider all facets of reproduction.

A new line of research is looking at the negative effects of male obesity on fertility [56,57]. Far fewer articles have been published on this topic; however, it is worth noting given the prevalence of obesity in the general population. There is also evidence that, in heterosexual couples, male BMI is positively associated with female BMI and vice versa [32,57]. Male obesity may be an important confounding variable in future research and it is important for clinicians to note from a health promotion perspective.

6.6 Weight loss

Just as obesity rates have grown, so too has the booming weight loss industry. This is due to the fact that losing weight is very challenging and the long-term maintenance of reduced weight is extremely difficult as well. Only 15% of subjects undergoing weight loss interventions maintain either their reduced weight or an overall reduction of 9 to 11 kg 14 years after the initial weight loss [42].

A recent systematic review in 2014 looked at the effect of weight loss on fertility in obese patients [9]. The authors identified seven studies that used a dietary intervention to achieve weight loss. Four of the studies found a statistically significant improvement in the pregnancy rate/live birth rate [10–13] whereas two reported a nonsignificant trend to increased pregnancy rates [14,15] and only one study showed a small decrease [16]. For example, Sim et al. [10] instituted a 3-month-long intervention period and noted an average weight loss of 6.6kg. At 12 months, the intervention group's pregnancy rate was 48% with 23% of those being conceived naturally. The control group pregnancy rate was 14% and none were conceived naturally. This was a statistically significant difference ($p = 0.014$). Also, the intervention group took, on average, 2.46 cycles of ART to achieve pregnancy whereas the control group took 4.33 cycles ($p = 0.01$). The studies also showed that weight loss was associated with regular menstrual cycles [11,12], a reduction in the number of ART cycles needed to achieve pregnancy [10,15], and a decrease in cancellation rates [15]. In addition, natural conception rates were increased after weight loss in five of the six studies that reported this outcome [10–13,15].

One of the only large-scale, randomized control trials (RCTs) looking at weight loss in obese, infertile women was recently published by Mutsaerts et al. [43]. They had 822 women with a BMI of 29 or greater randomized to either 24 months of infertility treatments or a 6-month lifestyle intervention including dieting and exercise preceding 18 months of infertility treatments. Their primary outcome was the vaginal birth of a healthy singleton at term within the 24-month study period. In the intervention group, 27.1% achieved this marker. However, 35.2% of the control group achieved this as well. Overall, significantly more women in the intervention group had ongoing pregnancies that resulted from natural conception. This study demonstrates that delaying infertility treatment, even for weight loss, can have a detrimental effect on outcomes. However, weight loss lessens the need for ART and can lead to a healthier pregnancy and delivery.

Weight loss by diet and lifestyle interventions significantly increased pregnancy rates by natural conception. There is also evidence that it may improve the success of ART cycles. However, the optimal amount of weight loss is not known. Also, weight loss takes time and elevated BMI must be balanced with increasing age and decreasing ovarian reserve to determine how best to proceed to achieve a live birth.

6.7 Bariatric surgery

For years, physicians have encouraged overweight and obese patients to lose weight through diet and exercise. The 1950s saw the birth of bariatric surgery. Initially very complex with significant complications, bariatric surgery now includes a number of different procedures with fewer adverse effects. As a result, the popularity of bariatric surgery has skyrocketed. The incidence of bariatric surgery has increased by 800% in the US between 1998 and 2005 (from 12,480 to 113,500 cases) [44]. Of all the procedures, 83% were being performed on women between the ages of 18 and 45 [44]. Bariatric surgery types include gastric banding, gastric bypass including Roux-en-Y, biliopancreatic diversion, and sleeve gastrectomy with varying mechanisms of action (restriction versus malabsorption), effectiveness, and complications.

Maggard et al. [44] performed a systematic review and found six articles related to fertility after bariatric surgery. One study ($n = 298$) found that after bariatric surgery, the need for fertility treatment was low (6.7%) but exceeded that of the control group (2.3%, $p < 0.001$) [47]. Three studies reported improvements in fertility by comparing pregnancy rates before and after surgery [45,46,48]. The authors also identified six studies that found a normalization of hormones and menstrual cycles and lessening of PCOS following surgery [46,49,51–54]. Unfortunately, most of the studies were observational and lacked complete data on total number of women attempting to become pregnant and eventual pregnancy rates.

In their systematic review, Sim et al. found two case report studies looking at ART outcomes after bariatric surgery [17,18]. In the first study, four out of five women underwent Roux-en-Y bypass surgery and one had a gastric band procedure done [17]. The average weight loss was 46 kg. They found a 100% pregnancy rate after nine IVF cycles.

Recently, Goldman et al. [55] published a retrospective cross-sectional survey study of 219 women. They found that different types of bariatric surgery have differing effects on reproductive outcomes. Fewer women reported menstrual cycle irregularity after Roux-en-Y bypass surgery than before (OR = 0.21, CI = 0.07–0.61), whereas women who underwent adjustable gastric banding did not have statistically significant improvements in menstrual cycle regularity postsurgery; however, it was trending in that direction. There was no significant difference in self-reported history of infertility among the groups. Among all women, 7.2% of women before Roux-en-Y and 4.6% of women before adjustable gastric banding reported that it took more than 12 months for them to conceive, compared with 1.8% and 4.6% after Roux-en-Y and after adjustable gastric banding, respectively. It is well described in the bariatric surgery literature that physiologic changes occurring after Roux-en-Y are distinct from those after adjustable gastric banding and involve gut hormone biology and changes in insulin resistance, which may play a role in ovulation and fertility.

In regards to fertility, it is important to note that patients are counseled to delay conception for the first year after surgery [19–21]. Although there is no evidence published to support this, the theory is that the most rapid rate of weight loss occurs at this time and it could negatively affect a pregnancy, for instance, through nutritional or caloric deficiency. In women with low ovarian reserve, 12 months could have a significant effect on the outcome of their ART cycles.

Bibliography

[1] Ng M, Fleming T, Robinson M, et al. Global, regional, and national prevalence of overweight and obesity in children and adults during 1980–2013: a systematic analysis for the Global Burden of Disease Study 2013. Lancet 2014;384:766–81.

[2] Ramlau-Hansen CH, Thulstrup AM, Nohr EA, Bonde JP, Sørensen TI, Olsen J. Subfecundity in overweight and obese couples. Hum Reprod 2007;22:1634–7.
[3] van der Steeg JW, Steures P, Eijkemans MJ, et al. Obesity affects spontaneous pregnancy chances in subfertile, ovulatory women. Hum Reprod 2008;23:324–8.
[4] Rich-Edwards JW, Goldman MB, Willett WC, et al. Adolescent body mass index and infertility caused by ovulatory disorder. Am J Obstet Gynecol 1994;171:171–7.
[5] Pasquali R, Pelusi C, Genghini S, Cacciari M, Gambineri A. Obesity and reproductive disorders in women. Hum Reprod Update 2003;9:359–372.
[6] Pasquali R, Patton L, Gambineri A. Obesity and infertility. Curr Opin Endocrinol Diabetes Obes 2007;14:482–7.
[7] Jensen TK, Scheike T, Keiding N, Schaumburg I, Grandjean P. Fecundability in relation to body mass and menstrual cycle patterns. Epidemiology 1999;10:422–8.
[8] Gesink Law DC, Maclehose RF, Longnecker MP. Obesity and time to pregnancy. Hum Reprod 2007;22:414–20.
[9] Sim KA, Partridge SR, Sainsbury A. Does weight loss in overweight or obese women improve fertility treatment outcomes? A systematic review. Obes Rev 2014;1:113–9.
[10] Sim KA, Dezarnaulds GM, Denyer GS, Skilton MR, Caterson ID. Weight loss improves reproductive outcomes for obese women undergoing assisted reproductive technology: a randomised controlled trial. Clin Obes 2014;14:792–805.
[11] Clark AM, Ledger W, Galletly C, et al. Weight loss results in significant improvement in pregnancy and ovulation rates in anovulatory obese women. Hum Reprod 1995;10:2705–12.
[12] Clark AM, Thornley B, Tomlinson L, Galletley C, Norman RJ. Weight loss in obese infertile women results in improvement in reproductive outcome for all forms of fertility treatment. Hum Reprod 1998;13:1502–5.
[13] Galletly C, Clark A, Tomlinson L, Blaney F. A group program for obese, infertile women: weight loss and improved psychological health. J Psychosom Obstet Gynaecol 1996;17:125–8.
[14] Moran L, Tsagareli V, Norman R, Noakes M. Diet and IVF pilot study: short-term weight loss improves pregnancy rates in overweight/obese women undertaking IVF. Aust N Z J Obstet Gynaecol 2011;51:455–9.
[15] Awartani KA, Al-Sahan N, Al-Hassan SH, Coskun S. Effect of weight loss in morbidly obese infertile women on IVF outcome. Fertil Steril 2012;98:S204.
[16] van Veen LJ, van den Dool GC, Rijnsaardt HGM, Lambers MDA. The development of a life style program aimed at weight reduction in obese patients with subfertility in a large district hospital, results after five years. European Society of Human Reproduction and Embryology: Stockholm, 2011.
[17] Doblado MA, Lewkowksi BM, Odem RR, Jungheim ES. In vitro fertilization after bariatric surgery. Fertil Steril 2010;94:2812–4.
[18] Hirshfeld-Cytron J, Kim HH. Empty follicle syndrome in the setting of dramatic weight loss after bariatric surgery: case report and review of available literature. Fertil Steril 2008;90:1199.
[19] Merhi ZO. Weight loss by bariatric surgery and subsequent fertility. Fertil Steril 2007;87:430–2.
[20] Catalano PM. Management of obesity in pregnancy. Obstet Gynecol 2007;109:419–33.
[21] Khan R, Bashir D, Chappatte O. Pregnancy outcome following bariatic surgery. Obstet Gynecol 2013;15:37–43.
[22] Koning AM, Mutsaerts MA, Kuchenbecker WK, Kuchenbecher WK, Broekmans FJ, Land JA, et al. Complications and outcome of assisted reproduction technologies in overweight and obese women. Hum Reprod 2012;27:457–67.
[23] Vilarino F, Bianco B, Christofolini D, Barbosa C. Impact of body mass index on in vitro fertilization outcomes. Rev Bras Ginecol Obstet 2005;32:536–40.
[24] Farhi J, Ben-Haroush A, Sapir O, Fisch B, Ashkenazi J. High-quality embryos retain their implantation capability in overweight women. Reprod Biomed Online 2010;21:706–11.

[25] Sathya A, Balasubramanyam S, Gupta S, Verma T. Effect of body mass index on in vitro fertilization outcomes in women. Hum Reprod 2010;3(3):135–8.
[26] Thum MY, El-Sheikhah A, Faris R, Parikh J, Wren M, Ogunyemi T, et al. The influence of body mass index to in vitro fertilization treatment outcome, risk of miscarriage and pregnancy outcome. J Obstet Gynaecol 2007;27(7):699–702.
[27] Bellver J, Ayllon Y, Ferrando M, Melo M, Goyri E, Pellicer, et al. Female obesity impairs in vitro fertilization outcome without affecting embryo quality. Fertil Steril 2010;93:447–54.
[28] Shah DK, Missmer SA, Berry KF, Racowsky C, Ginsberg ES. Effect of obesity on oocyte and embryo quality in women undergoing in vitro fertilization. Am J Obstet Gynecol 2011;118(1):63–70.
[29] Vilarino F, Bianco B, Christofolini D, Barbosa C. Impact of body mass index on in vitro fertilization outcomes. Rev Bras Gynecol Obstet 2005;32:536–40.
[30] Sathya A, Balasubramanyam S, Gupta S, Verma T. Effect of body mass index on in vitro fertilization outcomes in women. Hum Reprod 2010;3(3):135–8.
[31] Flegal KM, Carroll MD, Kit BK, Ogden CL. Prevalence of obesity and trends in the distribution of body mass index among US adults, 1999–2010. JAMA 2012;307:491–7.
[32] Schliep KC, Mumford SL, Ahrens KA, Hotaling JM, Carrell DT, Link M, Hinkle ST, Kissell K, Porucznik CA, Hammoud AO. Effect of male and female body mass index on pregnancy and live birth success after in vitro fertilization Fertil Steril 2015;103(2):388–95.
[33] Provost MP, Acharya KS, Acharya CR, Yeh JS, Steward RG, Eaton JL, Goldfarb JM, Muasher SJ. Pregnancy outcomes decline with increasing body mass index: analysis of 239,127 fresh autologous in vitro fertilization cycles from the 2008–2010 Society for Assisted Reproductive Technology registry. Fertil Steril 2016;105:663–9.
[34] Valckx SDM, de Pauw I, de Neubourg D, Inion I, Berth M, Fransen E, et al. BMI-related metabolic composition of the follicular fluid of women undergoing assisted reproductive treatment and the consequences for oocyte and embryo quality. Hum Reprod 2012;27:3531–9.
[35] Leroy JLMR, Vanholder T, Delanghe JR, Opsomer G, van Soom A, Bols PEJ, et al. Metabolic changes in follicular fluid of the dominant follicle in high-yielding dairy cows early post partum. Theriogenology 2004;62:1131–43.
[36] Leroy JLMR, Vanholder T, Mateusen B, Christophe A, Opsomer G, de Kruif A, et al. Nonesterified fatty acids in follicular fluid of dairy cows and their effect on developmental capacity of bovine oocytes in vitro. Reproduction 2005;130:485–95.
[37] Jungheim ES, MacOnes GA, Odem RR, Patterson BW, Lanzendorf SE, Ratts VS, et al. Associations between free fatty acids, cumulus oocyte complex morphology and ovarian function during in vitro fertilization. Fertil Steril 2011;95:1970–4.
[38] Assimakopoulos K, Panayiotopoulos S, Iconomou G, et al. Assessing sexual function in obese women preparing for bariatric surgery. Obes Surg 2006;16:1087091.
[39] Schwartz MB, Brownell KD. Obesity and body image. Body Image 2004;1:43–56.
[40] Mozafari M, Khajavikhan J, Jaafarpour M, et al. Association of body weight and female sexual dysfunction: a case control study. Iran Red Cresent Med J 2015;17:e24685.
[41] Nackers LM, Appelhans BM, Segawa E, Janssen I, Dugan SA, Kravitz HM. Associations between body mass index and sexual functioning in midlife women: the Study of Women's Health Across the Nation. Menopause 2015;22:1175–81.
[42] Ayyad C, Andersen T. Long-term efficacy of dietary treatment of obesity: a systematic review of studies published between 1931 and 1999. Obes Rev 2000;1:113–9.
[43] Mutsaerts MAQ, van Oers AM, Groen H, et al. Randomized trial of a lifestyle program in obese infertile women. N Engl J Med 2016;374:1942–53.
[44] Maggard MA, Yermilov I, Li Z, Maglione M, Newberry S, Suttorp M, Hilton L, Santry HP, Morton JM, Livingston EH, Shekelle PG. Pregnancy and fertility following bariatric surgery. JAMA 2008;300(19):2286–96.

[45] Bilenka B, Ben-Shlomo I, Cozacov C, Gold CH, Zohar S. Fertility, miscarriage and pregnancy after vertical banded gastroplasty operation for morbid obesity. Acta Obstet Gynecol Scand. 1995;74(1):42–4.
[46] Deitel M, Stone E, Kassam HA, Wilk EJ, Sutherland DJ. Gynecologic-obstetric changes after loss of massive excess weight following bariatric surgery. J Am Coll Nutr 1988;7(2):147–53.
[47] Sheiner E, Levy A, Silverberg D, et al. Pregnancy after bariatric surgery is not associated with adverse perinatal outcome. Am J Obstet Gynecol 2004;190(5):1335–40.
[48] Marceau P, Kaufman D, Biron S, et al. Outcome of pregnancies after biliopancreatic diversion. Obes Surg 2004;14(3):318–24.
[49] Teitelman M, Grotegut CA, Williams NN, Lewis JD. The impact of bariatric surgery on menstrual patterns. Obes Surg 2006;16(11):1457–63.
[50] Sheiner E, Menes TS, Silverberg D, et al. Pregnancy outcome of patients with gestational diabetes mellitus following bariatric surgery. Am J Obstet Gynecol 2006;194(2):431–5.
[51] Gerrits EG, Ceulemans R, van Hee R, Hendrickx L, Totte E. Contraceptive treatment after biliopancreatic diversion needs consensus. Obes Surg 2003;13(3):378–82.
[52] Escobar-Morreale HF, Botella-Carretero JI, Alvarez-Blasco F, Sancho J, San Millan JL. The polycystic ovary syndrome associated with morbid obesity may resolve after weight loss induced by bariatric surgery. J Clin Endocrinol Metab 2005;90(12):6364–9.
[53] Eid GM, Cottam DR, Velcu LM, et al. Effective treatment of polycystic ovarian syndrome with Roux-en-Y gastric bypass. Surg Obes Relat Dis 2005;1(2):77–80.
[54] Bastounis EA, Karayiannakis AJ, Syrigos K, Zbar A, Makri GG, Alexiou D. Sex hormone changes in morbidly obese patients after vertical banded gastroplasty. Eur Surg Res 1998;30(1):43–7.
[55] Goldman RH, Missmer SA, Robinson MK, Farland LV, Ginsburg ES. Reproductive outcomes differ following Roux-en-Y gastric bypass and adjustable gastric band compared with those of an obese non-surgical group. Obes Surg 2016;26(11):2581–9.
[56] Anifandis G, Dafopoulos K, Messini CI, Polyzos N, Messinis IE. The BMI of men and not sperm parameters impact on embryo quality and the IVF outcome. Andrology 2013;1:85–9.
[57] Petersen GL, Schmidt L, Pinborg A, Kamper-Jorgensen M. The influence of female and male body mass index on live-birth rates after assisted reproductive technology treatment—a nationwide register-based cohort study. Fertil Steril 2013;99:1654–62.
[58] Wang JX, Davies M, Norman RJ. Body mass index and probability of pregnancy during assisted reproduction treatment: retrospective study. Br Med J 2000;321:1320–1.
[59] Bellver J, Rossal LP, Bosch E, Zuñiga A, Corona JT, Melendez F, Gomez E, Simon C, Remohí J, Pellicer A. Obesity and the risk of spontaneous abortion after oocyte donation. Fertil Steril 2003;79:1136–40.
[60] Bellver J, Melo MAB, Bosch E, Serra V, Remohí J, Pellicer A. Obesity and poor reproductive outcome: the potential role of the endometrium. Fertil Steril 2007;88:446–51.
[61] Luke B, Brown MB, Stern JE, Missmer SA, Fujimoto VY, Leach R. Female obesity adversely affects assisted reproductive technology (ART) pregnancy and live birth rates. Human Reprod 2011;26(1):245–52.
[62] Gambineri A, Pelusi C, Vicennati V, Pagotto U, Pasquali R. Obesity and the polycystic ovary syndrome. Int J Obes Relat Metab Disord 2002;26:883–96.
[63] von Schoultz B, Carlstrom K. On the regulation of sex-hormone binding globulin—a challenge of an old dogma and outlines of an alternative mechanism. J Steroid Biochem 1989;32:327–34.
[64] Pasquali R, Casimirri F. The impact of obesity on hyperandrogenism and polycystic ovary syndrome in premenopausal women. Clin Endocrinol 1993;39:1–16.
[65] Poretsky L, Cataldo NA, Rosenwaks Z, Giudice LC. The insulin-related ovarian regulatory system in health and disease. Endocr Rev 1999;20:535–82.

[66] Clark AM, Ledger W, Galletly C, Tomlinson L, Blaney F, Wang X, Norman RJ. Weight loss results in significant improvement in pregnancy and ovulation rates in anovulatory obese women. Hum Reprod 1995;10:2705–12.
[67] Tamer Erel C, Senturk LM. The impact of body mass index on assisted reproduction. Curr Opin Obstet Gynecol 2009;21:228–35.
[68] Gosman GG, Katcher HI, Legro RS. Obesity and the role of gut and adipose hormones in female reproduction. Hum Reprod Update 2006;12:585–601.

Claire Jones and Crystal Chan

7 Obesity and contraception

7.1 Introduction

The World Health Organization (WHO) recognizes sexual and reproductive health care as a fundamental human right. Among other interventions, the WHO recommends that access to comprehensive contraceptive information and services be provided equally to all women, without discrimination [1]. Contraception enables women to have control over their fertility, the timing of starting a family, and their family size. Despite these recommendations and the existence of various forms of contraception, studies show an underutilization of contraception in obese women compared with women with normal body mass index (BMI) [2, 3]. This disparity extends to the adolescent population, as obese teenagers are less likely to use contraception or receive contraceptive counseling, compared with their healthy weight peers [4]. Whether this disparity is patient or provider-driven is unclear, but there are several possible barriers to contraceptive use in obese and overweight women. First, contraceptive efficacy has not been well studied in the obese population, as most trials have excluded women who are more than 130% of the ideal body weight [5, 6]. Some studies suggest that obesity may impair the effectiveness of hormonal contraceptives, but more research is needed to guide physicians and patients. In addition, medical comorbidities associated with obesity may contraindicate the use of certain forms of hormonal contraception. However, contraception is particularly important for women with chronic medical conditions associated with obesity, as these women are at greater risk of developing pregnancy-related complications. There are many safe hormonal and nonhormonal contraceptive options available for women, and counselling should be offered to prevent unplanned pregnancy in this population.

7.2 Combined hormonal contraceptives

The combined oral contraceptive pill, transdermal patch, vaginal ring, and injectables are all effective forms of contraception for most women with well-established safety profiles. However, there have been concerns raised about both the efficacy and safety of combined hormonal contraceptive (CHC) use among obese women.

https://doi.org/10.1515/9783110487817-007

7.2.1 Physiological differences in obese patients

Obesity may affect pharmacokinetics in many ways including the absorption, distribution, metabolism, and excretion of drugs [7]. Obese patients may have increased drug absorption due to delayed emptying and potentially a shorter time to maximum plasma concentration of a drug. Furthermore, drug distribution is known to be altered by changes in body mass, adipose tissue, and circulating plasma proteins, with a known higher volume of distribution for hydrophobic drugs, but less so for hydrophilic drugs such as steroids [8].

The pharmacological activity of steroids is known to be greatly affected by the level of circulating plasma proteins, specifically, the proportion that are in the protein-bound inactive form, compared with the free unbound form. In obesity, greater proportions of other lipoproteins may be bound to albumin, leaving fewer hormone binding sites for steroids. This coupled with reduced levels of sex hormone binding globulin within the circulation results in a higher proportion of unbound hormones in the circulation [8].

Hepatic metabolism of drugs may also be altered in obesity which could lead to increased, decreased, or unchanged metabolism depending on the enzymes affected within the liver [8]. Renal excretion of drugs is increased with increasing BMI, likely due to increased glomerular filtration rates [8]. The main resulting pharmacokinetic changes in obese women taking a 20 mg ethinyl estradiol (EE)/100 μg levonorgestrel (LNG) pill include a longer half-life and a longer time to reach steady state than normal weight controls [9]. These changes result in a longer time to reach sufficient states for ovulatory suppression, and therefore could lead to an increased risk of contraceptive failure during combined oral contraceptive (COC) initiation or after the 7-day hormone-free interval [7, 9]. Cherala and Edelman [10] have recommended the use of a continuous low dose COC without a pill-free interval or a slightly higher dose estrogen pill as two methods of reducing contraceptive failure in obese patients, as well as strict adherence to dosing time intervals.

In non-oral hormonal contraceptives, delivery of hormones through parenteral routes is less altered by obesity due to the rapid achievement of relatively constant plasma concentrations, but obesity may still affect the steady state of drugs through differential plasma protein binding and drug elimination [7]. Studies of serum levels of drugs administered through various methods including the vaginal ring and the transdermal patch and implant are inconsistent, with some showing no effect of BMI and others showing lower plasma concentrations of hormones, but most of these studies are limited by testing total hormone levels, rather than free unbound hormone levels and are therefore difficult to interpret [7].

7.2.2 Efficacy

CHCs primarily achieve contraceptive efficacy by suppression of ovulation through LH and FSH suppression at the level of the pituitary by both the synthetic progestin and EE. Several review articles and systematic reviews have been published reviewing contraceptive efficacy in obese patients with unclear recommendations.

A large systematic review on the effectiveness and failure rates of CHC use by body weight or BMI was published in October 2016 after including 15 reports, all of fair to poor quality [11]. Three fair quality studies and one poor quality study reported increased COC failure among a heterogeneous population of overweight and obese women compared with normal weight women, whereas eight fair quality studies and two poor quality studies did not find a difference. This review included the analysis of a level II-2 study, which analyzed pooled individual data derived from seven phase 3 clinical trials between 2000 and 2012, showing a Pearl Index (number of pregnancies per 100 women years of COC exposure) for obese COC users of 3.14 (95% CI, 2.33–4.22) and 2.53 (1.88–3.41) for nonobese users, giving a 44% higher relative risk for pregnancy in obese patients compared with nonobese COC users (adjusted hazards ratio, 1.44; 95% CI, 1.06–1.95) but the absolute rates on contraceptive failure are still low and thus these findings are of questionable clinical significance [12]. Furthermore, multiple large prospective cohort studies of tens of thousands of women have demonstrated no difference in pregnancy rates among obese and nonobese women as measured by body weight or BMI [11].

A Cochrane review of CHC for contraception in overweight and obese women was also published in 2016 and included 17 studies for a total of 63,813 women but focused the analysis on 12 studies of high, moderate, or low quality results [6]. These authors likewise summarized that the majority of studies showed no difference in pregnancy rates between obese and nonobese women. Of the six studies of COC users included in the analysis, four showed no difference in pregnancy rates among obese and nonobese users, one showed a higher pregnancy risk in obese women, and one demonstrated a lower pregnancy rate among obese women. The authors concluded that there was no association between higher BMI or weight and effectiveness of hormonal contraceptives, but that the overall quality of evidence is low [6].

Several studies have reported on the risk of pregnancy with specific COC formulations and doses, but overall, the results are conflicting. Some studies have shown a higher contraceptive failure risk among obese women using pills containing 35 μg of EE or less whereas others did not [11]. These studies are limited by pooling of multiple different COC formulations, making it unclear whether the type of progestin has an effect [7]. A study of an ultra-low dose COC with only 10 μg of EE and 1.0 mg of norethindrone acetate did not find any clinically important differences in contraceptive failure rates, adverse events, or bleeding profiles in women with increasing BMI, but the Pearl Indices were 2.49, 2.32, and 1.89 for women with a BMI of <25, 25–30, and >30 kg/m^2, respectively [13]. Given that oral LNG has a high level of binding to SHBG, this progestin would theoretically be at higher risk for reduced effectiveness in obesity, although this has not been studied [7]. Some strategies proposed to reduce the rate of contraceptive failure in obese patients is to reduce the hormone-free interval or use a higher-dose estrogen pill, but no studies have specifically addressed these strategies to date [7].

Only two fair quality pooled analysis studies have reported on contraceptive efficacy of transdermal patches in obese women [14, 15]. Body weight >90 kg was found to be statistically significantly associated with a higher chance of pregnancy in women taking the transdermal contraceptive patch containing EE and norelgestromin, although the proportion of patients at this weight was very low [14]. A BMI higher than 30 was also found to be significantly associated with contraceptive failure for this same transdermal patch (adjusted hazard ratio, 8.8; 95% CI, 2.5–30.5) [11]. There were no studies identified that compared contraceptive efficacy using the combined injectable [6, 11]. The only study to report on contraceptive failure of the EE/ENG vaginal ring in obese women compared with nonobese women was a secondary analysis of phase 3 efficacy trials, which showed a pregnancy rate of 12% in women in the highest decile of weight (>167 lb.) with no pregnancies reported in the heaviest women (189–272 lb.) [16].

There are major limitations to the studies of COC efficacy in obese patients including self-reporting of body weight, a lack of data on adherence to the COC regimen, inclusion of multiple different CHC formulations and dosing strategies into the analysis, under-reporting of unintended pregnancy, and exclusion of very obese patients [7, 11]. Although most studies have not found a difference in contraceptive efficacy in obese patients, a few studies have. Fortunately, the overall risk of contraceptive failure even among the studies that found a significant difference was still small (<5%), and therefore obese women can be reassured that COC's do provide a good form of contraception.

7.2.3 Risks and safety profile

The WHO considers CHC to have advantages that generally outweigh the theoretical or proven risks of the drug [17]. The primary risks of CHC use include cardiovascular risks from exogenous estrogen, including acute myocardial infarction (MI), stroke, and venous thromboembolism (VTE) [18].

The risk of acute MI and stroke in women of reproductive age is low, regardless of BMI [7]. Few studies have been performed on the risk of acute MI and stroke among obese CHC users with conflicting results [18]. One large case-control study showed no difference in the risk for acute MI and stroke, whereas another case-control study showed a significantly increased risk of acute MI and stroke among CHC users, particularly among women with a BMI of >27.3 kg/m^2 [18]. One case-control study examined the risk of stroke among obese women using CHC, finding an increased risk of stroke among CHC users, with increasing risks of stroke in patients with a higher BMI, but this was not statistically significant [19]. In the other pooled analysis of two case-control studies, there was no increased risk of stroke among CHC users at both normal and high BMI categories [20].

Obesity and CHC use are both independent risk factors for VTE with a threefold increased risk of VTE in CHC users, with rates of VTE correlating with the degree of obesity [7, 18]. However, it is unclear if the risks of CHC use and obesity are additive, multiplicative, or otherwise affect VTE rates. One systematic review showed a five to eight times increased risk of VTE in obese COC users compared with obese nonusers, and 10 times the risk compared with normal weight nonusers [18]. This elevated risk should be considered in context of a known fivefold increased risk of VTE during pregnancy and 60-fold increased risk during the postpartum period across all BMI categories compared with nonpregnant women [21].

Weight gain is a common concern among patients planning to use an oral contraceptive pill, although no clear relationship has been established between weight gain and COC use in several studies and meta-analyses, and therefore should not be a concern for obese patients considering using a CHC [22]. Other minor side effects of COC that are affected by obesity include a slight increased risk of unscheduled vaginal bleeding and reduced rates of amenorrhea in obese compared with nonobese ultra-low dose COC users [13].

7.3 Progestin-only contraception

Progestin-only contraception (POC) has several methods of administration, including oral, implant, injectable, and intrauterine. The mechanisms of action of POC include suppression of ovulation, thickening of cervical mucus, and alteration of endometrial receptivity [23–25]. From a safety perspective, POC does not increase the risk of arterial or venous thrombosis, which may favor its use in the obese population.

7.3.1 Progestin-only pill

Several oral progestins are available but only one progestin-only pill (POP) is approved for use as a contraceptive in Canada. Norethindrone 0.35 mg (Micronor) is taken daily, with no hormone-free interval. The failure rate of the POP with perfect use in the first year is estimated at 0.3% [26], but studies on obese women are lacking. There is no data to suggest decreased efficacy of the POP in obese women, and the WHO Medical Eligibility Criteria for POP do not restrict use in this population [17]. Although more studies on efficacy are needed in the obese population, the safety profile of the POP is advantageous. The POP has not been shown to increase the risk of VTE or cardiovascular disease and therefore may be considered a safer alternative to COC [22].

7.3.2 Progestin implant

Progestin-containing subdermal implants are reversible contraceptives that can provide reliable, long-acting contraception [27]. A Cochrane review of contraception in overweight and obese women reviewed the efficacy of progestin implants [6]. The most studied implant was the six-rod implant containing 216 mg of LNG (Norplant), now discontinued. Of four studies examining the rate of contraceptive failure with the LNG implant, two showed differences in pregnancy rates by weight. One of these studies showed that increased weight was associated with a higher pregnancy rate in years 6 and 7 of implant use [28]. The Pearl Index was 0.86 in those >70 kg, and was 0.26 in those <60 kg ($p < 0.05$). The other study demonstrated higher pregnancy rates in the fifth year of use in heavier women, although the rates for women more than 70 kg did not differ significantly from the group weighing 60 to 69 kg [29]. The two-rod LNG implant (Norplant-2/Jadelle/Sino-implant II) contains 150 mg of LNG and has a 3- to 5-year duration of effectiveness. Three studies on the newer LNG implant found few cases of contraceptive failure [30–32]. Due to the small number of cases, there is insufficient evidence to determine if the efficacy of the two-rod LNG implant is affected by weight. The etonogestrel-containing implant (Implanon/Nexplanon) contains 68 mg of etonogestrel, and has a three-year duration of effectiveness [27]. In a study of 1,168 women using the etonogestrel implant, only one pregnancy occurred over 3 years [33]. A total of 28% of the study subjects were overweight (BMI, 25–29.9) and 35% were obese (BMI ≥ 30). The subject who conceived with the implant had a BMI of 31 kg/m^2 and pregnancy occurred within 4 days of implant placement. This suggests an undiagnosed luteal phase pregnancy, rather than contraceptive failure. Overall the data are reassuring that contraceptive failure is rare with progestin implants in any weight class, particularly within the first 3 years of use.

7.3.3 Progestin injectables

Depo-medroxyprogesterone acetate (DMPA) is administered by intramuscular injection, at a dose of 150 mg/mL. It is an effective contraceptive given at 3-month intervals. Data on efficacy in the obese population are lacking, but existing studies do not suggest that pregnancy rates differ by body weight [7]. A study of 846 DMPA users reported a pregnancy rate of 0.7/100 woman-years across all weight classes, and body weight was not found to be a significant factor [34]. However, only 5% of study subjects were >80 kg, and the study was not designed to compare contraceptive failure in obese versus healthy weight women. DMPA is sometimes avoided in the overweight and obese population because its use has been associated with an average weight gain of 5 lb. in the first year of use. The association with weight gain is attributed to appetite stimulation and a possible anabolic effect [35]. In particular, for overweight or obese women who are trying to lose weight during the postpartum period, DMPA may not be a good choice as it may prevent them from returning to their prepregnancy weight [22]. Future fertility plans may also affect the decision to use this method, as DMPA use has been associated with a delay in the resumption of ovulation and menses [27].

7.3.4 Progestin-containing intrauterine contraceptives

Intrauterine contraceptives (IUC) are long-acting reversible contraceptives. The LNG-releasing intrauterine systems (LNG-IUS) have two modes of action. The first is progestin-mediated disruption of ovulation, cervical mucus, and endometrial receptivity. The second is mechanical interference with fertilization and implantation [36]. Because the latter mechanism reduces the reliance on systemic drug levels, body weight is unlikely to affect efficacy. A prospective randomized trial of LNG-IUS use demonstrated good contraceptive efficacy (Pearl Index of 0.3 at 3 years of use) and no association with BMI [37]. From a technical perspective, IUC placement in obese women may be difficult due to suboptimal visualization of the cervix. However, such challenges can often be overcome by appropriate speculum and instrument selection and vaginal retraction.

7.4 Emergency contraception

Emergency postcoital contraception (EC) is used to prevent unplanned pregnancy following unprotected intercourse. Options include oral LNG, COC, ulipristal acetate, or insertion of an IUC. Only four pooled secondary analyses of fair to poor quality have been published on the effectiveness of emergency contraception in obese patients, three studying LNG, and two studying ulipristal acetate [38]. Women with obesity (BMI >30 kg/m2) were at a fourfold increased risk of pregnancy after EC with LNG compared with normal weight women, whereas there was no statistically significant difference after ulipristal acetate use [7, 38]. Increasing the dose of LNG emergency contraceptive to 3 mg from 1.5 mg was found to normalize the PK parameters to that of normal weight women, and may therefore improve the efficacy of LNG EC in obese women so that it can be considered a reasonable option [39]. The copper IUC is still the most effective form of emergency contraception regardless of body weight with a failure rate of 0.09% when inserted within 5 days of unprotected intercourse [40].

7.5 Contraceptive use after bariatric surgery

Women are commonly recommended to wait 1 to 2 years after bariatric surgery before conception due to a theoretical risk of fetal malnourishment during the rapid weight loss following surgery [22]. However, rates of unintended pregnancy are high among patients after bariatric surgery due to improved fertility due to weight loss, and therefore contraceptive counseling is important [22, 41]. Unfortunately, studies of contraceptive use after bariatric surgery are limited to pharmacokinetic and poor-quality observational studies [41].

Although data is limited, oral contraceptive use and oral emergency contraceptive use is generally not recommended after malabsorptive bariatric surgery procedures such as the Roux-Y gastric bypass due to concerns with reduced absorption resulting in reduced COC efficacy [22, 41–43]. There are no contraindications to COC use in women undergoing strictly restrictive procedures with no malabsorption component such as a gastric band procedure [42]. However, there is a theoretical increased risk of VTE in obese patients planning major surgery that involves prolonged immobilization, in which COC use could theoretically further increase the risk of VTE during this thrombogenic period [41].

Concerns have been raised regarding bone loss and fracture risk with DMPA use in a women already losing bone mass from significant weight loss and nutritional deficiency after bariatric surgery [41]. Studies have shown the effectiveness of the etonogestrel subdermal implant and the LNG intrauterine device after bariatric surgery, and therefore they are considered to be excellent contraceptive options after bariatric surgery [22, 44].

7.6 Sterilization

Tubal ligation, bilateral salpingectomy, and hysteroscopic tubal occlusion with microinserts are permanent methods of contraception that render patients sterile. They are intended to be irreversible procedures, and patients should be counselled adequately before consenting. Tubal ligation and bilateral salpingectomy are procedures that can be performed abdominally (often at the time of caesarean section) or laparoscopically. The U.S. Collaborative Review of Sterilization studied 9,475 women who had interval laparoscopic tubal sterilization and reported that obesity was an independent predictor of surgical complications (OR 1.7; CI, 1.2–2.6) [45]. Smaller cohort studies have found an association between obesity and the incidence of surgical difficulties, technical failure of tubal interruption, and longer operating times [46]. Studies on hysteroscopic tubal occlusion in the obese population are lacking. However, similar to IUC insertion, hysteroscopic microinsert placement in obese women may be more challenging due to difficulty in visualizing and accessing the cervix.

7.7 Summary

Although concerns have been raised about the safety and efficacy of various contraceptives among obese women, there are still many contraceptive options available that provide reliable and safe methods for preventing unintended pregnancy. Obese women should be counselled thoroughly about contraceptive options including the risks, efficacy, and the importance of compliance. This is particularly important in the period following bariatric surgery, when women may be more fecund. CHCs offer good contraceptive efficacy despite changes in steroid metabolism in obesity. The biggest predictor of CHC failure in all patients across all BMI categories is compliance, and thus the importance of compliance should be stressed to patients. There may be lowered efficacy for obese women using the combined hormonal patch, but the overall efficacy is still good. Obese women should be counseled about the risks of CHC including VTE for which they are at an increased risk relative to nonobese women, but are still at a relatively lower risk than during pregnancy and the postpartum period. To avoid the VTE and cardiovascular risks associated with the CHC, POC is a good option for obese patients. However, studies on the efficacy of the POP are limited in this population. Other delivery systems of POC, including the implant, injection, and LNG-IUS, are good options for obese women, but DMPA injection is associated with further weight gain. Obese women are candidates to receive postcoital emergency contraception to avoid unplanned pregnancy, but failure rates with hormonal EC may be higher. Tubal sterilization may be more challenging in the obese population, but should be considered if women have completed childbearing and wish for a reliable and permanent method to prevent pregnancy.

Bibliography

[1] Ensuring human rights in the provision of contraceptive information and services: guidance and recommendations. Geneva: World Health Organization Press, 2014.

[2] Chuang, CH, et al. Contraceptive use by diabetic and obese women. Womens Health Issues 2005;15(4):167–73.

[3] Callegari LS, et al. Factors associated with lack of effective contraception among obese women in the United States. Contraception, 2014;90(3):265–71.

[4] Becnel JN, et al. Romantic, sexual, and sexual risk behaviours of adolescent females with severe obesity. Ped Obes 2016 may 30;DOI:10.1111/ijpo.12155 epub.

[5] Higginbotham S. Contraceptive considerations in obese women: release date 1 September 2009, SFP Guideline 20091. Contraception 2009;80(6):583–90.

[6] Lopez LM, et al. Hormonal contraceptives for contraception in overweight or obese women. Cochrane Database Syst Rev 2016;(8):CD008452.

[7] Simmons KB, Edelman AB. Hormonal contraception and obesity. Fertil Steril 2016;106(6): 1282–1288.

[8] Cho SJ, Yoon IS, Kim DD. Obesity-related physiological changes and their pharmacokinetic consequences. J Pharm Investig 2013;43(3):161–9.

[9] Edelman AB, et al. Prolonged monitoring of ethinyl estradiol and levonorgestrel levels confirms an altered pharmacokinetic profile in obese oral contraceptives users. Contraception 2013;87(2);220–6.

[10] Cherala G, Edelman A. How can we improve oral contraceptive success in obese women? Expert Rev Clin Pharmacol 2015;8(1);1–3.

[11] Dragoman MV, et al. Combined hormonal contraceptive (CHC) use among obese women and contraceptive effectiveness: a systematic review. Contraception 2017;95(2):117–129.

[12] Yamazaki M, et al. Effect of obesity on the effectiveness of hormonal contraceptives: an individual participant data meta-analysis. Contraception 2015;92(5):445–52.

[13] Nakajima ST, Pappadakis J, Archer DF. Body mass index does not affect the efficacy or bleeding profile during use of an ultra-low-dose combined oral contraceptive. Contraception 2016;93(1):52–7.
[14] Zieman M, et al. Contraceptive efficacy and cycle control with the Ortho Evra/Evra transdermal system: the analysis of pooled data. Fertil Steril 2002;77(2 Suppl 2):S13–8.
[15] Kaunitz AM, et al. Low-dose levonorgestrel and ethinyl estradiol patch and pill: a randomized controlled trial. Obstet Gynecol 2014;123(2 Pt 1):295–303.
[16] Westhoff CL, et al. Pharmacokinetics and ovarian suppression during use of a contraceptive vaginal ring in normal-weight and obese women. Am J Obstet Gynecol 2012;207(1):39 e1–6.
[17] Medical eligibility criteria for contraceptive use. Geneva: World Health Organization Press, 2015.
[18] Horton LG, Simmons KB, Curtis KM. Combined hormonal contraceptive use among obese women and risk for cardiovascular events: a systematic review. Contraception 2016;94(6):590–604.
[19] Kemmeren JM, et al. Risk of Arterial Thrombosis in Relation to Oral Contraceptives (RATIO) study: oral contraceptives and the risk of ischemic stroke. Stroke 2002;33(5):1202–8.
[20] Schwartz SM, et al. Stroke and use of low-dose oral contraceptives in young women: a pooled analysis of two US studies. Stroke 1998:29(11);2277–84.
[21] Pomp ER, et al. Pregnancy, the postpartum period and prothrombotic defects: risk of venous thrombosis in the MEGA study. J Thromb Haemost 2008;6(4):632–7.
[22] Mody SK, Han M. Obesity and contraception. Clin Obstet Gynecol 2014;57(3):501–7.
[23] Moghissi KS, Marks C. Effects of microdose norgestrel on endogenous gonadotropic and steroid hormones, cervical mucus properties, vaginal cytology, and endometrium. Fertil Steril 1971;22(7):424–34.
[24] Croxatto HB. Mechanisms that explain the contraceptive action of progestin implants for women. Contraception 2002;65(1):21–7.
[25] Petta CA, et al. Timing of onset of contraceptive effectiveness in Depo-Provera users. II. Effects on ovarian function. Fertil Steril 1998;70(5):817–20.
[26] Trussell J. Contraceptive failure in the United States. Contraception 2011;83(5):397–404.
[27] Black A, et al. Canadian contraception consensus (Part 3 of 4): Chapter 8 – Progestin-only contraception. J Obstet Gynaecol Can 2016;38(3):279–300.
[28] Gu S, et al. Effectiveness of Norplant implants through seven years: a large-scale study in China. Contraception 1995;52(2):99–103.
[29] Grubb GS, Moore D, Anderson NG. Pre-introductory clinical trials of Norplant implants: a comparison of seventeen countries' experience. Contraception 1995;52(5):287–96.
[30] Sivin I, et al. Levonorgestrel concentrations during use of levonorgestrel rod (LNG ROD) implants. Contraception 1997;55(2);81–5.
[31] Sivin I, et al. The performance of levonorgestrel rod and Norplant contraceptive implants: a 5 year randomized study. Hum Reprod 1998;13(12):3371–8.
[32] Sivin I, et al. Contraception with two levonorgestrel rod implants. A 5-year study in the United States and Dominican Republic. Contraception 1998;58(5):275–82.
[33] Xu H, et al. Contraceptive failure rates of etonogestrel subdermal implants in overweight and obese women. Obstet Gynecol 2012;120(1):21–6.
[34] Benagiano G, et al. Multinational comparative clinical evaluation of two long-acting injectable contraceptive steroids: norethisterone oenanthate and medroxyprogesterone acetate. Contraception 1977;15(5);513–33.
[35] Rees HD, Bonsall RW, Michael RP. Pre-optic and hypothalamic neurons accumulate [3H] medroxyprogesterone acetate in male cynomolgus monkeys. Life Sci 1986;39(15):1353–9.

[36] Black A, et al. Canadian contraception consensus (Part 3 of 4): Chapter 7 – Intrauterine contraception. J Obstet Gynaecol Can 2016;38(2):182–222.
[37] Gemzell-Danielsson K, et al. The effect of age, parity and body mass index on the efficacy, safety, placement and user satisfaction associated with two low-dose levonorgestrel intrauterine contraceptive systems: subgroup analyses of data from a phase III trial. PLoS One 2015;10(9):e0135309.
[38] Jatlaoui TC, Curtis KM. Safety and effectiveness data for emergency contraceptive pills among women with obesity: a systematic review. Contraception 2016;94(6):605–11.
[39] Edelman AB, et al. Impact of obesity on the pharmacokinetics of levonorgestrel-based emergency contraception: single and double dosing. Contraception 2016;94(1):52–7.
[40] Turok DK, et al. Emergency contraception with a copper IUD or oral levonorgestrel: an observational study of 1-year pregnancy rates. Contraception 2014;89(3):222–8.
[41] Paulen ME, et al. Contraceptive use among women with a history of bariatric surgery: a systematic review. Contraception 2010;82(1):86–94.
[42] Ostrowska L, et al. The use of contraception for patients after bariatric surgery. Ginekol Pol 2016;87(8):591–3.
[43] Buchwald H, et al. Bariatric surgery: a systematic review and meta-analysis. JAMA 2004;292(14):1724–37.
[44] Merhi ZO. Revisiting optimal hormonal contraception following bariatric surgery. Contraception 2013;87(2):131–3.
[45] Jamieson DJ, et al. Complications of interval laparoscopic tubal sterilization: findings from the United States Collaborative Review of Sterilization. Obstet Gynecol 2000;96(6):997–1002.
[46] Chi IC, Wilkens L. Interval tubal sterilization in obese women – an assessment of risks. Am J Obstet Gynecol 1985;152(3):292–7.

Dana Vitner, Kristin Harris, Cynthia Maxwell and Dan Farine

8 Obesity in pregnancy: a review of international guidelines

Developed nations have witnessed growing rates of obesity across all populations over recent years [1]. This translates to higher rates of obesity in reproductive aged women and their pregnancies. Maternal obesity has therefore become one of the most common risk factors in obstetric practice, and one of the most important challenges in obstetric care [2]. Obesity in pregnancy is associated with both short-term and long-term complications for mothers including miscarriage, thromboembolism, gestational diabetes, preeclampsia, dysfunctional labor, postpartum hemorrhage, and wound infection [1, 3–9]. Compared with women with a normal body mass index (BMI), obesity in pregnancy is associated with higher rates of cesarean section and lower rates of breastfeeding [9–11]. Furthermore, adverse health outcomes are noted in the offspring of obese women such as congenital anomalies, stillbirth, and neonatal death [12–18]. For these reasons, various esteemed committees from developed nations have made recommendations for the care of obese pregnant women and their babies. In this chapter, we will outline these recommendations to provide an understanding of the current evidence and identify areas of agreement, discord, and limitation within the existing international guidelines on obesity in pregnancy.

Currently, the American College of Obstetricians and Gynecologists (ACOG), Royal Australian and New Zealand College of Obstetricians and Gynecologists (RANZCOG), Royal College of Obstetrics and Gynecology (RCOG), and the Society of Obstetrics and Gynecologists of Canada (SOGC) offer published guidelines for the management of obesity in pregnancy [2, 19–21]. Each appointed committee reviewed the literature separately and made recommendations for their specific populations. The following themes were universally reviewed and are summarized: definition, preconception counseling, antenatal care, intrapartum management, and postpartum care.

8.1 Definition of obesity

The World Health Organization BMI classification system was used universally to define obesity in pregnancy as a BMI ≥30 kg/m^2 (see Table 8.1) [22].

https://doi.org/10.1515/9783110487817-008

Tab. 8.1: BMI and recommended weight gain in pregnancy.

	BMI (kg/m²)*	Suggested weight gain (kg)**
Underweight	<18.5	12.5–18
Normal weight	18.5–24.9	11.5–16
Overweight	25–29.9	7–11.5
Obese class I	30–34.9	5–9
Obese class II	35–39.9	5–9
Obese class III	≥40	5–9

* World Health Organization BMI references [22].
** Institute of Medicine on weight gain in pregnancy [34].

Maternal weight (kg) and height (m) at the first antenatal visit, or prepregnancy, if known, were recommended as the best measure of preexisting obesity [2, 19–21]. Of note, the SOGC guidelines included women who were 110% to 120% of their ideal body weight or >91 kg (200 lb.) as alternative criteria to the definition of obesity, as some regions in Canada do not routinely collect maternal height as part of the antenatal record, thus not permitting the calculation of BMI [21, 23].

The prevalence of obesity in pregnancy ranged from 11% to 50% across the developed nations reported [2, 19–21]. The differences in prevalence rates could result from variations in definitions and sampling within each population coupled with diversity in national diet and exercise patterns. For instance, the SOGC report of 10.2% is estimated from BMI data from a national survey of reproductive aged women [24], whereas the RCOG range of 16% to 19% is extracted from large cohort studies from two maternal centers in the United Kingdom [25, 26]. These guidelines did not specify between overweight and obese categories, so one can assume that they are referring to obese women alone given their low prevalence compared with the RANZCOG prevalence of 50% when overweight and obese women were combined [27]. ACOG reported the prevalence of obesity in women of reproductive age (20–39 years) in the United States at 58.5% but not the prevalence of obesity in pregnancy, which is difficult to compare with the previous studies [28, 29]. Overall, we can extract that there is a general increase in the rates of obesity across all reported populations, with at least 1 in 10 women identified with the risk factor of obesity in pregnancy.

8.2 Preconception counseling

All guidelines recommend identification of obesity prior to conception with encouragement and support of sustainable lifestyle changes [2, 19–21]. Primary care appointments are recognized as the optimal setting for identification of weight issues in reproductive aged obese women [30], as well as thorough counseling of potential adverse maternal and fetal outcomes in pregnancy (see Tables 8.2 and 8.3). If obesity is identified, a nutritional consultation should be offered prior to conception as weight loss prior to pregnancy has been reported as the most effective intervention to improve medical comorbidities [31]. RANZCOG and ACOG briefly discussed the implications of bariatric surgery as a method for weight loss, with recommendations for specialized advice given the rapidly evolving data in this area, as well as consultation with a nutritionist to help identify nutritional deficiencies and evaluate the need for vitamin supplementation such as vitamin B_{12}, iron, folate, vitamin D, and calcium due to issues with absorption [32].

Tab. 8.2: Maternal complications associated with obesity in pregnancy.

	ACOG	RANZCOG	RCOG	SOGC
Hypertensive disorders of pregnancy	Increased	5%–10%	OR 2.1–3.3	OR 2.38–3
Gestational diabetes	Increased	3%–7%	OR 2.4–3.6	OR 2.6–4
Thromboembolism	Increased	Increased	OR 9.7	–
Slow labor progression	Prolonged first stage	–	Increased	–
Shoulder dystocia	–	Increased	2.9–3.14	
PPH	–	Increased	OR 1.4–2.3	–
Assisted birth	–	5%–8%	–	–
Cesarean delivery	Increased	45%–52%	OR 2.05	OR 1.5–3.1
Emergency C/S	–	–	OR 1.8–2.0	–
C/S associated complications	Increased (consider higher dose of prophylactic antibiotics)	–	Increased	Increased
VBAC*	Inverse relationship between BMI and success rates of VBAC Greater rates of composite morbidity for class III obesity undergoing VBAC	Low success rate	Low success rate Greater risk for uterine rupture during trial of labor	Low success rate
Maternal death	–	Increased	–	–

* VBAC, vaginal birth after cesarean section.

Tab. 8.3: Fetal/neonatal complications described with obesity in pregnancy.

	ACOG	RANZCOG	RCOG	SOGC
Spontaneous abortion	OR 1.2	–	–	OR 1.2 Recurrent >3 OR 3.5
Congenital abnormalities	OR 1.2–2.2	–	OR 1.6	Increased
Preterm birth <37 weeks gestational age	–	9%–11%	OR 1.2	–
Small-for-gestational age (customized)	Increased	13%–19%	–	–

Tab. 8.3: (continued)

	ACOG	RANZCOG	RCOG	SOGC
Macrosomia >4,000 g	Increased	9%–11%	OR 2.4–3.1	OR 1.4–2
Macrosomia >4,500 g				OR 2–2.4
Neonatal mechanical ventilation	–	7%–10%	–	–
NICU admission	–	–	OR 1.3–1.5 in BMI ≥35 kg/m² advised to give birth in an obstetric unit*	–
Stillbirth	OR 1.4	Increased	OR 2.1	OR 2.79
Perinatal death	OR 1.16	1%–2%	OR 2.6	–
Childhood and adolescent obesity	Increased	–	Increased	–

* NICE clinical guideline No. 55.

8.3 Antenatal care

Standard antenatal care is recommended for obese women with particular attention to focused maternal and fetal surveillance based on assessments of risk. Recommendations for weight gain are an important piece that was touched on similarly by all groups. Studies have reported that women who gained the recommended amount of weight in pregnancy, regardless of BMI, had fewer adverse outcomes [33]. All guidelines referenced the Institute of Medicine gestational weight gain guidelines for recommendations of appropriate weight gain based on prepregnancy BMI (see Table 8.4) [34]. Weight loss during pregnancy is not recommended by the RANZCOG and ACOG guidelines given concerns regarding higher incidence of small-for-gestational age fetuses and associated adverse outcomes [2, 19, 35–37].

Tab. 8.4: Recommendations for antepartum, intrapartum, and postpartum care.

	ACOG	RANZCOG	RCOG	SOGC
Identification of obesity	Yes	Yes	Yes	Yes
Recommendation for exercise	Yes	Yes	Yes	Yes
Nutritional consult	Yes	Yes	Yes	Yes

Tab. 8.4: (continued)

	ACOG	RANZCOG	RCOG	SOGC
Nutritional supplementation (preconception)	No recommendation	5 mg/day folic acid 10 mg/day vitamin D for BMI ≥30 kg/m^2	5 mg/day folic acid For BMI >30 kg/m^2 at least 1 month before conception	No recommendation
Bariatric surgery	May require additional nutritional supplementation	Reduction in maternal risks with a possible increase in IUGR; may require additional supplementation	No recommendation	No recommendation
H1N1 vaccination	No recommendation	Yes	No recommendation	No recommendation
Antenatal facilities: appropriate bariatric equipment	Yes	Yes	Yes	yes
Early GDM testing	Yes	Yes	Yes	Yes
Referral to anesthesia	Yes	Yes	Yes	yes
Antenatal thromboprophylaxis (LMWH)	Risk should be evaluated individually	No data	Assessed at first visit. Should be considered in accordance with Green Top Guideline No. 37*	Risk should be evaluated individually
Preeclampsia surveillance	No recommendation	Yes	In accordance with the PRECOG, 2004**	No recommendation
Antenatal aspirin	No recommendation	No recommendation	Should be considered when BMI ≥30 kg/m^2 and one more moderate risk factor. In accordance to NICE Guideline Development Group***	No recommendation

Tab. 8.4: (continued)

	ACOG	RANZCOG	RCOG	SOGC
Limitations of fetal anatomic and weight assessment	Yes	No recommendation	No recommendation	Yes
Postpartum LMWH	Yes	No recommendation	Recommended when BMI ≥35 kg/m^2 and one additional risk factor. If two or more, then compression stockings in addition to LMWH	Individual risk assessment

* Green Top Guideline No. 37 – women with BMI ≥30 kg/m^2 who also have two or more additional risks factors for thromboembolism should be considered for low molecular weight heparin (LMWH) prophylaxis in the antenatal period. Prescribed doses should be appropriate for maternal weight. This should be started as early in pregnancy as practical. All women receiving LMWH should usually continue prophylactic doses of LMWH until 6 weeks postpartum, at which time a postnatal risk assessment should be made. All women with a BMI ≥40 kg/m^2 should be offered postnatal thromboprophylaxis regardless of their mode of delivery.

** Pre-eclampsia Community Guideline (PRECOG), 2004 – women with BMI ≥35 kg/m^2 and who also have at least one additional risks factor for preeclampsia should be referred early in pregnancy for specialist input in their care.

*** NICE Guideline Development Group – women with more than one moderate risk factor (obesity, first pregnancy, maternal age >40 years, family history of preeclampsia, multiple pregnancy) may benefit from taking aspirin at 75 mg daily from 12 weeks of gestation until delivery.

There is much discrepancy with respect to recommendations for supplementation for obese women in pregnancy. With respect to folic acid supplementation, studies have demonstrated obese women to have upward of a twofold increase in neural tube defects, with a dose–response noted [38]. Given this elevated risk, RANZCOG and RCOG recommend high dose preconception folic acid supplementation of 5 mg daily for women with a BMI ≥30 kg/m^2 with continuance through the antenatal period [2, 20]. However, ACOG and SOGC simply acknowledge the elevated risk without recommendation for additional supplementation [19, 22]. The SOGC guideline explains that current evidence is inconclusive in terms of whether folic acid provides protective effects for obese women and whether a higher dosage would reduce the risk compared with that of a lean woman [22, 39]. The Folic Acid Supplementation Guideline released by the SOGC in 2015 does not classify obesity as a risk factor for neural tube defects that would require adjustment in dosage from the standard of 0.4 mg daily; however, they acknowledge that this deserves further consideration [40].

RANZCOG and RCOG further recommend vitamin D supplementation at 10 mg daily, whereas there is no mention of vitamin D in ACOG and SOGC despite similar ecosystems [2, 20, 41]. RANZCOG is the only guideline to recommend iodine supplementation (150 µg daily) [42] and H1N1 vaccination antenatally for obese women [43].

All guidelines outline that proper maternal surveillance can only be achieved with appropriate equipment (including blood pressure cuffs and scales) calibrated for the obese population [2, 19–21]. They acknowledge the increased maternal risks as detailed in Tab. 8.2, which should be communicated to the patient and screened for routinely. With respect to preeclampsia, all guidelines recommended close monitoring of blood pressure at obstetrical visits with the appropriate cuff and further work-up with laboratory screening as necessary. The RCOG guideline goes on to recommend monitoring according to PRECOG, which outlines visits every 3 weeks from 24 to 32 weeks' gestation, followed by every other week minimum until delivery [44]. Furthermore, the RCOG guideline is unique in recommending the use of low-dose aspirin (75 mg daily) during pregnancy if more than one risk factor is present according to the NICE guidelines for the prevention of gestational hypertension and preeclampsia [45]. All guidelines recommend early screening for gestational diabetes mellitus with an oral glucose tolerance test, with repeat screens between 24 and 28 weeks if initially negative [2, 19–21].

There was no consensus on prophylaxis for venous thromboembolism in obese women. RCOG refers to the Clinical Green Top Guideline No. 37 for venous thromboembolism guidance, which recommends antenatal prophylaxis with LMWH for women with a BMI ≥30 kg/m^2 and two additional risk factors for thromboembolism [46]. A 1-week course of postpartum thromboprophylaxis is recommended regardless of the mode of delivery for women with a BMI ≥40 kg/m^2, and women ≥30 kg/m^2 with one persisting thrombotic risk factor [46]. SOGC and ACOG recommend LMWH in the antenatal period on an individually assessed basis [19,21]. All guidelines recommended weight-based dosing if LMWH is used [46].

Adverse health outcomes are noted in the offspring of obese women such as congenital anomalies, stillbirths, and neonatal death [12–18]. All guidelines acknowledge the difficulty of ultrasound surveillance in the obese patient given suboptimal visualization. However, repeat examinations are often necessary in 12% to 20% of patients in whom fetal anatomical structures are still poorly visualized [47–49]. The SOGC guideline recommends deferring the anatomy exam until 20 to 22 weeks of gestation to allow further structural development for better visualization [21]. The remaining guidelines simply acknowledge the decreased detection of congenital anomalies in the obese patient [2, 19–20]. The RANZCOG guideline recommends serial growth ultrasound examinations as symphysis-fundal height measurements are difficult to interpret in obese patients [2]. SOGC, on the other hand, states that ultrasound is not superior to clinical examination, and therefore no serial ultrasounds are required for growth alone [50]. Lastly, although obese women are at higher risk of stillbirths, all guidelines agree that there is no evidence showing improvements in pregnancy outcomes with antepartum surveillance, and therefore no formal recommendations are made for health care providers [2, 19–21].

8.4 Intrapartum

There are a few considerations for intrapartum care in the obese pregnant. First, all guidelines recommend having an experienced team available for management, as well as appropriate equipment for maternal and fetal monitoring in labor and surgical procedures [2, 19–21]. The SOGC guideline recommends that intrauterine pressure catheters be available given that contractions are often difficult to assess on tocometry [21]. Furthermore, all guidelines recommend having longer instruments available for cesarean section [2, 19–21]. Second, all guidelines recommend an anesthesia consult for obese patients as they are at a higher risk of anesthetic complications including re-siting of epidurals, epidural failure, aspiration, difficult intubation, and postoperative atelectasis [51–54]. At this assessment, potential difficulties with regional and/or general anesthesia can be acknowledged and addressed.

With respect to labor management, both ACOG and RCOG do not recommend induction based on obesity alone. ACOG recommends allowing for a longer first stage of labor before moving to a cesarean section as a prolonged first stage is common in obese women. Aside from recognizing the consideration of shoulder dystocia by SOGC and RANZCOG, there are no further recommendations from the guidelines for management of labor alone. Trial of labor after cesarean section (TOLAC) requires individual counseling based on risk factors and chance of success [20, 55]. All guidelines discussed that TOLAC are less successful in the obese patient, with greater risk of morbidity [55]. With respect to cesarean section, obese women are at increased risk of requiring surgical intervention and of subsequent wound infection than women of normal BMI [9, 10]. RCOG and ACOG recommend antibiotic prophylaxis for surgery without weight-based dosage as there is no evidence to support that higher doses lead to fewer infections [56]. RCOG recommends suturing of the subcutaneous space to help prevent collections in an effort to decrease postoperative wound infection [56].

8.5 Postpartum

There are important considerations for obese women in the postpartum period including venous thromboembolism prophylaxis, breastfeeding, and weight loss that should be addressed by the health care provider team. Similar to antepartum venous thromboembolism prophylaxis, SOGC and ACOG recommend individualized assessment given that studies are inconsistent in terms of benefit [19, 21]. RCOG refers to the Green Top Guideline, which recommends thromboprophylaxis for 1 week in all women with BMI ≥40 kg/m^2 regardless of mode of delivery. For women with a BMI ≥30 kg/m^2 and one persisting risk factor, thromboprophylaxis for 1 week is recommended, and if two or more risk factors are evident, then the addition of compression stockings is advised [46]. Weight-based dosing is advised for all obese women [46].

Breastfeeding rates are lower and challenges are common in the obese population [11], and consensus was seen across guidelines in recommendation of support in the postpartum period by nursing or lactation consultants.

Weight loss should be addressed after delivery with behavioral interventions using diet and exercise. All guidelines recommend providing information and support to patients in this endeavor, as interpregnancy weight loss in obese women may decrease the risks for mother and baby in a subsequent pregnancy [2, 19–21].

8.6 Conclusions

In summary, our review of four major national guidelines shows consensus for the following important recommendations regarding obesity in pregnancy (Table 8.4):

1. Identification of obesity prior to conception is advised. A nutritional consultation should be offered to all overweight or obese women and they should be encouraged to follow an exercise program.
2. Patients should be informed of the potential maternal complications related to high BMI (pregnancy induced hypertension and preeclampsia, gestational diabetes, thromboembolism, and death).
3. Patients should be informed of the increased fetal complications correlated with high BMI (macrosomia, preterm birth, small-for-gestational age, spontaneous abortion, stillbirth, congenital abnormalities, perinatal death). Fetal abnormalities are more difficult to detect in obese patients due to suboptimal visibility.
4. Weight gain in pregnancy should follow the Institute of Medicine's guidelines to help prevent adverse outcomes. Gaining more weight than recommended is associated with macrosomia, labor augmentation, gestational hypertension, and neonatal metabolic abnormalities.
5. Access to appropriately calibrated monitors and instruments is important in the surveillance of obese women in pregnancy.
6. Early testing for gestational diabetes mellitus is recommended, with a repeat screen at 24–28 weeks if the initial result is negative.
7. An anesthesia consult is recommended given the higher risk of anesthetic complications.
8. Induction of labor in patients with high BMI should not be recommended in the absence of other obstetric or medical indications.
9. Patients should be informed of an increased delivery and postpartum complications, especially increased rates of cesarean section, wound infection, and low success rate of VBAC.
10. Postpartum counseling and support regarding breastfeeding and weight loss is important.

Areas of debate that require further investigation include:
1. Terminology and definitions of clinical parameters including prevalence rates of obesity in pregnancy were inconsistent and made comparisons between groups difficult. An effort should be made for consensus.
2. The efficacy of higher dosage of folic acid supplementation in preventing neural tube defects.
3. Prophylaxis for venous thromboembolism is recommended on individual assessments based on most guidelines. An effort should be made for further standardization.

Overall, the management of obesity requires sustainable interventions ranging from population-based public health and economic initiatives to individual nutritional, behavioral, and surgical practices. Management should begin during preconception and continue through the postpartum period. Given the higher incidence of maternal and neonatal complications in obese women, it is important that all health care providers providing maternity care are aware of the strategies for minimizing the identified risks in an effort to provide optimal care for this growing population. Given the rapidly evolving literature in the field of obesity in pregnancy, a timely review of these guidelines will be necessary to reflect the standard of care.

Bibliography

[1] Huda SS, Brodie LE, Sattar N. Obesity in pregnancy: prevalence and metabolic consequences. Semin Fetal Neonatal Med 2010;15(2):70–6.

[2] Management of Obesity in Pregnancy – RANZCOG College statement. C-Obs 49.

[3] Bhattacharya S, Campbell DM, Liston WA, Bhattacharya S. Effect of body mass index on pregnancy outcomes in nulliparous women delivering singleton babies. BMC Public Health 2007;7:168.

[4] Heslehurst N, Simpson H, Ells LJ, et al. The impact of maternal BMI status on pregnancy outcomes with immediate short-term obstetric resource implications: a meta-analysis. Obes Rev 2008;9(6):635–83.

[5] Cedergren MI. Maternal morbid obesity and the risk of adverse pregnancy outcome. Obstet Gynecol 2004;103(2):219–24.

[6] Jacobsen AF, Skjeldestad FE, Sandset PM. Ante- and postnatal risk factors of venous thrombosis: a hospital-based case control study. J Thromb Haemost 2008;6(6):905–12.

[7] Sebire NJ, Jolly M, Harris JP, et al. Maternal obesity and pregnancy outcome: a study of 287,213 pregnancies in London. Int J Obes Relat Metab Disord 2001;25(8):1175–82.

[8] O'Brien TE, Ray JG, Chan W-S. Maternal body mass index and the risk of preeclampsia: a systematic overview. Epidemiology 2003;14(3):368–74.

[9] Nuthalapaty FS, Rouse DJ, Owen J. The association of maternal weight with cesarean risk, labor duration, and cervical dilation rate during labor induction [erratum appears in Obstet Gynecol 2004;103(5 Pt 1):1019]. Obstet Gynecol 2004;103(3):452–6.

[10] Chu SY, Kim SY, Schmid CH, et al. Maternal obesity and risk of cesarean delivery: a meta-analysis. Obes Rev 2007;8(5):385–94.

[11] Amir LH, Donath S. A systematic review of maternal obesity and breastfeeding intention, initiation and duration. BMC Pregnancy Childbirth 2007;7:9.

[12] Yao R, Ananth CV, Park BY, Pereira L, Plante LA, Perinatal Research Consortium. Obesity and the risk of stillbirth: population-based cohort study. Am J Obstet Gynecol 2014;210(5):457.

[13] Lashen H, Fear K, Sturdee DW. Obesity is associated with increased risk of first trimester and recurrent miscarriage: matched case-control study. Hum Reprod 2004;19(7):1644–6.

[14] Rasmussen SA, Chu SY, Kim SY, Schmid CH, Lau J. Maternal obesity and risk of neural tube defects: a metaanalysis. Am J Obstet Gynecol 2008;198(6):611–9.

[15] Chu SY, Kim SY, Lau J, et al. Maternal obesity and risk of stillbirth: a metaanalysis. Am J Obstet Gynecol 2007;197(3):223–8.

[16] Kristensen J, Vestergaard M, Wisborg K, Kesmodel U, Secher NJ. Pre-pregnancy weight and the risk of stillbirth and neonatal death. BJOG 2005;112(4):403–8.

[17] Aune D, Saugstad OD, Henriksen T, Tonstad S. Maternal body mass index and the risk of fetal death, stillbirth, and infant death: a systematic review and meta-analysis. J Am Med Assoc 2014;311(15):1536–46.

[18] Meehan S, Beck CR, Mair-Jenkins J, Leonardi-Bee J, Puleston R. Maternal obesity and infant mortality: a meta-analysis. Pediatrics 2014;133(5):863–71.

[19] ACOG Practice Bulletin No. 495. Obesity in pregnancy. American College of Obstetrics and Gynecologists. Obstet Gynecol 2011;118:197–8.

[20] CMACE/RCOG Joint Guideline. Management of women with obesity in pregnancy March 2010.

[21] Davies GA, Maxwell C, McLeod L, Gagnon R, Basso M, Bos H, et al. SOGC clinical practice guidelines: obesity in pregnancy. No. 239, February 2010. Int J Gynaecol Obstet 2010;110(2):167–73.

[22] World Health Organization. Global database on body mass index: BMI classification 2006. Available from: http://apps.who.int/bmi/index.jsp?introPage=intro_3.html.

[23] Robinson HE, O'Connell CM, Joseph KS, McLeod NL. Maternal outcomes in pregnancies complicated by obesity. Obstet Gynecol 2005;106:1357–64.

[24] Statistics Canada. Adult obesity in Canada: measured height and weight. 2005. Available at: http://www.statcan.gc.ca/pub/82-620-m/2005001/article/ adults-adultes/8060-eng.htm. Accessed January 6, 2010.

[25] Heslehurst N, Ells LJ, Simpson H, Batterham A, Wilkinson J, Summerbell CD. Trends in maternal obesity incidence rates, demographic predictors, and health inequalities in 36,821 women over a 15-year period. BJOG 2007;114(2):187–94.

[26] Kanagalingam MG, Forouhi NG, Greer IA, Sattar N. Changes in booking body mass index over a decade: retrospective analysis from a Glasgow maternity hospital. BJOG 2005;112(10):1431–3.

[27] National Institute of Health and Clinical Excellence. Weight management before, during and after pregnancy. 2010.

[28] Ogden CL, Carroll MD, Kit BK, Flegal KM. Prevalence of childhood and adult obesity in the United States, 2011–2012. JAMA 2014;311:806–14.

[29] National Center for Health Statistics. NCHS obesity data. Hyattsville (MD): NCHS 2014. Available at: http://www.cdc.gov/nchs/data/factsheets/factsheet_obesity.pdf. Retrieved September 2, 2015.

[30] Handbook for physical activity guide to healthy active living. Ottawa: Health Canada 1998. Available at: http://www.eatwellbeactive.gc.ca. Accessed December 1, 2009.

[31] Villamor E, Cnattingius S. Interpregnancy weight change and risk of adverse pregnancy outcomes: a population-based study. Lancet 2006;368(9542):1164–70.

[32] Buchwald H, Avidor Y, Braunwald E, Jensen MD, Pories W, Fahrbach K, et al. Bariatric surgery: a systematic review and meta-analysis [published erratum appears in JAMA 2005;293:1728]. JAMA 2004;292:1724–37.

[33] Crane JMG, White J, Murphy P, Burrage L, Hutchens D. The effect of gestational weight gain by body mass index on maternal and neonatal outcomes. J Obstet Gynaecol Can 2009;31:28–35.
[34] Institute of Medicine (US) and National Research Council (US) Committee to Reexamine IOM Pregnancy Weight Guidelines. Weight gain during pregnancy: reexamining the guidelines. Washington, DC: National Academy of Sciences, 2009.
[35] Hinkle SN, Sharma AJ, Dietz PM. Gestational weight gain in obese mothers and associations with fetal growth. Am J Clin Nutr 2010;92:644–51.
[36] Catalano PM, Mele L, Landon MB, et al. Inadequate weight gain in overweight and obese pregnant women: what is the effect on fetal growth? Eunice Kennedy Shriver National Institute of Child Health and Human Development Maternal-Fetal Medicine Units Network. Am J Obstet Gynecol 2014;211:137.e1–137.e7.
[37] Kapadia MZ, Park CK, Beyene J, Giglia L, Maxwell C, McDonald SD. Weight loss instead of weight gain within the guidelines in obese women during pregnancy: a systematic review and meta-analyses of maternal and infant outcomes. PLoS One 2015;10:e0132650.
[38] Nuthalapaty FS, Rouse DJ. The impact of obesity on obstetrical practice and outcome. Clin Obstet Gynecol 2004;47:898–913.
[39] Werler MM, Louik C, Shapiro S, Mitchell AA. Prepregnant weight in relation to risk of neural tube defects. JAMA 1996;275:1127–8.
[40] Wilson RD. Pre-conception folic acid and multivitamin supplementation for the primary and secondary prevention of neural tube defects and other folic acid sensitive congenital anomalies. JOGC 2015;37(6):534–49.
[41] Bodnar LM, Catov JM, Roberts JM, Simhan HN. Prepregnancy obesity predicts poor vitamin D status in mothers and their neonates. J Nutr 2007;137(11):2437–42.
[42] National Health and Medical Research Council. Iodine supplementation for pregnant and breastfeeding women: Public statement, 2010.
[43] The Royal Australian and New Zealand College of Obstetricians and Gynaecologists. Influenza vaccination during pregnancy (C-Obs 45). Melbourne, Australia 2011.
[44] The Pre-eclampsia Community Guideline Development Group. Pre-eclampsia Community Guideline (PRECOG). Middlesex: Action on Pre-Eclampsia (APEC), 2004.
[45] National Institute for Health and Clinical Excellence. Hypertensive disorders during pregnancy (draft, accessed January 2010). London: National Institute for Health and Clinical Excellence 2010.
[46] Royal College of Obstetricians and Gynaecologists. Green-top guideline no. 37. Reducing the risk of thrombosis and embolism during pregnancy and puerperium. London: Royal College of Obstetricians and Gynaecologists, 2009.
[47] Lantz ME, Chisholm CA. The preferred timing of second trimester obstetric sonography based on maternal body mass index. J Ultrasound Med 2004;23:1019–22.
[48] Wolfe HM, Sokol RJ, Martier SM, Zador IE. Maternal obesity: a potential source of error in sonographic prenatal diagnosis. Obstet Gynecol 1990;76:339–42.
[49] Dashe JS, McIntire DD, Twickler DM. Effect of maternal obesity on the ultrasound detection of anomalous fetuses. Obstet Gynecol 2009;113:1001–7.
[50] Field NT, Piper JM, Langer O. The effect of maternal obesity on the accuracy of fetal weight estimation. Obstet Gynecol 1995;86:102–7.
[51] Lewis G, editor. Confidential enquiry into maternal and child health. Saving mothers' lives – reviewing maternal deaths to make motherhood safer 2003–2005. London: CEMACH, 2007.
[52] Dresner M, Brocklesby J, Bamber J. Audit of the influence of body mass index on the performance of epidural analgesia in labour and the subsequent mode of delivery. BJOG 2006;113(10):1178–81.

[53] Hawkins JL, Koonin LM, Palmer SK, Gibbs CP. Anesthesia-related deaths during obstetric delivery in the United States, 1979–1990. Anesthesiology 1997;86(2):277–84.
[54] Hood DD, Dewan DM. Anesthetic and obstetric outcome in morbidly obese parturients. Anesthesiology 1993;79(6):1210–8.
[55] Induction of labor. ACOG Practice Bulletin No. 107. American College of Obstetricians and Gynecologists. Obstet Gynecol 2009;114:386–97.
[56] National Institute for Health and Clinical Excellence. Caesarean section. London: Royal College of Obstetricians and Gynaecologists, 2004.

Irene Cetin, Francesca Parisi and Martina I. Mazzocco

9 Diet and the obese pregnant patient

9.1 Introduction

Worldwide, the prevalence of obesity has reached epidemic proportions. The European Peristat Database and World Health Organization (WHO) identified maternal obesity rates in Europe ranging from the highest (25.2%) in the United Kingdom to the lowest (7.1%) in Poland. Furthermore, low-income and middle-income countries have experienced major changes in diet and physical activity patterns, with increased consumption of processed, energy-dense food groups and an overall transition to a sedentary lifestyle. The result is a progressive energy and nutrient imbalance, leading to a global shift from undernutrition to overnutrition and micronutrient deficiencies. The Developmental Origins of Health and Disease (DoHaD) hypothesis underlined that early prenatal exposures strongly affect subsequent risk of obesity and noncommunicable diseases throughout epigenetics modifications realizing as early as the periconceptional period, when gametogenesis and embryogenesis take place [1]. Thus, maternal obesity, nutritional exposures, and excessive weight gain are also major contributors to obesity and metabolic disturbances in the offspring. This means that early modifications of maternal lifestyle and nutrition could strongly affect short-term and long-term health outcomes, further interrupting the intergenerational effect on cardiovascular and metabolic risk profile in the offspring [2].

9.2 Maternal nutritional needs in pregnancy

A healthy pregnancy strongly depends on prepregnancy diet and body composition, as well as on nutrients consumed during pregnancy [3]. We define nutrition as the intake of food essential for optimal growth, function, and health. Good nutrition is defined as a well-balanced diet, providing all necessary nutrients in optimal amounts and proportions, whereas poor nutrition is defined as unbalanced diet in which all or some components are defective or excessive [4]. Adequate nutritional counseling, including dietary manipulations aiming to modify the body mass index as appropriate and to improve micronutrient intake, is essential to meet pregnancy needs, ensure adequate fetal growth and affect future health of the offspring [5, 6]. Unless prepregnancy nutrition is poor or inappropriate, macronutrient and energy intake do not substantially change during pregnancy compared with the nonpregnant state. In particular, energy intake should not increase during the first trimester of pregnancy, whereas an increase of 340 and 452 kcal/day is recommended in the second and third trimesters, respectively, to ensure adequate fetal growth and fat deposition [7]. Protein

https://doi.org/10.1515/9783110487817-009

needs increase during the second half of pregnancy to account for increased tissue formation for the fetus, placenta, and maternal tissues. Overall, the recommended increase in protein intake is 10 to 25 g/day above the prepregnancy recommendation of 60 g/day. As for the nonpregnant woman, fats should represent 15% to 30% of the overall energy intake. Because polyunsaturated fatty acid (PUFA) status (especially omega-3 fatty acid status) declines during pregnancy and is essential for fetal brain development, PUFA intake should be maintained or increased by consuming one to two meals per week of oily fish. Table 9.1 shows the main characteristics of a healthy dietary pattern during pregnancy (so-called Mediterranean or “Prudent diet”).

Tab. 9.1: Healthy dietary pattern during pregnancy.

Food group	Recommendation
Fruit and vegetables	At least five portions/day (400 mg)
Free sugars	<10% total energy intake (possibly <5%)
Fats	<30% total energy intake
Saturated fats	<10% total energy intake
PUFA	6% to 10% total energy intake, one to two portions of oily fish/week
Salt	<5 g/day, iodized salt

Conversely, micronutrient intake should substantially increase during pregnancy. Inadequate micronutrient intake during pregnancy has been associated with preterm, low birth weight, or small-for-gestational age babies in industrialized countries as well [8]. Insufficient iodine intake in pregnancy is considered the leading cause of preventable mental impairment. Nutrients of concern during pregnancy include iron, folate, vitamin B_{12}, calcium, vitamins A and D, and zinc. Currently, supplementation efforts are focused on the provision of iron, folic acid, iodine, calcium, and multiple micronutrient formulations. International organizations have advocated routine iron and folic acid supplementation for all pregnant women. Current recommendations for pregnancy include supplementation with a standard daily dose of 30 to 60 mg of elemental iron and 400 µg of folic acid to reduce the risk of neural tube defects, anemia, and low birth weight, starting preconceptionally and continuing throughout pregnancy. The WHO recommends that in populations in which calcium intake is low, women receive 1.5 and 2.0 mg of elemental calcium per day from 20 weeks of pregnancy until the end of pregnancy to prevent preeclampsia. Current global guidance recommends iodine supplementation in pregnant and lactating women in settings in which large proportions of the population do not have access to iodized salt (single annual dose of 400 mg or a daily dose of 250 µg). Recent evidence suggests that multiple micronutrient supplements could be the option of choice in countries with high incidence of low birth weight or small-for-gestational age babies because the benefits on birth outcomes seem to outweigh those observed with iron and folic acid alone. Table 9.2 summarizes the current supplementation guidelines for pregnant women.

Tab. 9.2: Summary of supplementation guidelines.

Micronutrient	Supplementation dosage	Target population
Iron	30–60 mg	All pregnant women
Folic acid	400 µg 5 mg (high risk population)	All pregnant women, starting 3 months before conception
Iodine	250 µg/day	Iodine deficient areas
Vitamin D	600 UI/day	Darkly pigmented skin, low or no sun exposure, obesity, vitamin D <30 ng/mL
Calcium	1.5–2.0 mg	High risk for preeclampsia, low calcium intake
Vitamin B_{12}	2.6 µg/day	Vegetarian/vegan diet
DHA	200 mg/day	High risk of preterm birth

9.3 Diet and low-grade inflammation in obese pregnancy

Pregnancy is considered a natural inflammatory state in which inflammatory cytokines have a pivotal role in placental function throughout pregnancy. Of interest, in early pregnancy, coordinated release of interleukin IL-10 and IL-11 regulate trophoblast differentiation and invasion, being therefore crucial in the establishment of pregnancy [9]. Moreover, pregnancy is a state of profound metabolic changes characterized by increased fat mass, insulin resistance, and mild hyperlipidemia in which phospholipids, total LDL and HDL cholesterol, and triglycerides significantly increase [10]. Potentially, these metabolic changes become pathologically exacerbated by pregestational obesity, leading to increased risks of short-term and long-term adverse outcomes [11]. In this regard, maternal obesity has been associated with several maternal, perinatal, and long-term adverse outcomes, including gestational hypertension and diabetes, preterm delivery, congenital anomalies, and impaired fetal growth (Fig. 9.1) [2].

Obesity is a well-known chronic low-grade inflammation state, characterized by raised concentrations of inflammatory markers in the systemic circulation [12]. Significantly increased concentrations of inflammatory cytokines have been detected in maternal plasma and placenta of obese pregnancies, probably stimulated by end toxin, lipids, reactive oxygen species, or oxidized lipids released by the adipose tissue [13, 14]. The preexisting chronic low-grade inflammation in obese women initiates a cascade of events leading to inflammatory environment *in uteri*, significant accumulation of placental macrophages and increased production of proinflammatory cytokines and adipokines (i.e., IL-6, leptin, TNF-α, monocyte chemotactic protein 1, and TLR4) [15]. Finally, uncontrolled placental inflammation leads to impaired placental function, increased free fatty acid delivery to the fetus, mitochondrial dysfunction, and altered fetal growth and development [16]. TNF-α, used to simulate the inflammatory milieu of obesity in animal models, decreases trophoblast mitochondrial respiration in a sexually dimorphic manner [17]. This reduction in placental

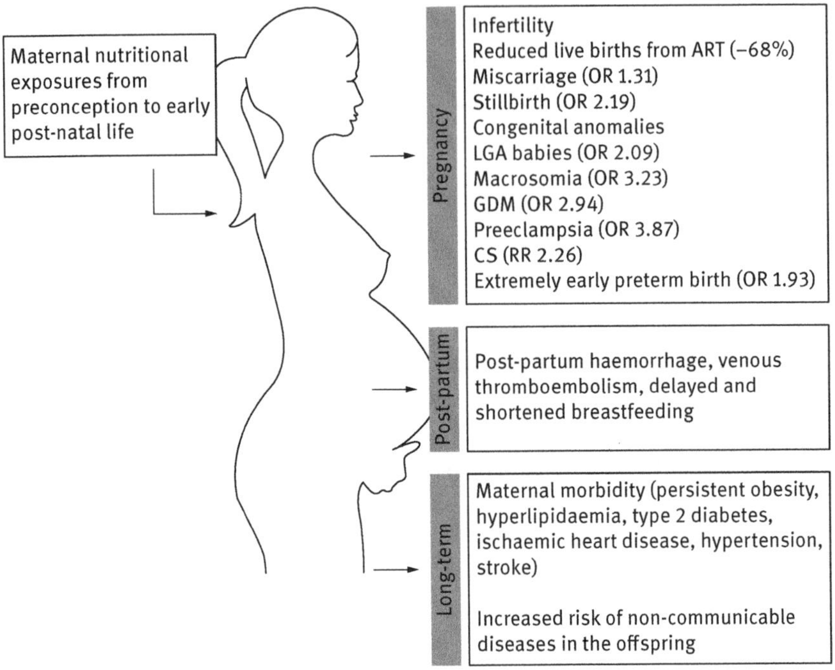

Fig. 9.1: Short-term and long-term outcomes associated with maternal obesity [2]. ART, assisted reproductive technology; LGA, large-for-gestational age; GDM, gestational diabetes mellitus; CS, cesarean section; OR, odds ratio.

mitochondrial respiration in pregnancies complicated by maternal obesity could compromise placental function, further explaining the increased susceptibility to fetal demise in obese late gestation [18].

Diet is an important regulatory factor of immune response. There is considerable evidence to suggest that overnutrition leads to immune-activation due to susceptibility to an inflammatory condition. Therefore, optimal nutrition is required for a healthy immune balance [19].

9.3.1 Macronutrients, micronutrients, and low-grade inflammation

Carbohydrates are a main dietary energy source and can be evaluated according to glycemic index (GI) and glycemic load (GL) values. Large cross-sectional studies have shown a positive association between dietary GI and inflammatory cytokines, including plasma adiponectin and C-reactive protein (CRP). Instead, whole grain intake seems inversely associated with markers of inflammation [20].

Saturated fat acid stimulates inflammatory response by a pathway involving Toll-like receptors (TLR), a class of pattern recognition receptors that play a crucial role in the innate immune system. Saturated fat acids also stimulate proinflammatory mechanisms through the TLR-independent pathway by producing reactive oxygen species, finally leading to the release of IL-1 [21].

The omega-6 (*n*-6) PUFA and omega-3 (*n*-3) PUFA families are precursors of eicosanoids, which play an important role in the immune response. A number of reviews reported the anti-inflammatory mechanisms of *n*-3 PUFA [22]. The down-regulation of proinflammatory cytokines in adipose tissue such as TNF-α, IL-6, and CRP is an example. Furthermore, the EPA and DHA were found to inhibit the TLR-4 signaling pathway [23]. Alpha-lipoic acid (ALA) is a mitochondrial PUFA with antioxidant function. Animal models showed that ALA significantly enhances the capacity of the insulin-dependent glucose transport system and inhibits the TNF-α pathway [24]. Human studies confirmed that ALA reduces body weight in obese subjects [25], plasma nonesterified fatty acid concentrations, and plasma levels of interleukin-6 and plasminogen activator-1 [26].

A recent randomized intervention trial on the inflammatory state in obese individuals revealed that total protein and meat protein intake were positively associated with inflammation, whereas neither vegetable- nor fish-derived proteins were found to influence the inflammatory status [27]. Current evidence for specific effects of single vegetable and fruit varieties is not convincing whereas a high overall intake of vegetables and fruits seems to be associated with a lower state of inflammation [28].

A recent study shows the association between maternal macronutrient intake and markers of inflammation in lean pregnant women [29]. Selenium, copper, zinc, manganese, vitamins C and E are antioxidant micronutrients found to reduce oxidative stress associated with obesity, preeclampsia, and intrauterine growth restriction.

9.3.2 Dietary patterns and low-grade inflammation

Many studies suggest that healthy eating patterns are associated with lower concentrations of markers of chronic low-grade inflammation. The Mediterranean diet has been inversely associated with markers of inflammation (circulating IL-6 and CRP), as well as markers of endothelial dysfunction [30, 31]. Large intervention studies strongly suggest that Mediterranean diets can lead to reductions in chronic low-grade inflammation and improvement in endothelial function, thereby offering cardioprotective effects. Cross-sectional studies suggest that a vegetarian-style diet can lower chronic inflammation compared with an omnivorous diet, but bias related to lifestyle other than diet, such as physical activity, smoking behavior, and socioeconomic class should be considered [32]. Whole grain intake and fish consumption have been "dose-dependently" associated with lower inflammation markers, including CRP, IL-6, and TNF-α concentrations [20, 33].

9.4 Nutritional recommendations in obese pregnancy to improve pregnancy outcomes

Maternal obesity is characterized by insulin resistance, hyperglycemia, hyperlipidemia, and a low-grade chronic inflammation, which in turn have been documented to influence nutrient availability and transfer to the developing fetus [34]. Research focused on the effects of dietary and lifestyle interventions to limit gestational weight gain among overweight or obese women. The Institute of Medicine recommends a weight gain of 5 to 9.1 kg in obese pregnancies [7]. The diet should be tailored for women of different classes of obesity by recommending a nutrient-dense caloric intake in the range of 2,000 to 2,500 kcal/day. Despite recommendations, conclusive evidence on the effects of interventions limiting gestational weight gain on birth outcomes are lacking and controversial [35–37].

Consumption of carbohydrates with low GI has been associated with reduced postprandial hyperglycemia. Furthermore, a low GI diet has been associated with improved weight loss through potential effects on hunger and energy intake [38]. It is known that maternal hyperglycemia is associated with increased placental transfer of glucose, resulting in fetal hyperglycemia, increased insulin production and finally increased insulin-mediated fetal growth. Therefore, reducing maternal hyperglycemia could potentially modulate fetal growth and development. Nevertheless, a systematic review on the influence of lowering dietary GI in nondiabetic pregnancies reported controversial results, showing both reduced risk of large-for-gestational age infants and increased risk of small-for-gestational age infants [39]. Until larger scale intervention trials are not completed, a low GI diet should not replace the current dietary recommendations. Fatty acids represent important fuel substrates for obese pregnant women who demonstrated increased reliance on lipid metabolism to meet the energy requirements of pregnancy [40, 41]. Increased consumption of dietary fibers and reduced saturated fat intake could improve maternal insulin resistance [42] and substantially contribute to the reduction in high birth weight, following antenatal dietary and physical activity advices [35]. Moreover, high maternal PUFA intake has been associated with a reduction in early childhood adiposity and improved body composition [43, 44].

These reports highlight the potential effect of relatively modest changes in maternal diet quality on *in utero* growth, birth weight, and future childhood adiposity. Recently, in the UPBEAT randomized controlled trial (Pregnancies Better Eating and Activity Trial), pregnant obese women were randomly assigned to receive a diet/physical activity intervention or standard antenatal care [45]. The dietary intervention aims to promote a healthier pattern of eating, but does not aim to restrict energy intake, focusing mainly on achieving two dietary goals: a reduction in dietary GL (50 unit reduction) and a reduction in saturated fat intake (<10% of energy). In the intervention group, GI was reduced, as was mean intake of total energy, carbohydrate, saturated fat, and total fats whereas protein and fiber intake was increased. To reduce saturated fat intake participants were encouraged to use low-fat dairy products and replace fatty meats and meat products with lean meat or fish. The trial suggests that only a complex intervention addressing both diet and physical activity in obese pregnant women is effective in improving diet quality and lifestyle, reducing gestational weight gain, and decreasing surrogate measures of maternal body fatness. However, the intervention did not prevent the development of gestational diabetes nor change the incidence of large-for-gestational age infants. Although gestational diabetes was not prevented, the behavioral intervention has the potential to reduce the risk of obesity and adverse metabolic risk in the child, because excessive gestational weight gain, high maternal fat mass, and increased GL are all associated independently with greater adiposity in the offspring, potentially through epigenetic pathways [46, 47].

9.5 Epigenetics in obese pregnancy

Nutrition plays a major role in maternal and child health, and dietary interventions in pregnancy have been shown to influence maternal, fetal, and infant health, with relevant effects across future generations (Fig. 9.2). Epigenetic processes, including DNA methylation or histone acetylation, describe heritable changes in gene expression not mediated by alterations of the DNA sequence [48], but susceptible to environmental influences, including nutrition, inflammation, lifestyle, and

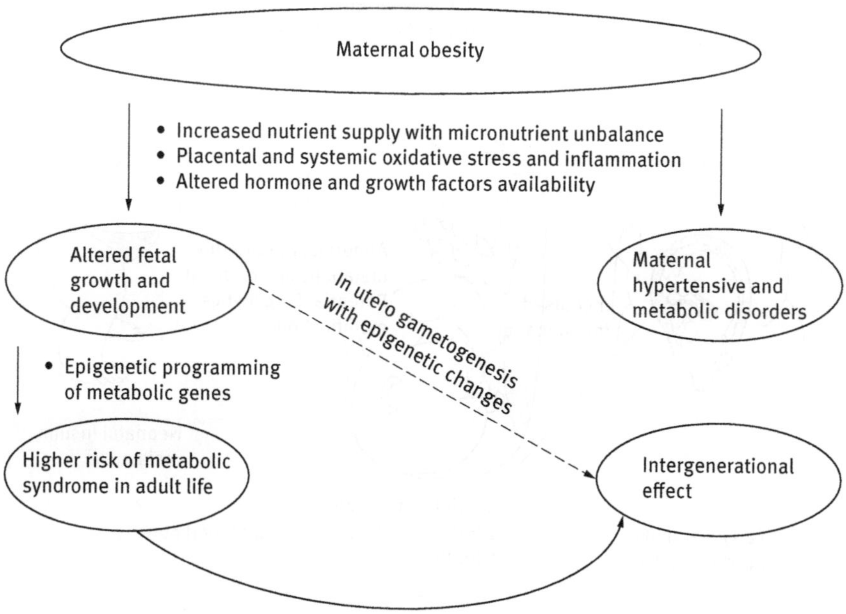

Fig. 9.2: The intergenerational cycle of obesity.

nonmodifiable characteristics (i.e., age and gender) [49]. Macro- and micronutrients affect the availability of methyl donors, substrates, and transcription factors, which are direct regulators of DNA stability and gene expression. In this way, nutrients are able to influence the complex biological pathways involved in gametogenesis, embryogenesis, as well as in placental and fetal growth, not only with short-term effects on pregnancy outcome as previously seen but also affecting future health status by permanently modulating gene expression [50].

Such *in utero* perturbations may alter developmentally plastic systems and predispose the fetus to noncommunicable diseases in later life (Fig. 9.3) by compromising physiological thresholds of energy balance regulation [51–53]. As extensively described, obesity induces a chronic, low-grade intrauterine inflammation with overexpression of maternal cytokines and nutrient imbalance [54, 55]. Chronic exposure to energy surplus, hormones, and growth factors *in utero* may potentially increase susceptibility to chronic diseases. Considerable animal models illustrated that maternal diet (i.e., high-fat or Western style diet) can program an obesogenic phenotype through epigenetic changes of metabolic control genes that play central roles in body composition and metabolism [56, 57]. A proposed mechanism explaining the increased adiposity is a permanent state of hyperphagia in offspring exposed to overnutrition *in utero* possibly through programming of central pathways involved

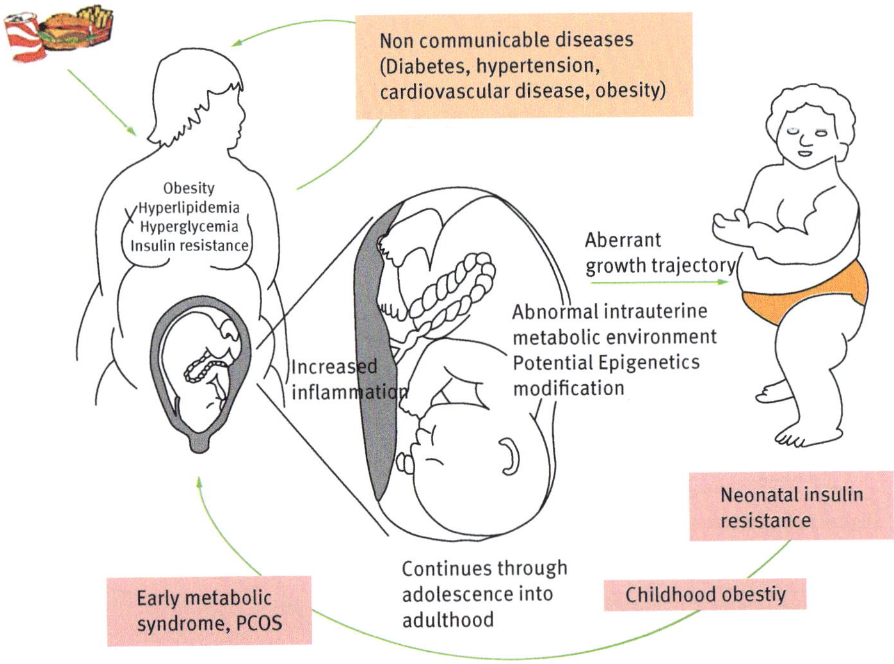

Fig. 9.3: The vicious cycle of noncommunicable diseases.

in appetite control [58]. In this context, a balanced maternal diet high in fruit and vegetables is beneficial for both the mother and developing child. Furthermore, supplementation of antioxidants to the maternal diet may decrease adiposity and glucose intolerance in the offspring [59].

9.6 Conclusions

It is increasingly clear that obesity is already programmed *in utero* at an early stage of development, and inflammation and oxidative stress, as a result of maternal obesity, play important roles. Obese mothers are at risk of delivering large babies who become obese during childhood and adulthood, and subsequently obese parents, thus creating a vicious intergenerational effect. Interventions based on diet alone and mixed interventions resulted in a reduction of gestational weight gain, whereas no effect was found on birth weight and outcome. However, no data are available on long-term effects.

Bibliography

[1] Cetin I, Berti C, Calabrese S. Role of micronutrients in the periconceptional period. Hum Reprod Update 2010;16:80–95.

[2] Poston L, Caleyachetty R, Cnattingius S, Corvalán C, Uauy R, Herring S, Gillman MW. Preconceptional and maternal obesity: epidemiology and health consequences. Lancet Diabetes Endocrinol 2016;4(12):1025–36.

[3] Berti C, Cetin I, Agostoni C, Desoye G, Devlieger R, Emmett PM, Ensenauer R, Hauner H, Herrera E, Hoesli I, Krauss-Etschmann S, Olsen SF, Schaefer-Graf U, Schiessl B, Symonds ME, Koletzko B. Pregnancy and infants' outcome: nutritional and metabolic implications. Crit Rev Food Sci Nutr 2016;56:82–91.

[4] Hanson MA, Bardsley A, De-Regil LM, Moore SE, Oken E, Poston L, Ma RC, McAuliffe FM, Maleta K, Purandare CN, Yajnik CS, Rushwan H, Morris JL. The International Federation of Gynecology and Obstetrics (FIGO) recommendations on adolescent, preconception, and maternal nutrition: "Think Nutrition First". Int J Gynaecol Obstet 2015;131(S4):S213–53.

[5] Berti C, Biesalski HK, Gartner R, Lapillonne A, Pietrzik K, Poston L, Redman C, Koletzo B, Cetin I. Micronutrients in pregnancy: current knowledge and unresolved questions. Clin Nutr 2011;30:689–701.

[6] Steegers-Theunissen RP, Twigt J, Pestinger V, Sinclair KD. The periconceptional period, reproduction and long-term health of offspring: the importance of one-carbon metabolism. Hum Reprod Update 2013;19(6):640–55. Review.

[7] Institute of Medicine (US) and National Research Council (US) Committee to Reexamine IOM Pregnancy Weight Guidelines. Weight gain during pregnancy: reexamining the guidelines. Washington, DC: National Academies Press, 2009.

[8] Parisi F, Laoreti A, Cetin I. Multiple micronutrient needs in pregnancy in industrialized countries. Ann Nutr Metab 2014;65:13–21.

[9] Guzeloglu-Kayisli O, Kayisli UA, Taylor HS. The role of growth factors and cytokines during implantation: endocrine and paracrine interactions. Semin Reprod Med 2009;27(1):62–79.

[10] Ghio A, Bertolotto A, Resi V, Volpe L, Di Cianni G. Triglyceride metabolism in pregnancy. Adv Clin Chem 2011;55:133–53.
[11] Cetin I, Laoreti A. The importance of maternal nutrition for health. JPNIM 2015;4(2):e040220.
[12] Ramsay JE, Ferrell WR, Crawford L, Wallace AM, Greer IA, Sattar N. Maternal obesity is associated with dysregulation of metabolic, vascular, and inflammatory pathways. J Clin Endocrinol Metab 2002;87(9):4231–7.
[13] Basu S, Haghiac M, Surace P, et al. Pregravid obesity associates with increased maternal endotoxemia and metabolic inflammation. Obesity (Silver Spring) 2011;19(3):476–82.
[14] Aye IL, Lager S, Ramirez VI, et al. Increasing maternal body mass index is associated with systemic inflammation in the mother and the activation of distinct placental inflammatory pathways. Biol Reprod 2014;90(6):129.
[15] Challier JC, Basu S, Bintein T, et al. Obesity in pregnancy stimulates macrophage accumulation and inflammation in the placenta. Placenta 2008;29(3):274–81.
[16] Lager S, Jansson N, Olsson AL, Wennergren M, Jansson T, Powell TL. Effect of IL-6 and TNF-α on fatty acid uptake in cultured human primary trophoblast cells. Placenta 2011;32(2):121–7.
[17] Muralimanoharan S, Guo C, Myatt L, Maloyan A. Sexual dimorphism in miR-210 expression and mitochondrial dysfunction in the placenta with maternal obesity. Int J Obes 2015;39(8):1274–81.
[18] Mele J, Muralimanoharan S, Maloyan A, Myatt L. Impaired mitochondrial function in human placenta with increased maternal adiposity. Am J Physiol Endocrinol Metab 2014;307(5):E419–25.
[19] Calder PC, Ahluwalia N, Brouns F, Buetler T, Clement K, Cunningham K, Esposito K, Jönsson LS, Kolb H, Lansink M, Marcos A, Margioris A, Matusheski N, Nordmann H, O'Brien J, Pugliese G, Rizkalla S, Schalkwijk C, Tuomilehto J, Wärnberg J, Watzl B, Winklhofer-Roob BM. Dietary factors and low-grade inflammation in relation to overweight and obesity. Br J Nutr 2011;106 Suppl 3:S5–78.
[20] Masters RC, Liese AD, Haffner SM, et al. Whole and refined grain intakes are related to inflammatory protein concentrations in human plasma. J Nutr 2010;140:587–94.
[21] Wong SW, Kwon MJ, Choi AM, Kim HP, Nakahira K, Hwang DH. Fatty acids modulate Toll-like receptor 4 activation through regulation of receptor dimerization and recruitment into lipid rafts in a reactive oxygen species-dependent manner. J Biol Chem 2009;284:27384–92.
[22] Calder PC. *n*-3 polyunsaturated fatty acids, inflammation, and inflammatory diseases. Am J Clin Nutr 2006;83:1505S–19S.
[23] Lee JY, Ye J, Gao Z, Youn HS, Lee WH, Zhao L, Sizemore N, Hwang DH. Reciprocal modulation of Toll-like receptor-4 signaling pathways involving MyD88 and phosphatidylinositol 3-kinase/AKT by saturated and polyunsaturated fatty acids. J Biol Chem 2003;278:37041–51.
[24] Jacob S, Streeper RS, Fogt DL, Hokama JY, Tritschler HJ, Dietze GJ, Henriksen EJ. The antioxidant alpha-lipoic acid enhances insulin-stimulated glucose metabolism in insulin-resistant rat skeletal muscle. Diabetes 1996;45(8):1024–9.
[25] Koh EH, Lee WJ, Lee SA, Kim EH, Cho EH, Jeong E, Kim DW, Kim MS, Park JY, Park KG, Lee HJ, Lee IK, Lim S, Jang HC, Lee KH, Lee KU. Effects of alpha-lipoic acid on body weight in obese subjects. Am J Med 2011;124(1):85.e1–8.
[26] Sola S. Irbesartan and lipoic acid improve endothelial function and reduce markers of inflammation in the metabolic syndrome. Results of the Irbesartan and Lipoic Acid in Endothelial Dysfunction (ISLAND) study. Circulation 2005;111:343–8.
[27] Lopez-Legarrea P, de la Iglesia R, Abete I, Navas-Carretero S, Martinez JA, Zulet MA. The protein type within a hypocaloric diet affects obesity-related inflammation: the RESMENA project. Nutrition 2014;30(4):424–9.
[28] Wannamethee SG, Lowe GD, Rumley A, et al. Associations of vitamin C status, fruit and vegetable intakes, and markers of inflammation and hemostasis. Am J Clin Nutr 2006;83:567–74.

[29] Hrolfsdottir L, Schalkwijk CG, Birgisdottir BE, Gunnarsdottir I, Maslova E, Granström C, Strøm M, Olsen SF, Halldorsson TI. Maternal diet, gestational weight gain, and inflammatory markers during pregnancy. Obesity (Silver Spring) 2016;24:2133–9.
[30] Fung TT, McCullough ML, Newby PK, et al. Diet-quality scores and plasma concentrations of markers of inflammation and endothelial dysfunction. Am J Clin Nutr 2005;82:163–73.
[31] Chrysohoou C, Panagiotakos DB, Pitsavos C, et al. Adherence to the Mediterranean diet attenuates inflammation and coagulation process in healthy adults: The ATTICA Study. J Am Coll Cardiol 2004;44:152–8.
[32] Szeto YT, Kwok TC, Benzie IF. Effects of a long-term vegetarian diet on biomarkers of antioxidant status and cardiovascular disease risk. Nutrition 2004;20:863–6.
[33] Zampelas A, Panagiotakos DB, Pitsavos C, et al. Fish consumption among healthy adults is associated with decreased levels of inflammatory markers related to cardiovascular disease: the ATTICA study. J Am Coll Cardiol 2005;46:120–4.
[34] Catalano PM, Hauguel-De Mouzon S. Is it time to revisit the Pedersen hypothesis in the face of the obesity epidemic? Am J Obstet Gynecol 2011;204:479–87.
[35] Dodd JM, Turnbull DA, McPhee AJ, Deussen AR, Grivell RM, Yelland LN, Crowther CA, Wittert G, Owens JA, Robinson JS. Antenatal lifestyle advice for women who are overweight or obese: the LIMIT randomised trial. BMJ 2014;348:g1285.
[36] Oteng-Ntim E, Varma R, Croker H, Poston L, Doyle P. Lifestyle interventions for overweight and obese pregnant women to improve pregnancy outcome: systematic review and meta-analysis. BMC Med 2012;10:47.
[37] Gardner B, Wardle J, Poston L, Croker H. Changing diet and physical activity to reduce gestational weight gain: a meta-analysis. Obes Rev 2011;12:e602–20.
[38] Thomas DE, Elliott EJ, Baur L. Low glycaemic index or low glycaemic load diets for overweight and obesity. Cochrane Database Syst Rev 2007;3:CD005105.
[39] Louie JCY, Brand-Miller JC, Markovic TP, Ross GP, Moses RG. Glycemic index and pregnancy: a systematic literature review. J Nutr Metab 2010;2010:1–8.
[40] Okereke NC, Huston-Presley L, Amini SB, Kalhan S, Catalano PM. Longitudinal changes in energy expenditure and body composition in obese women with normal and impaired glucose tolerance. Am J Physiol Endocrinol Metab 2004;287:E472–9.
[41] Butte NF, King JC. Energy requirements during pregnancy and lactation. Public Health Nutr 2005;8:1010–27.
[42] Ley SH, Hanley AJ, Retnakaran R, Sermer M, Zinman B, O'Connor DL. Effect of macronutrient intake during the second trimester on glucose metabolism later in pregnancy. Am J Clin Nutr 2011;94:1232–40.
[43] Donahue SM, Rifas-Shiman SL, Gold DR, Jouni ZE, Gillman MW, Oken E. Prenatal fatty acid status and child adiposity at age 3 y: results from a US pregnancy cohort. Am J Clin Nutr 2011;93:780–8.
[44] Moon RJ, Harvey NC, Robinson SM, Ntani G, Davies JH, Inskip HM, Godfrey KM, Dennison EM, Calder PC, Cooper C, SWS Study Group. Maternal plasma polyunsaturated fatty acid status in late pregnancy is associated with offspring body composition in childhood. J Clin Endocrinol Metab 2013;98:299–307.
[45] Poston L, Bell R, Croker H, Flynn AC, Godfrey KM, Goff L, Hayes L, Khazaezadeh N, Nelson SM, Oteng-Ntim E, Pasupathy D, Patel N, Robson SC, Sandall J, Sanders TA, Sattar N, Seed PT, Wardle J, Whitworth MK, Briley AL. UPBEAT Trial Consortium. Effect of a behavioural intervention in obese pregnant women (the UPBEAT study): a multicentre, randomised controlled trial. Lancet Diabetes Endocrinol 2015;3(10):767–77.
[46] Robinson SM, Crozier SR, Harvey NC, et al. Modifiable early-life risk factors for childhood adiposity and overweight: an analysis of their combined impact and potential for prevention. Am J Clin Nutr 2015;101:368–75.

[47] Okubo H, Crozier SR, Harvey NC, et al. Maternal dietary glycemic index and glycemic load in early pregnancy are associated with off spring adiposity in childhood: the Southampton Women's Survey. Am J Clin Nutr 2014;100:676–83.
[48] Bird A. DNA methylation patterns and epigenetic memory. Genes Dev 2002;16(1):6–21.
[49] Alegría-Torres JA, Baccarelli A, Bollati V. Epigenetics and lifestyle. Epigenomics 2011;3(3):267–77.
[50] Cetin I, Mandò C, Calabrese S. Maternal predictors of intrauterine growth restriction. Curr Opin Clin Nutr Metab Care 2013;16(3):310–9.
[51] Barker DJ. The fetal and infant origins of adult disease. Br Med J 1990;301:1111.
[52] Gluckman PD, Lillycrop KA, Vickers MH, et al. Metabolic plasticity during mammalian development is directionally dependent on early nutritional status. Proc Natl Acad Sci U S A 2007;104:12796–800.
[53] McMillen IC, Rattanatray L, Duffield JA, et al. The early origins of later obesity: pathways and mechanisms. Adv Exp Med Biol 2009;646:71–81.
[54] Cetin I, Parisi F, Berti C, Mandò C, Desoye G. Placental fatty acid transport in maternal obesity. J Dev Orig Health Dis 2012;3(6):409–14.
[55] Zhu MJ, Du M, Nathanielsz PW, Ford SP. Maternal obesity up-regulates inflammatory signaling pathways and enhances cytokine expression in the mid-gestation sheep placenta. Placenta 2010;31(5):387–91.
[56] Levin BE. Epigenetic influences on food intake and physical activity level: review of animal studies. Obesity (Silver Spring) 2008;16:S51–4.
[57] Shankar K, Harrell A, Liu X, Gilchrist JM, Ronis MJ, Badger TM. Maternal obesity at conception programs obesity in the offspring. Am J Physiol Regul Integr Comp Physiol 2008;294(2):R528–38.
[58] Kirk SL, Samuelsson AM, Argenton M, Dhonye H, Kalamatianos T, Poston L, Taylor PD, Coen CW. Maternal obesity induced by diet in rats permanently influences central processes regulating food intake in offspring. PLoS One 2009;4(6):e5870.
[59] Sen S, Simmons RA. Maternal antioxidant supplementation prevents adiposity in the offspring of Western diet-fed rats. Diabetes 2010;59(12);3058–65.

Sean Wharton MD and Rebecca A.G. Christensen MSc

10 Medical and surgical management of obesity prior to planned pregnancy

10.1 Introduction

In 2014, 6.1 million women in Canada (46.2%) self-identified as overweight or obesity, which was an increase of 4.9% from 2003 [1]. Pregnant women with obesity have a higher risk of maternal and fetal complications [2]. Fortunately, a moderate weight loss of 5% to 10% in nonpregnant women has been shown to improve metabolic conditions associated with obesity [3], and has the potential to improve maternal and fetal outcomes during pregnancy [4]. However, greater amounts of weight loss may be needed to decrease the risk of certain fertility procedures, such as in vitro fertilization [5].

10.2 Treatment options for obesity

The cornerstone of weight management is lifestyle intervention, which includes increasing physical activity and decreasing caloric intake [3]. However, there is considerable interindividual variability in response to lifestyle interventions (range: 2%–13% of initial body weight loss) [6, 7], and patients are often unable to maintain their weight loss over the long-term [7–9]. Despite the modest weight loss, many trials have demonstrated significant metabolic benefits from lifestyle interventions, including improved renal function [10,11] and decreased blood sugars [12–14]. Greater effects on weight loss and maintenance can be achieved with medication and surgery. Pharmacotherapy is recommended as an adjunct to lifestyle intervention for the treatment of overweight and obesity in patients with a BMI ≥30 kg/m^2 or a BMI ≥27 kg/m^2 with comorbidities [3]. Bariatric surgery is also an alternative option for patients with a BMI ≥40 kg/m^2 or a BMI ≥35 kg/m^2 with comorbidities [3].

It is important to note that the treatment recommendations below focuses on weight loss and weight loss maintenance related to pregnancy planning (nonpregnant women), and are not treatments during pregnancy. There are no approved pharmacotherapy options for weight management during pregnancy nor is surgery recommended during pregnancy. Contraceptive methods should be used when taking these medications and medications should be stopped prior to planned pregnancy, with adequate time for the medication to clear the system.

https://doi.org/10.1515/9783110487817-010

10.3 Pharmacotherapies

Within Canada, there are two main pharmacotherapies used to treat overweight or obesity: orlistat and liraglutide 3.0 mg. Additional pharmacotherapies are available throughout the world, and some of these agents are being considered for approval in Canada.

10.3.1 Orlistat

Orlistat (Xenical) is currently recommended for weight reduction and weight loss maintenance in many countries, including Canada [15]. It was approved by Health Canada in 1999 [15]. Orlistat is taken in conjunction with a hypocaloric diet and exercise regimen during or up to 1 hour after meals, three times per day at 120 mg [15]. Orlistat decreases caloric intake by blocking lipase activity, which prevents approximately 30% of dietary fat from being broken down into free fatty acids and results in them being excreted in the feces rather than absorbed in the intestine [16].

Several large-scale randomized control trials have evaluated the efficacy of orlistat in weight reduction in populations with overweight and/or obesity [17, 18], as well as type 2 diabetes (T2D) [19]. After approximately 1 year of treatment, patients taking orlistat lost significantly more weight than those taking the placebo [17–19]. In populations with T2D, patients lost an average of 6.2% [19] and patients without T2D lost 5.8% [18] to 8.5% [20] of their initial body weight.

Side effects are primarily gastrointestinal in nature and include loose fatty stools, oily spotting, and fecal incontinence [15]. These adverse effects may decrease rates of patient compliance. A meta-analysis suggests that those taking orlistat were at a 1.59-fold greater risk of dropping out of the study due to side effects compared with those taking the placebo [21]. Orlistat has also been associated with rare cases of liver damage and failure [15].

10.3.2 Liraglutide 3.0 mg

Liraglutide 3.0 mg was approved to be prescribed for weight reduction by Health Canada in 2015 [22]. Liraglutide 3.0 mg is a glucagon-like peptide-1 (GLP-1) receptor stimulator. GLP-1 is secreted naturally by the body when glucose or fat is ingested, signaling satiety through various mechanisms [23]. GLP-1 can bind to receptors in the hypothalamus, which suppresses appetite [24], and can also reduce gastric emptying thereby slowing the digestion of food and lessening postprandial surges in blood glucose [25].

Large-scale randomized control trials called the Satiety and Clinical Adiposity – Liraglutide Evidence in Non-diabetic and diabetic people (SCALE) trials have explored the efficacy of liraglutide 3.0 mg as an adjunct lifestyle intervention for weight management. Two of these trials examined the use of liraglutide 3.0 mg in addition to a hypocaloric diet and physical activity for 56 weeks in populations with moderate obesity with [26] or without [27] T2D. Patients with T2D lost 6.0% [27] and patients without T2D lost 8.0% [26] of their initial body weight taking liraglutide 3.0 mg.

Side effects for liraglutide 3.0 mg tend to be gastrointestinal in nature, such as nausea, vomiting, diarrhea, and constipation [26, 27]. Due to the use of liraglutide as a T2D medication, unsurprisingly, hypoglycemic episodes have also been reported [26, 27].

10.3.3 Options available outside of Canada

There are several other medications for weight management available in the United States, but these are not currently available in most of the worldwide market. These options include a phentermine and topiramate combination, a bupropion and naltrexone combination, and lorcaserin. The latter two medications are currently under review for approval in both Canada and Europe.

Briefly, the mechanisms for these weight loss medications are as follows: phentermine is a sympathomimetic agent that exerts anorectic effects [28]. Topiramate is a neurostabilizer prescribed for seizures and migraines, and the exact mechanism of action for weight reduction remains unclear [28].

Bupropion is a weak dopamine, norepinephrine-dopamine reuptake inhibitor that is currently prescribed as an antidepressant and smoking cessation aid [29]. Naltrexone is an opioid receptor-antagonist and is currently indicated for opioid and alcohol dependence [30]. These medications are thought to work by stimulating the release of anorexic hormones from the proopiomelanocortin (POMC) neurons in the hypothalamus while inhibiting the release of hormones responsible for inactivating these anorectic effects [31].

Lorcaserin is a selective serotonin (5-hydroxytryptamine 2C) receptor agonist [32]. This serotonin receptor is found in many locations of the brain, most notably the hypothalamus, and activation of this receptor in the hypothalamus increases satiety [32].

In comparing the weight loss reported from phase 3 trials examining the efficacy of these three weight reduction pharmaceuticals as an adjunct to lifestyle intervention in populations with overweight and obesity, phentermine/topiramate seems to result in the greatest weight loss (9.8%) [33], followed by bupropion/naltrexone (8.1%) [34], and then lorcaserin (5.81%) [35].

10.4 Considerations for medication cessation before attempting to become pregnant

Weight loss is not recommended for women during pregnancy [4], thus all women should discontinue the use of these medications before attempting to conceive or once pregnancy becomes known. Although little to no human data exists, accidental exposure to these medications during pregnancy has suggested that some may be associated with pregnancy complications. For example, in a study examining the outcomes of 109 pregnancies exposed to orlistat, three of the babies were born with congenital abnormalities [36]. Additionally, research examining the effects of taking topiramate during the first trimester of pregnancy found that it is associated with a 5.4 times greater risk of children being born with a cleft lip [37]. The phentermine/topiramate combination has a risk evaluation and mitigation strategy program as a result of the high risk of orofacial clefts in the third trimester of pregnancy [38]. Healthcare professionals should consider the half-life of the medication in question, and can check-in with a pharmacist or programs such as Motherisk in Canada to ensure that sufficient time has passed for the medication to have left the patient's system prior to recommending planned pregnancy.

10.5 Bariatric surgery

Bariatric surgery has the best long-term success in the amount of weight lost, and weight loss maintained compared with existing alternatives [39]. Nonetheless, there are potential adverse effects [40], complications [39, 41, 42], and lifelong dietary changes, including vitamin supplementation [43], which are required. Bariatric surgery is recommended for patients with obesity who have been unsuccessful with other weight management options. Roux-en-Y gastric bypass is currently the most common procedure performed worldwide (45%), followed by sleeve gastrectomy (45%), and adjustable gastric banding (10%) [44]. For images related to these procedures, please see Chapter 5 of this textbook.

10.5.1 Roux-en-Y gastric bypass

During a Roux-en-Y gastric bypass, a small portion of the stomach is used to create a 15-mL pouch, which is attached to the jejunum to bypass the remaining portion of the stomach and start of the small intestine [39]. The mechanism by which this procedure reduces weight goes beyond the physical restriction of the size of the stomach. There are often alterations in key hunger hormones such as ghrelin and GLP that result in patients having decreased hunger [39].

The American Society for Metabolic and Bariatric Surgery suggest that the rate of mortality from this procedure is rather low, ranging from 0.2% to 0.5% in expert centers [39]. Results from several studies suggest an average weight loss ranging from 68% to 77% of excess body weight within the first year [45–47]. Beyond the amount of weight loss associated with this procedure, there are many comorbidities that may be improved or even resolved by the Roux-en-Y gastric bypass such as T2D, hypertension, and obstructive sleep apnea [39, 45, 47].

10.5.2 Sleeve gastrectomy

During sleeve gastrectomy, a bougie of approximately 32–36F is used to size the sleeve, and then the stomach is stapled to the new smaller size [48]. Research suggest that there may be even greater reductions in ghrelin levels from this procedure than the Roux-en-Y gastric bypass, which may contribute to the weight loss experienced by patients who have had this procedure [49]. A significant weight loss ranging from 38% to 70% of excess weight can be expected 12 months following surgery [49–51]. A report from the American College of Surgeons suggest that patients have low rates of complications from sleeve gastrectomy, with 5.6% experiencing complications within 30 days of their procedure, and only 0.2% of patients dying [42].

10.5.3 Adjustable gastric banding

During gastric banding, a small pouch is created using the upper stomach [39]. This restriction of the stomach decreases the amount of food a patient can consume as well as slows food transportation [39]. A silicone band that contains a balloon is used to create this pouch to allow for band adjustment should pouch dilatation occur [39].

In 2003, gastric banding was the second most popular bariatric surgery procedure and accounted for 25.6% of bariatric surgeries performed worldwide [44]. However, this procedure is being abandoned in favor of those with better long-term outcomes. The gastric band is not as effective for weight loss, and has a high rate of reoperation compared with gastric bypass or sleeve gastrectomy [39, 42].

10.6 Considerations post-surgery prior to attempting to become pregnant

There are clear guidelines regarding when patients should try to conceive following bariatric surgery. During the first year to 18 months following bariatric surgery, the amount of food a patient can eat is severely restricted, and the patient is typically still losing significant amounts of weight [39, 52]. Therefore, patients should wait a minimum of 18 months following any type of bariatric surgery before trying to conceive.

Research has also examined the rate of complications during pregnancy in women who have had bariatric surgery. Women who have had bariatric surgery have lower rates of maternal complications such as gestational diabetes and hypertension compared to women with obesity; however, women who have had bariatric surgery may have a slightly higher risk of cesarean delivery [52–54]. Furthermore, due to the potential complications of malabsorption following surgery, vitamin and iron supplementation may be even more important than in other pregnancies, and should be prescribed during pregnancy in addition to the supplements that women who have had bariatric surgery are already taking [52].

Bibliography

[1] Overweight and obese adults (self-reported) 2014 (Accessed March 26, 2016, http://www.statcan.gc.ca/pub/82-625-x/2015001/article/14185-eng.htm).

[2] Cedergren MI. Maternal morbid obesity and the risk of adverse pregnancy outcome. Obstet Gynecol 2004;103(2):219–24.

[3] Lau DCW, Douketis JD, Morrison KM, Hramiak IM, Sharma AM, Ur E. Canadian clinical practice guidelines on the management and prevention of obesity in adults and children. Can Med Assoc J 2007;176(8 Suppl):s1–13.

[4] Davies GAL, Maxwell C, McLeod L, et al. Obesity in pregnancy. Int J Gynecol Obstet 2010;110(2):167–73.

[5] Clark AM, Thornley B, Tomlinson L, Galletley C, Norman RJ. Weight loss in obese infertile women results in improvement in reproductive outcome for all forms of fertility treatment. Hum Reprod 1998;13(6):1502–5.

[6] Dakour Aridi HN, Wehbe M-R, Shamseddine G, Alami RS, Safadi BY. Long-term outcomes of Roux-en-Y gastric bypass conversion of failed laparoscopic gastric band. Obes Surg 2017;1–8.

[7] Curioni CC, Lourenço PM. Long-term weight loss after diet and exercise: a systematic review. Int J Obes 2005;29(10):1168–74.

[8] Brownell KD, Jeffery RW. Improving long-term weight loss: pushing the limits of treatment. Behav Ther 1987;18(4):353–74.

[9] Jeffery RW, Drewnowski A, Epstein LH, et al. Long-term maintenance of weight loss: current status. Health Psychol 2000;19(1):5–16.

[10] Cohen JB, Cohen DL. Cardiovascular and renal effects of weight reduction in obesity and the metabolic syndrome. Curr Hypertens Rep 2015;17(5):34.

[11] Morales E, Praga M. The effect of weight loss in obesity and chronic kidney disease. Curr Hypertens Rep 2012;14(2):170–6.

[12] Wing RR, Lang W, Wadden TA, et al. Benefits of modest weight loss in improving cardiovascular risk factors in overweight and obese individuals with type 2 diabetes. Diabetes Care 2011;34(7):1481–6.

[13] Wing RR, Koeske R, Epstein LH, Nowalk MP, Gooding W, Becker D. Long-term effects of modest weight loss in type II diabetic patients. Arch Intern Med 1987;147(10):1749.

[14] Anderson JW, Konz EC. Obesity and disease management: effects of weight loss on comorbid conditions. Obes Res 2001;9(S11):326S–334S.

[15] Xenical product monograph (Accessed March 28, 2017, at www.rochecanada.com).

[16] McNeely W, Benfield P. Orlistat. Drugs 1998;56(2):241–9.

[17] Finer N, James WP, Kopelman PG, Lean ME, Williams G. One-year treatment of obesity: a randomized, double-blind, placebo-controlled, multicentre study of orlistat, a gastrointestinal lipase inhibitor. Int J Obes Relat Metab Disord 2000;24(3):306–13.

[18] Broom I, Wilding J, Stott P, Myers N, UK Multimorbidity Study Group. Randomised trial of the effect of orlistat on body weight and cardiovascular disease risk profile in obese patients: UK Multimorbidity Study. Int J Clin Pract 2002;56(7):494–9.

[19] Hollander PA, Elbein SC, Hirsch IB, et al. Role of orlistat in the treatment of obese patients with type 2 diabetes: a 1-year randomized double-blind study. Diabetes Care 1998;21(8):1288–94.

[20] Finer N, James W, Kopelman P, Lean M, Williams G. One-year treatment of obesity: a randomized, double-blind, placebo-controlled, multicentre study of orlistat, a gastrointestinal lipase inhibitor. Int J Obes 2000;24(24):306–13.

[21] Johansson K, Neovius K, DeSantis SM, Rössner S, Neovius M. Discontinuation due to adverse events in randomized trials of orlistat, sibutramine and rimonabant: a meta-analysis. Obes Rev 2009;10(5):564–75.
[22] Saxenda product monograph (Accessed March 27, 2017, at http://www.novonordisk.ca/content/dam/Canada/AFFILIATE/www-novonordisk-ca/OurProducts/PDF/Saxenda_PM_English.pdf).
[23] Torekov SS, Madsbad S, Holst JJ. Obesity—an indication for GLP-1 treatment? Obesity pathophysiology and GLP-1 treatment potential. Obes Rev 2011;12(8):593–601.
[24] Woods SC, D'Alessio DA. Central control of body weight and appetite. J Clin Endocrinol Metab 2008;93(11 Suppl 1):S37–50.
[25] Delgado-Aros S, Kim D-Y, Burton DD, et al. Effect of GLP-1 on gastric volume, emptying, maximum volume ingested, and postprandial symptoms in humans. Am J Physiol Gastrointest Liver Physiol 2002;282(3):G424–31.
[26] Pi-Sunyer X, Astrup A, Fujioka K, et al. A randomized, controlled trial of 3.0 mg of liraglutide in weight management. N Engl J Med 2015;373(1):11–22.
[27] Davies MJ, Bergenstal R, Bode B, et al. Efficacy of liraglutide for weight loss among patients with type 2 diabetes: the SCALE Diabetes randomized clinical trial. JAMA 2015;314(7):687–99.
[28] Shin JH, Gadde KM. Clinical utility of phentermine/topiramate (Qsymia™) combination for the treatment of obesity. Diabetes, Metab Syndr Obes Targets Ther 2013;6:131–9.
[29] Mucklow JC. Martindale: the complete drug reference. Br J Clin Pharmacol 2000;49:613.
[30] Revia Monograph (Accessed March 30, 2017, at http://shoppers-healthcare-portal-a88a1f4b.s3.amazonaws.com/AgilityUGC/bd7cfe4d-a0ae-4496-a4e4-f2ebdbaf6f5d/EN_PM00003584.PDF).
[31] Ornellas T, Chavez B. Naltrexone SR/bupropion SR (Contrave): a new approach to weight loss in obese adults. Pharmacy and Therapeutics 2011;36(5):255–62.
[32] Thomsen WJ, Grottick AJ, Menzaghi F, et al. Lorcaserin, a novel selective human 5-hydroxytryptamine 2C agonist: in vitro and in vivo pharmacological characterization. J Pharmacol Exp Ther 2008;325(2):577–87.
[33] Gadde KM, Allison DB, Ryan DH, et al. Effects of low-dose, controlled-release, phentermine plus topiramate combination on weight and associated comorbidities in overweight and obese adults (CONQUER): a randomised, placebo-controlled, phase 3 trial. Lancet 2011;377:1341–52.
[34] Greenway FL, Plodkowski RA, Greenway FL. Effect of naltrexone plus bupropion on weight loss in overweight and obese adults (COR-I): a multicentre, randomised, double-blind, placebo-controlled, phase 3 trial. Lancet 2010;376(376):595–605.
[35] Smith SR, Weissman NJ, Anderson CM, et al. Multicenter, placebo-controlled trial of lorcaserin for weight management. N Engl J Med 2010;363:245–56.
[36] Acharya NV, Wilton LV, Shakir SAW. Safety profile of orlistat: results of a prescription-event monitoring study. Int J Obes 2006;30(11):1645–52.
[37] Margulis AV, Mitchell AA, Gilboa SM, et al. Use of topiramate in pregnancy and risk of oral clefts. Am J Obstet Gynecol 2012;207(5):405.e1–7.
[38] Fala L. Qsymia: combination oral therapy. A new weight-loss option for obese or overweight patients. Am Health Drug Benefits 2013;6(3):81–6.
[39] Story of obesity surgery (Accessed March 27, 2017, at https://asmbs.org/resources/story-of-obesity-surgery).
[40] After your gastric bypass surgery (Accessed March 28, 2017, at http://www.uhn.ca/PatientsFamilies/Health_Information/Health_Topics/Documents/After_Your_Gastric_Bypass_Surgery.pdf).
[41] Garb J, Welch G, Zagarins S, Kuhn J, Romanelli J. Bariatric surgery for the treatment of morbid obesity: a meta-analysis of weight loss outcomes for laparoscopic adjustable gastric banding and laparoscopic gastric bypass. Obes Surg 2009;19(10):1447–55.

[42] Hutter MM, Schirmer BD, Jones DB, et al. First report from the American College of Surgeons Bariatric Surgery Center Network: laparoscopic sleeve gastrectomy has morbidity and effectiveness positioned between the band and the bypass. Ann Surg 2011;254(3):410–20–2.
[43] Eating For health before and after bariatric surgery (Accessed March 28, 2017, at http://www.uhn.ca/PatientsFamilies/Health_Information/Health_Topics/Documents/Eating_for_Health_after_Gastric_Bypass_Surgery.pdf).
[44] Angrisani L, Santonicola A, Iovino P, Formisano G, Buchwald H, Scopinaro N. Bariatric surgery worldwide 2013. Obes Surg 2015;25(10):1822–32.
[45] Schauer PR, Ikramuddin S, Gourash W, Ramanathan R, Luketich J. Outcomes after laparoscopic Roux-en-Y gastric bypass for morbid obesity. Ann Surg 2000;232(4):515–29.
[46] Sugerman HJ, Kellum JM, Engle KM, et al. Gastric bypass for treating severe obesity. Am J Clin Nutr 1992;55(2 Suppl):560S–6S.
[47] Wittgrove AC, Clark W. Laparoscopic gastric bypass, Roux en-Y—500 patients: techniques and results, with 3–60 month follow-up. Obes Surg 2000;(10):233–9.
[48] Rosenthal RJ. International Sleeve Gastrectomy expert panel consensus statement: best practice guidelines based on experience of >12,000 cases. Surg Obes Relat Dis 2012;8(1):8–19.
[49] Karamanakos SN, Vagenas K, Kalfarentzos F, Alexandrides TK. Weight loss, appetite suppression, and changes in fasting and postprandial ghrelin and peptide-YY levels after Roux-en-Y gastric bypass and sleeve gastrectomy. Ann Surg 2008;247(3):401–7.
[50] Bohdjalian A, Langer FB, Shakeri-Leidenmühler S, et al. Sleeve gastrectomy as sole and definitive bariatric procedure: 5-year results for weight loss and ghrelin. Obes Surg 2010;20(5):535–40.
[51] Cottam D, Qureshi FG, Mattar SG, et al. Laparoscopic sleeve gastrectomy as an initial weight-loss procedure for high-risk patients with morbid obesity. Surg Endosc 2006;20(6):859–63.
[52] Wittgrove AC, Jester L, Wittgrove P, Clark GW. Pregnancy following gastric bypass for morbid obesity. Obes Surg 1998;8(4):461–4.
[53] Weintraub AY, Levy A, Levi I, Mazor M, Wiznitzer A, Sheiner E. Effect of bariatric surgery on pregnancy outcome. Int J Gynecol Obstet 2008;103(3):246–51.
[54] Willis K, Lieberman N, Sheiner E. Pregnancy and neonatal outcome after bariatric surgery. Best Pract Res Clin Obstet Gynaecol 2015;29(1):133–44.

Shital Gandhi

11 Maternal obesity and medical complications

11.1 Introduction

The prevalence of obesity in females in their reproductive years has skyrocketed in recent decades, an effect that is in evidence globally. In parallel with the increase in adult obesity, there has also been an alarming increase in the rates of childhood obesity over the last few decades. The World Health Organization's (WHO) report on Ending Childhood Obesity documents that the prevalence in all age groups (infant, childhood, and adolescent) is increasing; there are an estimated 42 million children under the age of 5 who are overweight or obese. There are more overweight/obese children in low- and middle-income countries than in high-income countries, with a rate of increase in these areas being 30% more than in developed nations. The WHO emphasizes the importance of reducing rates of childhood obesity. As girls enter their reproductive years, coupled with the already high rates of adult onset obesity, there is increasing awareness of the potential effects on pregnancy outcomes, both from a fetal and maternal perspective.

The fact that many obstetric societies worldwide have developed specific guidelines regarding the optimal management of obese women in the preconception and antenatal periods is proof of the growing need for health care workers to be skilled in the management of their specific needs. Being overweight or obese is associated with a higher risk of diabetes (both pregestational and gestational), chronic hypertension and preeclampsia, and venous-thromboembolic disease. These conditions are addressed in more detail in separate chapters. In this chapter, other medical conditions that are important to address when managing obese women will be reviewed, such as cardiac and respiratory conditions. There is also a growing body of literature suggesting that these women are at higher risk of dying in pregnancy when compared with women with a normal body mass index (BMI).

11.2 Obesity and increased risk of mortality

The recent increase in rates of obesity worldwide over the last few decades has had a major effect on the health of individuals, as well as increasing socioeconomic costs. Obesity is associated with chronic medical conditions such as diabetes, hypertension and dyslipidemia, all of which in turn contribute to atherosclerotic diseases such as ischemic heart disease and stroke. In addition, obesity is associated with an increased risk of certain malignancies such as breast cancer (postmenopausal), colon, and pancreatic cancer. As such, obesity is now recognized as an independent risk factor for

https://doi.org/10.1515/9783110487817-011

mortality. Population studies have demonstrated a trend toward increased risk of death; as the level of obesity increases in adults, so too does the risk of death. In a large prospective study in the United States in overweight and obese men and women between the ages of 50 and 71, there was an overall trend toward increased mortality across all ages and ethnic groups, even when correcting for preexisting disease and smoking [1]. In Canada, a similar study of 10,725 adults from the Canadian Fitness Survey demonstrated that the relative risk of mortality was almost threefold higher in class II and III obesity, when compared to the general population, corrected for age, gender, smoking, and alcohol [2].

11.3 Increased mortality in obese pregnant women

Increased weight may carry a significant risk of death compared with normal weighing individuals. Evaluating maternal mortality with accuracy can be challenging at the best of times. Systems for effective data collecting are often lacking. In 2013, the WHO estimated that 289,000 women still die annually in pregnancy or afterward. Rates of maternal mortality globally have declined by nearly 50% in the last 20 years, with most of this gain occurring in developing nations. However, maternal mortality in many developed nations has mostly stabilized, with maternal mortalities ratios of fewer than 15 deaths per 100,000 pregnancies; in some countries such the United States, rates have doubled in the same period.

In several analyses, obesity has been shown to be one of the risk factors for mortality in pregnancy. In the Eighth report of the Confidential Enquiries into Maternal Deaths in the United Kingdom [3], information on BMI was available in 87% of all mortalities occurring between 2006 and 2008. Of these women, 49% were either overweight or obese, in stark contrast to the estimated prevalence of obesity in women of reproductive age of approximately 24%. An astounding 78% of the women who died of venous thromboembolism had a high BMI. Another important cause of death was found to be cardiac disease, of which 61% were either overweight or obese. Prevalence of obesity among women who died from suicide, hemorrhage, and sepsis were not higher than expected.

In a national cohort in the United Kingdom using two data sources (the Centre for Maternal and Child enquiries maternal database and the United Kingdom Obstetric Surveillance System database),100 cases of maternal death due to pregnancy-specific causes were identified. Conditions that were examined included amniotic fluid embolism, eclampsia, antenatal pulmonary embolism, acute fatty liver of pregnancy, and antenatal stroke. Cases of fatal events were compared with women who survived the events. Women with a BMI greater than 30 were found to have an almost threefold increased risk of death in the years 2006 to 2008 [4]. The correlation was also seen for other periods, but the findings were not statistically significant.

In the United States, national data are lacking, but there is evidence for a correlation between maternal obesity and mortality in pregnancy. In the state of Michigan, a retrospective analysis of maternal mortality between 2004 and 2006 was conducted [5]. There were a total of 384,765 births recorded in the state, with a total of 205 women dying in pregnancy, of which 61 were concluded to be a direct result of pregnancy. Thirty-six of these deaths occurred in obese women, which was higher than the estimated expected rate of 17 based on the rates of obesity among women of reproductive age in Michigan. There were 25 deaths among nonobese women, indicating a threefold increased risk of mortality among obese women, similar to the risk established by the British cohort. Stated differently, the maternal mortalities ratio was 34/100,000 for obese women compared with 9/100,000 in the nonobese. The most common cause of death was cardiovascular disease and diabetes, adding to the evidence that this is a major problem in pregnancy. Postpartum hemorrhage and sepsis together accounted for another 40% of deaths. Similarly, in a retrospective review of mortality and "near-miss" morbidity among 25,837 pregnancies between 1995 and 2001 in a single center in New York, there were 8 deaths and 84 near-misses identified. Race and ethnicity were the strongest predictors of an adverse event; of the medical factors identified, obesity was associated with a threefold increased risk [6].

Medical complications due to obesity in pregnant women are seen worldwide, and obesity is recognized as a contributing factor in developing nations as well. In Africa, the prevalence of obesity in pregnant women is increasing; for instance, in Tanzania, rates of obesity (as defined by BMI documented in the first trimester) increased from 2.4% to 7.3% over a 9-year period [7]. Methods of reporting weight can vary: in a systematic review, if using first trimester or prepregnancy weight, rates of obesity across African countries varied between 9% and 18%, whereas rates in the third trimester ranged between 14% and 50% [8]. This study demonstrated that obese pregnant women across Africa were more likely to experience complications in pregnancy, including wound infection, gestational diabetes, hypertensive disorders, hemorrhage, hospitalization, and urinary tract infections. There was a trend toward increased risk of mortality among obese women that wasn't statistically significant, but it should be noted that very few of these studies actually reported on maternal mortality. This emphasizes the need for more studies.

The mechanism by which weight affects obstetric morbidity and mortality needs to be further examined. Generally, the risks of obesity in adults are manifested over the course of decades rather than months, and are mediated indirectly through developing chronic medical conditions. It is hypothesized that the combination of obesity, plus delaying childbearing until later in life, increases the prevalence of medical conditions prior to pregnancy, which can lead to maternal and fetal complications. Even though pregnancy itself is a relatively short time frame in a woman's life, the metabolic and vascular changes of pregnancy increase the likelihood of developing new onset conditions, such as diabetes, hypertension, and venous thromboembolic diseases.

11.4 Obesity and medical complications

11.4.1 Cardiac disease

Pregnancy is inherently a physiologic stress for all women. The cardiovascular changes are impressive: as early as 5 to 8 weeks after conception, blood volume starts to increase, and does so progressively until the late second trimester, with a net change of 40% to 50% compared with the nonpregnant state. As a consequence, cardiac output must necessarily increase by a similar amount, reaching a peak at the same time, and then remaining at that high level plateau until delivery. This change in cardiac output is facilitated by an increase in heart rate and a decrease in afterload pressures; systemic vascular resistance decreases due to hormonal effects in reducing systolic blood pressure, plus the redirection of blood through the new placental vascular bed.

In addition to the above changes in the cardiovascular system, pregnancy also is a hypercoagulable state, with increased risk for both arterial and venous thrombotic events. Procoagulant factors increase gradually in pregnancy, and the gravid uterus causes compression of the inferior vena cava, both of which conspire to increase rates of venous thrombosis. Presumably, from an evolutionary standpoint, this developed to prevent hemorrhage at the time of labor and delivery, but does conspire to increase the risk of venous thromboses. Unfortunately, arterial events, although overall rare in pregnancy, also do occur three to four times more frequently when compared with age-matched nonpregnant women.

The time of labor and delivery is associated with further hemodynamic changes: with each uterine contraction, there is an "auto-bolus" of 300 to 500 mL of blood back into the systemic circulation. The cardiac compensation is to increase stroke volume; cardiac output, which is already increased compared with the nonpregnant state, increases by a dramatic 50% with each contraction. Additional cardiovascular stressors include an increase in blood pressure due to pain, as well as blood loss. Estimates of blood loss for vaginal deliveries are typically 300 to 400 mL, and for caesarean sections, it could be 500 to 800 mL; however, in obesity, there may be an increased risk of postpartum hemorrhage compared with women who are of normal weight.

After delivery, relief of compression of the inferior vena cava then leads to a further increase in venous return. The ongoing increase in cardiac output results in an increase in renal perfusion and subsequent diuresis. All of the above vascular alterations resolve postpartum, eventually returning to normal 4 to 6 weeks later.

As a result of the above physiological changes, pregnant women often develop symptoms that are very similar to heart disease: shortness of breath, fatigue, and decreased exercise capacity are frequent complaints. Other expected changes include mild pedal edema, a systolic murmur that is physiologic due to the increased blood flow, and an S3 heart sound from increased blood volume. Objective cardiac tests are also affected by normal pregnancy: the electrocardiogram may show a leftward shift in the axis, especially closer to term when the uterus is pushing up against the diaphragm. The echocardiogram often shows an increase in left ventricular mass and left ventricular dilation. Brain natriuretic peptide, also known as B-type natriuretic peptide (BNP) levels are not affected by pregnancy.

In the obese pregnant woman, evaluating for actual cardiac disease can be especially challenging because the physical exam becomes difficult in many ways. As arm circumference increases, even the basic assessment of blood pressure can be problematic. With increasing arm circumference, larger sizes of blood pressure cuffs are needed, occasionally needing a thigh cuff. Assessing for jugular venous distension can be hampered by increased neck circumference. Precordial auscultation for heart sounds and murmurs is impeded by the chest wall thickness. Peripheral edema is often exaggerated in these women. Finally, objective evaluation with echocardiogram can also be technically difficult as clear images may be challenging to obtain.

The overall risk of acute coronary syndrome (ACS) is low, estimated to be 3 to 6 per 100,000 pregnancies, but as discussed earlier, heart disease is now consistently the most common indirect cause of mortality in pregnancy. The proportion of deaths due to congenital heart disease and valvular disease is decreasing but the rates of acute myocardial infarction are increasing. Women who are obese may already have atherosclerotic disease as they enter pregnancy. Traditional causes of atherosclerotic disease, such as chronic hypertension, smoking, diabetes, and hyperlipidemia play important roles in the pathogenesis of vascular heart disease. Advanced maternal age and preeclampsia are also independent risk factors. Given the increased physiologic stress that pregnancy and the puerperium exerts on the cardiovascular system, and the fact that women are delaying childbearing until later in life, obese women may be at particular risk for ACS.

Pregnancy-related myocardial ischemic events can occur at all time points in pregnancy and postpartum. In addition to a ruptured atherosclerotic plaque as the classic cause of the ACS, coronary dissection and coronary vasospasm need to be considered in the differential diagnosis in the pregnant woman, no matter what their BMI is. Spontaneous coronary rupture is more common in pregnant compared with nonpregnant women, and is thought to be related to a weakening of the vessel wall due to hormonal changes; ACS caused by spontaneous coronary rupture occurs most commonly during labor and delivery or shortly thereafter. Coronary vasospasm may be associated with ergotamine administration.

The diagnostic criteria for acute myocardial infarction in pregnancy and postpartum are no different than the general population: the triad of the presence of chest pain, abnormal electrocardiogram, and elevated cardiac biomarkers, should alert health care workers to the possibility. Preeclampsia can lead to an elevated troponin level, but clinicians should still suspect and evaluate for myocardial ischemia. For ST segment elevation myocardial infarction, pregnant women should be referred for immediate diagnostic angiogram and primary percutaneous coronary intervention. This approach is preferred over thrombolysis, as it can also evaluate for possible coronary dissection. Bare metal stents should be chosen over drug-eluting stents because the latter has not been evaluated in pregnancy, and would require long-term dual antiplatelet therapy, which should ideally be avoided in pregnancy. Recombinant tissue plasminogen activator should be reserved only for cases of life-threatening ischemia or if percutaneous coronary intervention is not available; recombinant tissue plasminogen activator does not cross the placenta, but can lead to significant bleeding in the placental vasculature. Non-ST segment elevated ischemia should also be evaluated by coronary angiogram, whereas stable angina can be monitored clinically during pregnancy. Radionuclide testing is not recommended to avoid the potential fetal effects of radiation, and because there is an alternative test (i.e., angiogram).

Aspirin and beta-blockers are considered safe in pregnancy. The treatment of coronary artery disease in pregnancy otherwise differs from nonpregnancy in a few respects. There is a paucity of data on the safety of clopidogrel; hence, it should be used after stenting only, and for the shortest amount of time possible. ACE inhibitors, angiotensin blockers, and direct renin inhibitors are teratogenic and cannot be used. The effect of glycoprotein IIb/IIIa inhibitors and ticagrelor are unknown and should be avoided.

Obese women who are already known to have coronary disease may seek medical advice regarding pregnancy. In an international registry of 1,321 women undergoing pregnancy with a variety of different types of heart disease, 2% (or 25) had ischemic heart disease [9]. These women were older, and were more likely to have metabolic disease. All women survived, although there was a higher rate of prematurity, growth restriction, and low APGAR scores; this may be related to the higher maternal age, and other exposures such as smoking, medications, and others.

Whether pregnancy itself increases the risk of heart disease is an intriguing question. Several studies have shown that women who develop a "maternal-placental syndrome," such as preeclampsia and/or fetal growth restriction, are at an increased risk of vascular heart disease. Women who develop early-onset preeclampsia seem to be at particularly high risk. Women who are obese are more likely to develop preeclampsia, and are more likely to have metabolic disease, and so it would be plausible to anticipate that obese pregnant women are at higher risk for future heart disease. The British Women's Heart and Health Study showed an interesting correlation between parity, the risk of obesity, and the risk of heart disease [10]. In both men and women, waist to hip ratio increased as the number of children increased; but when controlled for socioeconomic status, smoking, and alcohol, the correlation was no longer seen in men, whereas it remained for women. Hence, it would seem that pregnancy itself may increase the risk of heart disease. This raises the importance of aggressive lifestyle modification in the postpartum or inter-pregnancy period to blunt the development of heart disease.

11.4.2 Respiratory disease

Pregnancy alters pulmonary function in anatomic and functional aspects, regardless of body habitus. First, the upper airways become hyperemic and hence symptoms of nasal obstruction and epistaxis occur commonly. The diaphragm is progressively pushed upward by the enlarging uterus, typically by approximately 4 cm, although diaphragmatic excursion remains constant. The thoracic cage expands outward by approximately 2 cm in anteroposterior and transverse diameters. The elevation of the diaphragm diminishes residual volume and respiratory reserve volume, and so functional residual capacity (FRC) is reduced. Minute ventilation increases by 30% to 50%, and most of this is accommodated by a change in tidal volume by approximately 40%; this increase in respiratory drive is mediated by the central effect of progesterone on the medulla. Pregnancy has no effect on forced expiratory volume in 1 s, forced vital capacity or flow rates, nor does it affect lung compliance.

Obesity can have a marked effect on lung mechanics, and is often further compounded by the effects of pregnancy. In nonpregnant obese individuals, spirometry confirms that as BMI increases, lung volumes do decrease: forced expiratory volume in 1 s, forced vital capacity, and FRC are all reduced. In those with a BMI greater than 40, total lung capacity and residual volume can also be affected.

Putting the two conditions of obesity and pregnancy together, the most important net effect is the lack of compliance due to the increased weight of the chest wall. These women need to compensate by increasing their respiratory rate. Spirometric data in obese pregnant women are limited but it seems that FRC and expiratory reserve volume decrease more dramatically with even modest increases in the BMI.

Common respiratory conditions that occur with increasing weight include obstructive sleep apnea (OSA), obesity hypoventilation syndrome, and asthma. OSA is characterized by repetitive narrowing and/or occlusion of upper airways during sleep, leading to reduced airflow and hypoxemia, poor quality sleep and sympathetic activation, and is mostly a disorder of the overweight/obese. Understanding the prevalence, course, and effects of OSA in pregnancy is still evolving. Many of the normal physiologic changes that occur in pregnancy (narrowing of the nasal passages, edema of the airways, and increased ventilator drive), can worsen preexisting OSA. In a prospective study of 105 pregnant women (obese and nonobese), sleep disordered breathing occurred in 10.5% of women in the first trimester, and increased to 26.7% in the third trimester [11]. Increasing maternal age and obesity were the strongest predictors. In a prospective study of 175 pregnant obese women who underwent in-home portable polysomnogram (sleep study) testing, 14% were found to have OSA; these women were older, had a higher BMI (46.8 vs. 38.1, $p = 0.002$), and were more likely to have asthma and chronic hypertension. There were six severe complications in all women, including two maternal deaths; one woman in the OSA group had intrapartum cardiac arrest during caesarean section, and one without OSA had an amniotic fluid embolism [12].

This would suggest that pregnant women with OSA are at higher risk of complications. In a large, national database study in the US between 1998 and 2009, the diagnosis of OSA was seen to increase over time [13]. Women with OSA were more likely to develop pregnancy-specific conditions such as preeclampsia/eclampsia, and more worrisome still, were found to have a fivefold increased odds of dying in hospital, when adjusted for age, ethnicity, income, and medical comorbidities. Reporting of fetal risks in small case series included prematurity, stillbirth, and growth restriction; however, these outcomes may be a consequence of preeclampsia rather than the direct effect of nocturnal hypoxemia itself.

There are many practical challenges when it comes to OSA. One of the difficulties is in the poor performance of screening questionnaires in identifying such women in pregnancy. When compared with polysomnography in 100 pregnant women between 26 and 39 weeks of gestation, the sensitivity and specificity using the Berlin questionnaire was 35% and 63%, respectively [14]. Second, the gold standard test is an overnight in-laboratory polysomnogram that is costly and not necessarily readily available. In-home testing is still under evaluation; it is likely accurate in moderate-severe disease, but data in pregnancy is still in its infancy. A pragmatic approach is to screen high-risk obese women who have diabetes or hypertension, as well as those who snore or report daytime somnolence. These women should be referred for in-laboratory polysomnography.

Management of OSA in pregnancy is mainly by way of continuous positive airway pressure (CPAP). It should be noted that there have been no studies demonstrating that treatment prevents adverse fetal or maternal outcomes. There are no pharmacologic treatments for this condition; modafanil has been used to treat daytime sleepiness in nonpregnant individuals. Its use in pregnancy is not recommended, as safety data is lacking. Limiting weight gain in pregnancy should be emphasized; weight loss should be emphasized postpartum as an effective adjunctive method of reducing the severity of disease. Surgical approaches such as uvulopalatopharyngoplasty can be effective for mild to moderate disease, but given the surgical risk, is not really a viable option in pregnancy.

11.4.3 Hepatobiliary disease

Other medical conditions that are more likely to occur in obese pregnant women include higher rates of cholelithiasis. Pregnancy itself is acknowledged as a state that favors the formation of gallstones, and it seems that being obese accentuates that risk: in an analysis of 128 northern plains pregnant women in the United States, data were collected at 14 and 26 weeks of gestation, and 4 weeks postpartum. Three conditions were found to increase the risk of gallstone attacks during pregnancy/postpartum: a known history of gallstones prior to pregnancy, elevated BMI, and decreased physical activity [15]. In another prospective study of 3,254 women who were screened for sludge and gallstones in pregnancy, an overall incidence of the development of new stones, new sludge or else progression from sludge to stones was 10.2%. Prepregnancy obesity was found to be very strongly correlated with cholelithiasis, with an odds of 4.45 times higher compared to women with normal weight. Other risk factors were parity and HDL levels [16]. Therefore, overweight and obese women who develop upper abdominal pain should be given particular consideration for having cholelithiasis, sludge, or cholecystitis.

Bibliography

[1] Adams KF, Schatzkin A, Harris TB, et al. Overweight, obesity, and mortality in a large prospective cohort of persons 50 to 71 years old. N Engl J Med 2006;(355):763–78.
[2] Katzmarzyk PT, Ardern CI. Overweight and obesity mortality trends in Canada, 1985–2000. Can J Public Health 2004;95(1):16–20.
[3] Centre for Maternal and Child Enquiries (CMACE). Maternal obesity in the UK: findings from a national project. London: CMACE, 2010.
[4] Kayem G, Kurinczuk J, Lewis G, Golightly S, Brocklehurst P, Knight M. Risk factors for progression from severe maternal morbidity to death: a national cohort study. PLoS One 6(12):e29077. doi:10.1371/journal.pone.0029077.
[5] Mariona F. Does maternal obesity impact pregnancy-related deaths? Michigan experience. J Matern Fetal Neonatal Med. 2017;30(9):1060–5.
[6] Goffman D, Madden RC, Harrison EA, Merkatz IR, Chazotte C. Predictors of maternal mortality and near-miss maternal morbidity. J Perinatol 2007;(27):587–601.
[7] Villamor E, Msamanga G, Urassa W, et al. Trends in obesity, underweight, and wasting among women attending prenatal clinics in urban Tanzania, 1995–2004. Am J Clin Nutr 2006;83(6):1387–94.
[8] Onubi OJ, Marais D, Aucott L, Okonofua F, Poobalan AS. Maternal obesity in Africa: a systematic review and meta-analysis. J Public Health 2015;38(3):e218–31. doi: 10.1093/pubmed/fdv138.
[9] Roos-Hesselink JW, Ruys TP, Stein JI, et al. Outcome of pregnancy in patients with structural or ischemic heart disease: results of a registry of the European Society of Cardiology. Eur Heart J 2013;(34):657–65.
[10] Lawlor DA, Emberson JR, Ebrahim S. Is the association between parity and coronary heart disease due to biological effects of pregnancy or adverse lifestyle risk factors associated with child-rearing? Findings from the British Women's Heart and Health Study and the British Regional Heart Study. Circulation 2003;107:1260–4.
[11] Pien GW, Pack AI, Jackson N, Maislin G, Macones GA, Schwab RJ. Risk factors for sleep-disordered breathing in pregnancy. Thorax 2014;69(4):371–7. Epub 2013 Nov 21.
[12] Louis J, Auckley D, Miladinovic B, et al. Perinatal outcomes associated with obstructive sleep apnea in obese pregnant women. Obstet Gynecol 2012;120:1085–92.
[13] Louis J, Mogos MF, Salemi JL, Redline S, Salihu HM. Obstructive sleep apnea and severe maternal-infant morbidity/mortality in the United States, 1998–2009. Sleep 2014;37:843–9A.
[14] Olivarez SA, Maheshwari B, McCarthy M, et al. Prospective trial on obstructive sleep apnea in pregnancy and fetal heart rate monitoring. Am J Obstet Gynecol 2010;202(6):552.e1.
[15] Lindseth G, Bird-baker MY. Risk factors for cholelithiasis in pregnancy. Res Nurs Health 2004;27:382–91.
[16] Ko CW, Beresford SA, Schulte SJ, Matsmuto AM, Lee SP. Incidence, natural history, and risk factors for biliary sludge and stones during pregnancy. Hepatology 2005;41:359–365.

Section II: **Pregnancy management**

Karim D. Kalache, Balbir Bola and Daniel Kamil

12 Second trimester fetal ultrasonography in the obese pregnant patient

12.1 Introduction

Worldwide, there continues to be a rapid increase in the incidence of overweight and obesity. In 2014, more than 1.9 billion adults aged 18 years and older were overweight. Of these, more than 600 million adults were obese, as defined by a body mass index (BMI) of >30 kg/m^2, according to the World Health Organization (WHO).

Being overweight or obese are major risk factors for cardiovascular diseases, diabetes, musculoskeletal disorders, and some cancers (including endometrial, breast, and ovarian). Another important challenge of obesity for healthcare providers is the effect on obstetrical ultrasound. In this chapter, we will review some of the important aspects on the topic.

12.2 Overweight and obesity in pregnancy

In pregnancy, BMI is calculated using prepregnant weight or the weight measured during the initial visit at the prenatal care provider. In the United States, the incidence of obesity in pregnancy has increased over the past two decades [1] with 32% of white women and 59% of black women being affected. Slightly lower rates have been reported in the UK and in Germany where 25% of women are obese [2]. The problem was once considered to affect only high-income countries, but now seems to be dramatically on the rise in low- and middle-income countries as well [2].

12.3 Obesity and being overweight and the increased risk of congenital anomalies

For overweight and obese women, increased weight gain between pregnancies and excess gestational weight gain are all associated with an increased risk for maternal and fetal complications [3–6], including stillbirths [7,8]. The association between maternal and fetal pregnancy complications and the degree of obesity was clearly demonstrated in a retrospective study reviewing over a quarter of a million pregnancies [9].

Obesity is also proven to heighten the risk for several fetal malformations including neural tube defects and heart defects. This is covered in detail in Chapter 13. These risks are summarized in Tab. 12.1 [10]. A significant increased risk for neural tube defect (OR, 1.87) was described with the strongest correlation for open spina bifida

https://doi.org/10.1515/9783110487817-012

(OR, 2.24) [10]. The incidence of congenital heart defects is doubled in fetuses of obese women [11], and the higher the BMI, the higher the incidence of the malformations. A relative risk of 1.18 was observed with a BMI of >29 kg/m^2 and 1.40 for BMI >35 kg/m^2. For severe cardiovascular defects, the adjusted OR was 1.69.

Tab. 12.1: Risk of congenital anomalies in maternal overweight and obesity (adapted from Stothard et al. [10]).

Anomaly	Odds ratio (OR)	95% CI
Spina bifida	2.24	1.86–2.69
Cardiovascular	1.3	1.12–1.51
Cleft lip and palate	1.20	1.03–1.40
Anorectal atresia	1.48	1.12–1.97
Hydrocephaly	1.68	1.19–2.36
Limb reduction	1.34	1.03–1.73
Gastroschisis	0.17	0.10–0.30

A large study examining the associations between prepregnancy BMI and congenital heart defects found an increased risk in the overweight and adipose groups compared with the nonobese women showing an odds ratios for all congenital heart defects of 1.16, 1.15, and 1.31 for overweight status, moderate obesity, and severe obesity, respectively [12]. Phenotypes that were associated with elevated BMI included conotruncal defects (e.g. Tetralogy of Fallot), total anomalous pulmonary venous return, hypoplastic left heart syndrome, right ventricular outflow tract defects (pulmonary valve stenosis), and septal defects.

The reason for the higher fetal malformation incidence is not yet fully understood. One possible cause might be the metabolic abnormalities of obesity, as the increased serum insulin, triglycerides, uric acid, and endogenous estrogens, may have the same teratogenic effect as with maternal insulin-dependent diabetes [13]. Another explanation could be the folic acid supplementation dose that is needed to reduce the incidence of neural tube defect (NTDs) in the normal-weight pregnant woman that may be insufficient in the overweight and obese pregnant woman [14].

12.4 Obesity and being overweight as a significant cause of failed ultrasound examinations

Despite the tremendous advances in ultrasound technology since its introduction and its worldwide availability, obesity and being overweight in pregnancy are considered as significant causes of failed examinations due to inadequate diagnostic information [15]. The fact that visualization of fetal anatomy is decreased with increasing BMI was well recognized soon after the introduction of high-resolution ultrasound technology [16]. Since then, several studies have come to a similar conclusion.

In the FaSTER (First and Second Trimester Evaluation of Risk) trial, the detection rate of congenital anomalies in obese and overweight pregnant women was significantly decreased (by 30%) when compared with the normal population [17]. Another study also demonstrated the reduced detection rate of fetal anomalies in obese women with a detection rate of 66% in women with a normal BMI compared with 25% in morbidly obese women [18]. More recently, it has been shown that being overweight and obese is associated with a 23% reduced detection rate of congenital when compared with normal weight pregnant women [15]. In another study, optimal visualization of the fetal four-chamber and outflow-tract views was achieved in less than 50% of morbidly obese women, compared with almost 90% in nonobese women [19]. It has been shown that obesity is the main cause of missed prenatal diagnosis of fetal transposition of the great arteries and that obese patients with suboptimal prenatal scans may benefit from reassessment of fetal cardiac anatomy and/or from referral for fetal echocardiography [20]. The inadequate sonographic visualization of fetal organ structures is not necessarily improved by the use of high-end ultrasound technology [21].

12.5 Technical tips to overcome the challenge

In this section, we will provide a selection of important steps we feel are suitable and helpful to overcome the challenges when scanning a technically difficult pregnant woman and achieve a comprehensive routine second trimester anatomy screening examination.

An essential component when scanning a patient with a thick abdominal pannus is the frequency of the transducer. Low-frequency transducers are more efficient as they allow for improved penetration and thus improve the ability to image the fetus. The thicker adipose layer can cause absorption and reflection with a negative effect on the transmission of sound waves resulting in decreased visualization of fetal organ structures [16]. By using preprocessing and postprocessing filters such as harmonic imaging [22], compound imaging, and speckle reduction filters, it is sometimes possible to improve the diagnostic information (see Fig. 12.1) [23–26].

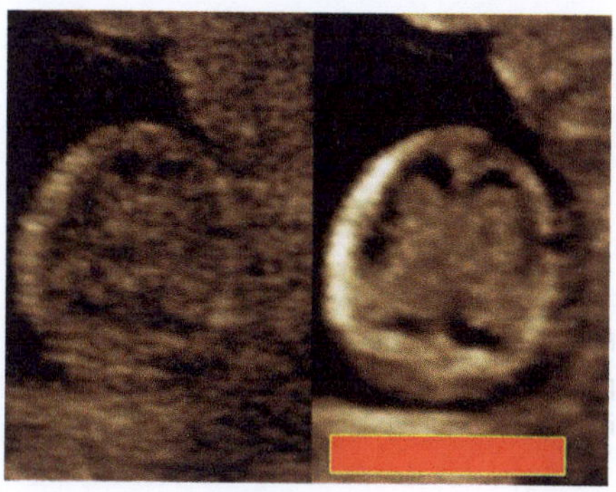

Fig. 12.1: Illustrative images of potential advantages of advanced technology such as harmonic imaging to improve image resolution.

The signal and image quality can be improved by reducing the distance between the transducer and the fetal anatomical structure to be examined. Elevating and retracting the pannus toward the patient's head and locating the transducer below the pannus will result in improved scan conditions as in Figures 12.2A and B.

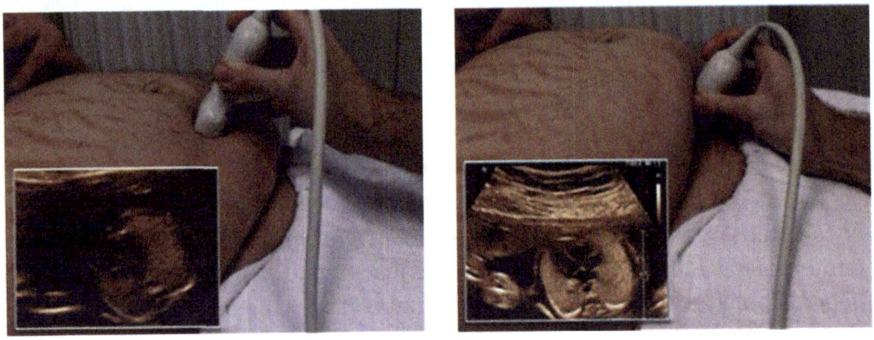

(a) (b)

Fig. 12.2: (A) Imaging the fetal heart through the abdominal pannus provided limited details. (B) Scanning below the abdominal pannus provides good anatomic detail.

Because the abdominal adipose tissue tends to accumulate in the area between the umbilicus and the pubis on the midline, the iliac fossae, similar to the area just above the symphysis and the umbilical region, are less prone to fat accumulation and can serve as acoustic windows. As shown in Fig. 12.3, some radiologists therefore recommend to ask the patient to lie in the left or right Sims position (whichever assures an optimal access to the uterus) almost to the point of being prone, with the upper leg flexed at the knee and the lower leg extended. This shifts the pannus and the pregnant abdomen onto the examining table and enables to scan the patient from the flank and from the side of the uterus, with the transducer aimed ventrally [27].

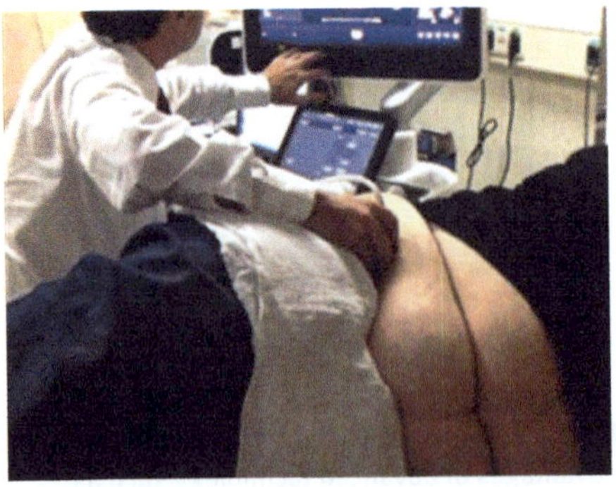

Fig. 12.3: Super obese patient in the Sims position. The abdominal transducer is over the iliac fossa, which is used as an acoustic window.

Using the endovaginal transducer with a narrower field of view through the umbilical region as in Fig. 12.4 can be of benefit providing clearer images [28, 29]. Paladini [30] reported improved fetal heart visualization (for fetuses in breech presentation) when a filled maternal urinary bladder is pushing the uterus cephalad, which enables the examination of the fetal heart transumbilically.

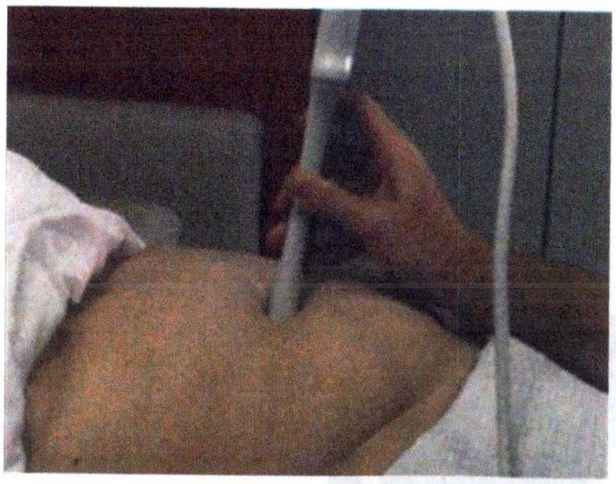

Fig. 12.4: Using the endovaginal transducer with a narrower field of view through the umbilical region.

Delaying the initial survey until 20 weeks of gestation may improve the capacity to complete the examination in a single visit [31] A recent study found no relationship between gestation and completion of the second trimester routine anatomy scan, suggesting that delaying the anomaly scan to 20 + 6 weeks (or even beyond) would not provide a solution to reducing the requirement for repeat scans [32].

Obese and overweight women required more attempts to complete the anomaly scan. Additionally, spending more time (10 additional minutes) for scanning, as well as moving the fetus so that the back is in a posterior or lateral position may improve the scan results [33]. One should bear in mind that studies on factors affecting feasibility and quality of second trimester ultrasound scans in obese pregnant women were mainly conducted in tertiary referral centers, and therefore may not reflect community experience.

In response to repetitive stress injury concerns, new ultrasound transducers have been designed that are lightweight and easy to hold to reduce operator fatigue. A highly flexible and optimal transducer balance adds to scanning comfort during extended or difficult exams that are common with technically challenging patients. However, it is sometimes necessary to use increased pressure on the transducer toward abdomen to reduce the depth of insonation.

It is of great importance that prior to the scanning of the obese patient, a clear and sensitive discussion of the expectations for the ultrasound should take place, reviewing potential scan constraints, association between abdominal thickness and impaired acoustic window, and consequent increased risk of missing fetal malformations. With increasing maternal BMI, decreased detection of anomalous fetuses using either standard or targeted ultrasonography is decreased by at least 20% when compared with normal weight [18, 34]. A fulsome discussion prior to the examination will result in more realistic expectations for the patient and her family, and may potentially reduce future conflicts and lawsuits [18, 35–37].

At our institution, we do not routinely obtain a written consent for the abovementioned issues, but rather have the discussion and document areas of concern, such as the distance between the maternal skin to the intrauterine region of interest. This way, we are able to document the degree of obesity and effect on ultrasound quality as shown in Fig. 12.5. We also recommend that a detailed explanation of the anticipated effect of obesity on the reduction in the detection rate of congenital anomalies be included in the ultrasound report.

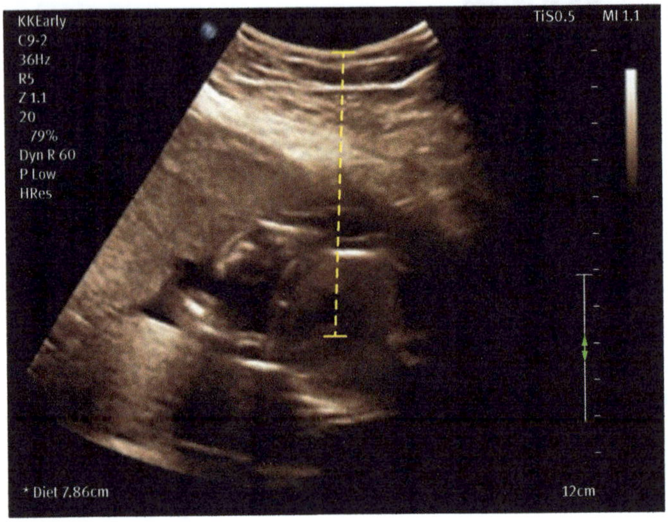

Fig. 12.5: Distance between the maternal skin to the intrauterine region of interest.

12.6 Conclusion

Increasing rates of worldwide obesity present a multifaceted challenge to healthcare providers. One of the major challenges of obesity in obstetrics is the challenge in providing accurate images and interpretation of findings for prenatal ultrasound scans. Taking into consideration the increased risk of congenital anomalies in obese and overweight pregnant women, and the difficulties of detecting common anomalies in this population, we believe that all obese pregnant women should be advised of these challenges and that providers consider referral to a center that is experienced in this type of scanning if the ultrasound results are unsatisfactory.

Bibliography

[1] Reece EA. Perspectives on obesity, pregnancy and birth outcomes in the United States: the scope of the problem. Am J Obstet Gynecol 2008;198(1):23–7.
[2] James PT, Leach R, Kalamara E, Shayeghi M. The worldwide obesity epidemic. Obes Res 2001;9(Suppl 4):228S–33S.
[3] Abrams B, Parker J. Overweight and pregnancy complications. Int J Obes 1988;12(4):293–303.
[4] Abrams B, Altman SL, Pickett KE. Pregnancy weight gain: still controversial. Am J Clin Nutr 2000;71(5 Suppl):1233S–41S.
[5] Cedergren MI. Maternal morbid obesity and the risk of adverse pregnancy outcome. Obstet Gynecol 2004;103(2):219–24.
[6] Villamor E, Cnattingius S. Interpregnancy weight change and risk of preterm delivery. Obesity (Silver Spring)2016;24(3):727–34.
[7] Chu SY, Kim SY, Lau J, Schmid CH, Dietz PM, Callaghan WM, Curtis KM. Maternal obesity and risk of stillbirth: a metaanalysis. Am J Obstet Gynecol 2007;197(3):223–8.
[8] Yao R, Ananth CV, Park BY, Pereira L, Plante LA, Perinatal Research Consortium. Obesity and the risk of stillbirth: a population-based cohort study. Am J Obstet Gynecol 2014;210(5):457 e451–9.
[9] Sebire NJ, Jolly M, Harris JP, Wadsworth J, Joffe M, Beard RW, Regan L, Robinson S. Maternal obesity and pregnancy outcome: a study of 287, 213 pregnancies in London. Int J Obes Relat Metab Disord 2001;25(8):1175–82.
[10] Stothard KJ, Tennant PW, Bell R, Rankin J. Mater´nal overweight and obesity and the risk of congenital anomalies: a systematic review and meta-analysis. JAMA 2009;301(6):636–50.
[11] Watkins ML, Rasmussen SA, Honein MA, Botto LD, Moore CA. Maternal obesity and risk for birth defects. Pediatrics 2003;111(5 Pt 2):1152–8.
[12] Gilboa SM, Correa A, Botto LD, Rasmussen SA, Waller DK, Hobbs CA, Cleves MA, Riehle-Colarusso TJ, National Birth Defects Prevention Study. Association between prepregnancy body mass index and congenital heart defects. Am J Obstet Gynecol 2010;202(1):51 e51–51e10.
[13] Metzger BE. Biphasic effects of maternal metabolism on fetal growth. Quintessential expression of fuel-mediated teratogenesis. Diabetes 1991;40(Suppl 2):99–105.
[14] Mojtabai R. Body mass index and serum folate in childbearing age women. Eur J Epidemiol 2004;19(11):1029–36.
[15] Best KE, Tennant PW, Bell R, Rankin J. Impact of maternal body mass index on the antenatal detection of congenital anomalies. BJOG 2012;119(12):1503–11.
[16] Wolfe HM, Sokol RJ, Martier SM, Zador IE. Maternal obesity: a potential source of error in sonographic prenatal diagnosis. Obstet Gynecol 1990;76(3 Pt 1):339–42.
[17] Aagaard-Tillery KM, Flint Porter T, Malone FD, Nyberg DA, Collins J, Comstock CH, Hankins G, Eddleman K, Dugoff L, Wolfe HM, D'Alton ME. Influence of maternal BMI on genetic sonography in the FaSTER trial. Prenat Diagn 2010;30(1):14–22.
[18] Dashe JS, McIntire DD, Twickler DM. Effect of maternal obesity on the ultrasound detection of anomalous fetuses. Obstet Gynecol 2009;113(5):1001–7.
[19] Adekola H, Soto E, Dai J, Lam-Rachlin J, Gill N, Leon-Peters J, Puder K, Abramowicz JS. Optimal visualization of the fetal four-chamber and outflow tract views with transabdominal ultrasound in the morbidly obese: are we there yet? J Clin Ultrasound 2015;43(9):548–555.
[20] Bertagna F, Rakza T, Vaksmann G, Ramdane-Sebbane N, Devisme L, Storme L, Francart C, Vaast P, Houfflin-Debarge V. Transposition of the great arteries: factors influencing prenatal diagnosis. Prenat Diagn 2014;34(6):534–7.
[21] Hendler I, Blackwell SC, Treadwell MC, Bujold E, Sokol RJ, Sorokin Y. Does advanced ultrasound equipment improve the adequacy of ultrasound visualization of fetal cardiac structures in the obese gravid woman? Am J Obstet Gynecol 2004;190(6):1616–9; discussion 1619–20.

[22] Tranquart F, Grenier N, Eder V, Pourcelot L. Clinical use of ultrasound tissue harmonic imaging. Ultrasound Med Biol 1999;25(6):889–94.
[23] Choudhry S, Gorman B, Charboneau JW, Tradup DJ, Beck RJ, Kofler JM, Groth DS, Comparison of tissue harmonic imaging with conventional US in abdominal disease. Radiographics 2000;20(4):1127–35.
[24] Treadwell MC, Seubert DE, Zador I, Goyert GL, and Wolfe HM. Benefits associated with harmonic tissue imaging in the obstetric patient. Am J Obstet Gynecol 2000;182(6):1620–3.
[25] Kovalchin JP, Lewin , Bezold LI, Altman CA, Ayres NA. Harmonic imaging in fetal echocardiography. J Am Soc Echocardiogr 2001;14(10):1025–9.
[26] Zhao BW, Tang FG, Shou JD, Xu HS, Lu JH, Fan MY, Fan XM, Pan M. Comparison study of harmonic imaging (HI) and fundamental imaging (FI) in fetal echocardiography. J Zhejiang Univ Sci 2003;4(3):374–7.
[27] Benacerraf B. The use of obstetrical ultrasound in the obese gravida. Semin Perinatol 2013;37(5):345–7.
[28] Davidoff A, Reuter K, Karellas A, Baker SP, Raptopoulos V. Maternal umbilicus: ultrasound window to the gravid uterus. J Clin Ultrasound 1994;22(4):263–7.
[29] Rosenberg JC, Guzman ER, Vintzileos AM, Knuppel RA. Transumbilical placement of the vaginal probe in obese pregnant women. Obstet Gynecol 1995;85(1):132–4.
[30] Paladini D. Sonography in obese and overweight pregnant women: clinical, medicolegal and technical issues. Ultrasound Obstet Gynecol 2009;33(6):720–9.
[31] Thornburg LL, Miles K, Ho M, Pressman EK. Fetal anatomic evaluation in the overweight and obese gravida. Ultrasound Obstet Gynecol 2009;33(6):670–5.
[32] Hunsley C, Farrell T. The influence of maternal body mass index on fetal anomaly screening. Eur J Obstet Gynecol Reprod Biol 2014;182:181–4.
[33] Fuchs F, Houllier M, Voulgaropoulos A, Levaillant JM, Colmant C, Bouyer J, Senat MV. Factors affecting feasibility and quality of second-trimester ultrasound scans in obese pregnant women. Ultrasound Obstet Gynecol 2013;41(1):40–6.
[34] Eastwood KA, Daly C, Hunter A, McCance D, Young I, Holmes V. The impact of maternal obesity on completion of foetal anomaly screening. J Perinat Med 2017;pii: /j/jpme.ahead-of-print/jpm-2016-0048/jpm-2016-0048.xml.
[35] Hershey D. Effect of maternal obesity on the ultrasound detection of anomalous fetuses. Obstet Gynecol 2009;114(3):694–5; author reply 695.
[36] Khoury FR, Ehrenberg HM, Mercer BM. The impact of maternal obesity on satisfactory detailed anatomic ultrasound image acquisition. J Matern Fetal Neonatal Med 2009;22(4):337–41.
[37] Weichert J, Hartge DR. Obstetrical sonography in obese women: a review. J Clin Ultrasound 2011;39(4):209–16.

Tim Van Mieghem, Johannes Keunen, Rory Windrim and Greg Ryan

13 Fetal anomalies in obese women

13.1 Introduction

Worldwide, the prevalence of obesity has doubled since the 1980s. Thirty-nine percent of adults are overweight and 13% are obese [1]. It is therefore not surprising that the incidence of maternal obesity in pregnancy is also on the rise. In Canada, the rate of obesity among women of reproductive age was 15% to 20% in 2014 [2]. Fifteen percent of obese pregnant women will be morbidly obese (body mass index (BMI) >40 kg/m²) and 2% will be superobese (BMI >50 kg/m²) [3]. The maternal obstetric risks of obesity are well-known and include gestational diabetes, hypertension, sleep disordered breathing, cesarean section, failed anesthesia, and venous thromboembolism [4]. From the fetal perspective, the increased incidence of macrosomia and ensuing shoulder dystocia is the most feared complication. The risk of prematurity, fetal anomalies, and intrauterine death is also increased.

The aim of this chapter is to review the current knowledge regarding the association between maternal obesity and fetal anomalies, and to describe how obesity may limit the detection and therapy of such anomalies.

13.2 Maternal obesity and incidence of fetal anomalies

Fetal anomalies occur in 2% to 3% of pregnancies overall, yet increasing evidence is available showing that obesity is an important independent risk factor. A recent systematic review, summarizing 12 studies looking at the incidence of fetal neural tube defects in relation to maternal weight [5], showed a 70% increase in the risk of fetal neural tube defects in obese women when compared with normal weight women (odds ratio (OR) 1.7; 95% confidence interval (95% CI) 1.34–2.15). A clear weight-dependent trend could be seen as overweight women had a smaller risk increase (OR 1.2; 95% CI 0.99–1.49) than women with severe obesity (OR 3.1; 95% CI 1.75–5.46). Strikingly, and for still unclear reasons, the effect seems to be more pronounced for spina bifida than for anencephaly [6].

Similar to what is seen for spina bifida, a systematic review of fetal heart defects in obese women [7], excluding those with pregestational diabetes, demonstrated an increased risk of fetal cardiac anomalies with increasing maternal BMI. This is in line with the finding that the population risk of fetal heart defects over the last decade increased almost in parallel with the incidence of obesity [8]. The OR for a fetal cardiopathy in overweight women is 1.08 (95% CI 1.02–1.15), when compared with normal weight women. Obese women have an OR of 1.15 (95% CI 1.09–1.21), and severe obesity is associated with an OR of 1.39 (95% CI 1.31–1.47).

https://doi.org/10.1515/9783110487817-013

Besides spina bifida and heart defects, increased risk of cleft lip and palate, isolated cleft palate, anorectal atresia, omphalocele, limb reduction, and hydrocephalus have been observed [6]. In contrast, the risk of gastroschisis seems to be lower in the obese gravida.

At present, the underlying reason for the increased incidence of certain anomalies is still unclear. Certainly, an increased prevalence of undiagnosed type II diabetes, and its associated metabolic dysregulation could play a role [9]. Additionally, there is evidence that the incidence of malnutrition and resulting micronutrient deficiencies are increased in maternal obesity [10]. Indeed, a higher BMI is associated with lower serum folate levels, independent of intake [11]. Moreover, obese women may be nutrient-deficient due to diet lacking a variety of macronutrients as well micronutrients.

Given our lack of understanding of the disease process, it is still unclear how we can prevent these anomalies. Increasing folic acid intake may not be the preferred strategy as studies have shown that folic acid supplementation does not decrease the risk of neural tube defects in an obese population to the same extent that was seen in the normal weight population [12]. Another strategy might be to encourage women to lose weight before pregnancy. Indeed, a large study comparing pregnancies of women who underwent bariatric surgery (n = 9,587) with morbidly obese women (n = 221,580) showed a trend toward a lower incidence of fetal anomalies (OR 0.74; 95% CI 0.52–1.04) [13] in the bariatric surgery group. Whether this is a truly causal relationship is unclear at present.

Further research into the link between obesity and fetal anomalies and into methods of prevention is certainly required. These studies, however, are difficult because although the above-mentioned increased ORs are compelling, the overall incidence of fetal anomalies remains low. As a consequence, large numbers are needed to demonstrate statistically (and clinically) significant benefit from interventions.

13.3 Screening and prenatal diagnosis of fetal anomalies in obese women

13.3.1 Aneuploidy screening

The higher incidence of fetal anomalies in the obese population certainly raises the question of screening and treatment. It is clear that routine prenatal ultrasound is more challenging in obese women. Starting in the first trimester, dating a pregnancy is more difficult due to the abdominal adipose pannus [14]. This leads to an increased number of underestimated crown-rump lengths and hence incorrectly dated pregnancies. Similarly, more complex first trimester measurements, including nuchal translucency measurement and assessment of the nasal bone [15], become more difficult. As a consequence, the need for conversion from transabdominal examination to transvaginal imaging in the first trimester almost doubles (from 23% to 42%), and the incidence of incomplete nasal bone exams increases from 2% to 12% [15] when comparing an obese population to a group of women of normal weight. Moreover, failure to obtain a reliable nuchal translucency (NT) measurement in the first scanning session in class III obese women is 22% rather than the usual 2% in normal weight women [16]. Even with repeat measurements, scanning in obese women will result in up to 12% failing to receive a valid measurement, thereby limiting the usefulness of first trimester screening in this population [16]. Nevertheless, when a valid nuchal translucency measurement can be achieved, and when this is combined with serum markers (PAPP-A and free β-hCG), the false-positive and false-negative detection rates for Down syndrome seem to be similar in the obese and the normal weight population [17].

It is worth noting that a higher maternal BMI does lead to lower PAPP-A and free β hCG levels due to a dilutional effect of the higher maternal blood volume [18], and as such these markers need to be adjusted for maternal weight. This becomes especially relevant when screening for trisomy 18 [17] as a combination of low PAPP-A and low free β hCG would significantly increase the risk of a false-positive test for this condition. In screening for trisomy 21, on the other hand, a low PAPP-A (which would increase the risk of trisomy 21) would be counterbalanced by a low free β-hCG (which would decrease the risk of trisomy 21), thereby not affecting the final risk significantly [17].

Aneuploidy screening in the second trimester of pregnancy, by a "genetic sonogram" aimed at identifying soft markers is similarly hampered by maternal obesity. A secondary analysis of the results of the FaSTER trial shows that the risk of "missed" soft markers is higher in obese women, thereby leading to a higher risk of missed prenatal diagnoses of aneuploidy [19].

Unfortunately, noninvasive prenatal aneuploidy screening using cell-free fetal DNA (NIPT) in maternal serum does not overcome the problem of more difficult ultrasound-based aneuploidy screening. Indeed, the incidence of a low fetal DNA fraction in maternal blood and hence an unreliable NIPT result is significantly increased in obese women. This is probably the consequence of a combination of a higher maternal blood volume [18] and a higher maternal adipocyte cellular turnover rate. The latter results in large amounts of maternal cell-free DNA being shed into the circulation and hence a decrease in the fetal fraction of circulating cell-free DNA [20]. A fetal fraction below the clinically used threshold of 4% is seen in 1% of women weighing less than 70 kg, but in 10% of women weighing more than 110 kg and in up to 25% of women weighing more than 130 kg [21]. A repeat blood draw at a later gestational age can sometimes overcome this technical problem, but the chance of a successful second test is still as low as 30% in women more than 120 kg [22].

Ultimately, these lower detection rates of fetal aneuploidy result in a higher risk of delivering a baby with trisomy 21 and this should be discussed with obese women, ideally preconceptionally or prior to initiating aneuploidy screening [23, 24].

13.3.2 Fetal anomaly screening

The limitations for fetal aneuploidy screening also apply for second trimester fetal anomaly screening. Maternal serum screening for open spina bifida and abdominal wall defects using alpha-fetoprotein is less sensitive in the obese gravida and requires adjustment for maternal weight [25]. Moreover, there is clear evidence that completion of a fetal anatomy screen by ultrasound is more difficult and less successful in the obese population than in a normal weight group. A study of more than 10,000 women showed that complete visualization of all 10 components of a fetal anomaly screen in one single visit was feasible in 72% of women with a BMI of less than 25 kg/m² but only in 68%, 57%, 41%, and 30% of overweight women, class I, class II, and class III obese women, respectively [26]. The organ systems most at risk of suboptimal assessment are the fetal heart (Fig. 13.1) and spine [27, 28], which are also the organ systems that are at higher risk of anomalies in obese women.

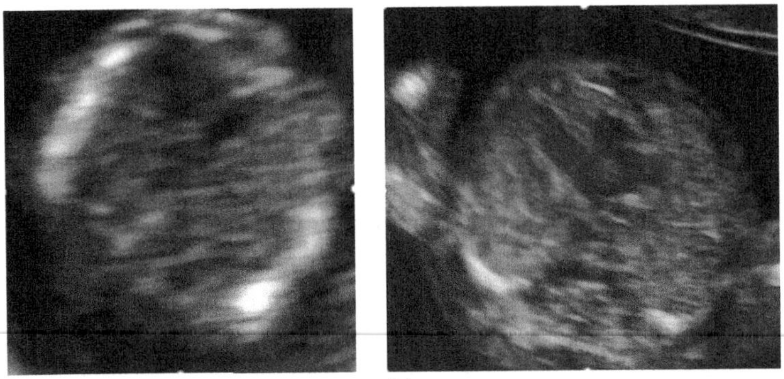

(a) (b)

Fig. 13.1: Axial view of the fetal chest and heart at 12 weeks of gestation in a gravida with BMI 35 kg/m²: **(a)** transabdominal; **(b)** transvaginal. Note the significant increase in resolution by using the transvaginal approach.

As a consequence of the lower completion rate of fetal anatomy screening ultrasounds, the risk of missed anomalies is higher [29, 30]. The detection rate of fetal anomalies reaches a low of 25% in class III obesity, compared with 66% in normal weight women after a standard screening exam [29]. Even in experienced hands, obese women undergoing a targeted organ screening will only achieve a 75% anomaly detection rate, compared with a 97% detection rate in normal weight women [29]. Additionally, the poorer image resolution increases the risk of a false-positive diagnosis, especially for fetal heart defects [19].

Different strategies have been suggested to improve the detection rate of fetal anomalies in obese women. Current ultrasound technology allows for considerable image optimization. Judicious use of tissue harmonic imaging [31], speckle reduction software, compound imaging, and Doppler ultrasound [32] can certainly increase image quality. Once the image has been optimized, the sonographer should try to image the fetus through areas with the least adipose tissue. It is clear that maternal adipose tissue tends to accumulate in the lower abdomen, at the level of the pannus. Therefore, avoiding this area is key. Different strategies include scanning through the suprapubic area underneath the pannus, or accessing the uterus from the maternal inguinal or periumbilical areas. Access through the flank or inguinal region can be facilitated by positioning the patient in lateral decubitus position [33]. Some authors prefer a transumbilical approach with a transvaginal probe, after filling the umbilicus with ultrasound gel [34]. Finally, waiting for spontaneous filling of the maternal bladder, which elevates the fetus, may be helpful as this will bring the fetus in closer reach of a transfundal ultrasound approach [32].

Given the need for a combination of image optimization and choosing the most appropriate ultrasound approach, sonographer expertise plays a crucial role in obtaining adequate images. Assigning more senior staff can triple the chance of achieving the required images when compared with junior staff [35]. One should nevertheless be careful not to overload experienced sonographers as the risk of repetitive strain injury is considerable among sonographers [36]. Fortunately, if regular breaks are implemented and observed, the risk of repetitive strain injury is not higher among those scanning obese women compared with those scanning normal weight patients [37].

If the above described methods are insufficient to achieve complete imaging, another logical approach would be to repeat the ultrasound examination at a later gestational age. A study by Hendler et al. [38] shows that when anatomy screening ultrasound is repeated for suboptimal visualization at the initial attempt, adequate visualization will be achieved in almost 99% of repeat exams in the normal weight population. In the obese population, however, imaging will still be suboptimal in 10% to 20% [38]. Moreover, by postponing completion of fetal anomaly screening, and thereby postponing detection of possible fetal anomalies, management options and especially the option of termination of pregnancy in the presence of severe anomalies, may be affected in some countries. An alternative approach, which overcomes the risk of late diagnosis, would be to perform an early fetal anatomy ultrasound, either in the late first trimester (12–13 weeks of gestation) [39,40] or in the early second trimester (15–16 weeks of gestation) [41]. Some organ systems, including the spine, limbs, and heart, will already be sufficiently developed for (at least a partial) assessment at this gestational age. Moreover, this early in pregnancy, a transvaginal ultrasound with higher resolution probes is often still an option and allows the probe to be brought closer to the fetus (Fig. 13.2).

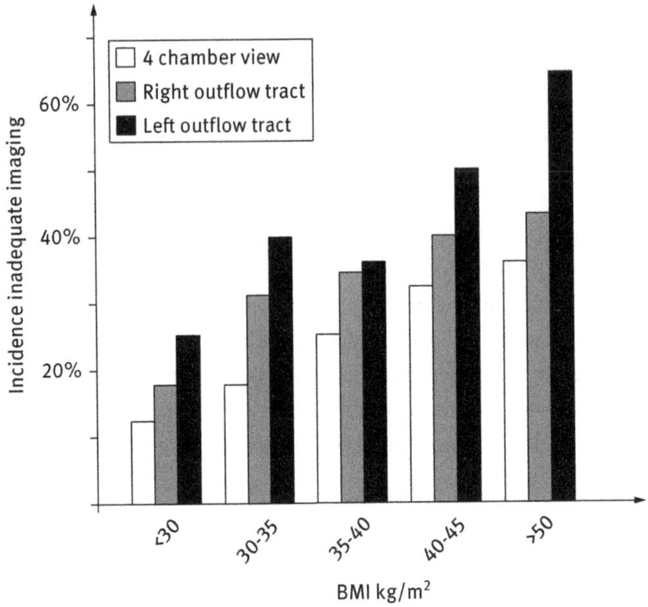

Fig. 13.2: Incidence of suboptimal imaging of cardiac structures at the 20-week anatomy ultrasound per BMI class. Adapted from Pasko et al. [27].

Finally, if all the above methods are insufficient, choosing an alternative imaging strategy by means of magnetic resonance imaging (MRI) may be a solution. Non-contrast-enhanced MRI is considered safe for fetal imaging [42], and is less affected by the maternal structures surrounding the fetus. MRI, however, is still limited by maternal abdominal circumference as the maximal diameter, even of the newer magnets, is only 70 cm. The table typically has an upper weight limit of approximately 250 kg [43]. "Open" MRIs may be less limited by abdominal circumference and are more patient-friendly yet high-end devices allowing 1.5 Tesla scans are not widely available yet.

13.4 Invasive procedures and fetal therapy in obese women

For some fetal anomalies, further fetal investigation by invasive genetic testing (amniocentesis or chorion villus biopsy; CVS) or fetal therapy is an option. As these procedures are often done under ultrasound guidance, poor imaging due to obesity may make the procedure more difficult and hence increase failure and complication rates.

In the only large study looking into complication rates after amniocentesis and CVS, class III obesity (BMI >40 kg/m^2) was associated with a doubling of the risk of fetal loss after the procedure when compared with normal weight women (OR 2.2; 95% CI 1.2–3.9) [44]. This was most likely due to the higher need for multiple needle insertions in this group. In this study, obesity was not associated with a higher loss rate after transvaginal CVS.

The potential effects of obesity on open fetal surgery for spina bifida are unknown, as all protocols for this procedure have thus far considered a BMI of <35 kg/m² as a crucial selection criterion [45]. Theoretically, maternal abdominal adiposity could hamper uterine and fetal exposure and thereby complicate the procedure. Moreover, obesity could affect the maternal safety of the general anesthesia required for the procedure. Within the 25 to 35 kg/m² BMI-range, however, overweight and obesity does not seem to be a significant predictor of adverse short-term obstetric outcome [46]. We are aware of two ongoing studies investigating an expansion of the inclusion criteria for open fetal therapy to women with a BMI between 35 and 40 kg/m² (www.clinicaltrials.gov – NCT02664207 and NCT02509377).

Little is known regarding the effect of obesity on outcomes of fetoscopic procedures or on complication rates of fetal shunting procedures or intrauterine needle procedures. Current literature seems to support the concept that, although obesity can make procedures more difficult [47], it does not seem to affect fetal outcomes significantly [48].

13.5 Conclusion

In summary, maternal obesity significantly increases the risk of fetal anomalies, through as yet unknown mechanisms. Detection of these anomalies by routine ultrasound screening is suboptimal, even in expert hands, and obese women should be counseled about the limitations of ultrasound. New imaging strategies should be explored in an attempt to increase the yield of fetal anomaly screening in this high-risk population. Further studies looking at the effect of obesity on invasive fetal diagnosis and therapy are needed.

Bibliography

[1] WHO. Obesity and overweight. http://www.who.int/mediacentre/factsheets/fs311/en/ last accessed 22-12-2016.
[2] Statistics Canada. Overweight and obese adults (self-reported), 2014. http://www.statcan.gc.ca/pub/82–625–x/2015001/article/14185 last accessed 22-12-2016.
[3] Marshall NE, Guild C, Cheng YW, et al. Maternal superobesity and perinatal outcomes. Am J Obstet Gynecol 2012;206(5):417.e1–6.
[4] Simhan HN. Antepartum care of the obese patient. Clin Obstet Gynecol 2016;59(1):148–57.
[5] Rasmussen SA, Chu SY, Kim SY, et al. Maternal obesity and risk of neural tube defects: a metaanalysis. Am J Obstet Gynecol 2008;198(6):611–9.
[6] Stothard KJ, Tennant PWG, Bell R, et al. Maternal overweight and obesity and the risk of congenital anomalies. Am Med Assoc 2009;301(6):636–50.
[7] Cai G-J, Sun X-X, Zhang L, et al. Association between maternal body mass index and congenital heart defects in offspring: a systematic review. Am J Obstet Gynecol 2014;211(April):91–117.
[8] N.L. M, S.M. S, M.B. L, et al. Prepregnancy body mass index and congenital heart defects among offspring: a population-based study. Congenit Heart Dis 2013;8(2):131–41.

[9] Mitanchez D. Foetal and neonatal complications in gestational diabetes: perinatal mortality, congenital malformations, macrosomia, shoulder dystocia, birth injuries, neonatal complications. Diabetes Metab 2010;36(6 Pt 2):617–27.
[10] Peterson LA, Cheskin LJ, Furtado M, et al. Malnutrition in bariatric surgery candidates: multiple micronutrient deficiencies prior to surgery. Obes Surg 2016;26(4):833–8.
[11] Mahabir S, Ettinger S, Johnson L, et al. Measures of adiposity and body fat distribution in relation to serum folate levels in postmenopausal women in a feeding study. Eur J Clin Nutr 2008;62(5):644–50.
[12] Ray JG, Wyatt PR, Vermeulen MJ, et al. Greater maternal weight and the ongoing risk of neural tube defects after folic acid flour fortification. Obstet Gynecol 2005;105(2):261–5.
[13] Abenhaim HA, Alrowaily N, Czuzoj-Shulman N, et al. Pregnancy outcomes in women with bariatric surgery as compared with morbidly obese women. J Matern Neonatal Med 2016;7058(March):1–22.
[14] Bak GS, Sperling L, Källén K, et al. Prospective population-based cohort study of maternal obesity as a source of error in gestational age estimation at 11–14 weeks. Acta Obstet Gynecol Scand 2016;95:1281–7.
[15] Gandhi M, Fox NS, Russo-Stieglitz K, et al. Effect of increased body mass index on first-trimester ultrasound examination for aneuploidy risk assessment. Obstet Gynecol 2009;114(4):856–9.
[16] Thornburg LL, Mulconry M, Post A, et al. Fetal nuchal translucency thickness evaluation in the overweight and obese gravida. Ultrasound Obstet Gynecol 2009;33(6):665–9.
[17] Krantz DA, Hallahan TW, Macri VJ, et al. Maternal weight and ethnic adjustment within a first-trimester Down syndrome and trisomy 18 screening program. Prenat Diagn 2005;25(8):635–40.
[18] Neveux LM, Palomaki GE, Larrivee DA, et al. Refinements in managing maternal weight adjustment for interpreting prenatal screening results. Prenat Diagn 1996;16(12):1115–9.
[19] Aagaard-Tillery KM, Flint Porter T, Malone FD, et al. Influence of maternal BMI on genetic sonography in the FaSTER trial. Prenat Diagn 2010;30(1):14–22.
[20] Haghiac M, Vora NL, Basu S, et al. Increased death of adipose cells, a path to release cell-free DNA into systemic circulation of obese women. Obesity (Silver Spring) 2012;20(11):2213–9.
[21] Ashoor G, Syngelaki A, Poon LCY, et al. Fetal fraction in maternal plasma cell-free DNA at 11–13 weeks' gestation: relation to maternal and fetal characteristics. Ultrasound Obstet Gynecol 2013;41(1):26–32.
[22] Wang E, Batey A, Struble C, et al. Gestational age and maternal weight effects on fetal cell-free DNA in maternal plasma. Prenat Diagn 2013;33(7):662–6.
[23] Hildebrand E, Källén B, Josefsson A, et al. Maternal obesity and risk of Down syndrome in the offspring. Prenat Diagn 2014;34(4):310–5.
[24] Ghidini A. Maternal obesity and Down syndrome in the offspring: is there a link? Prenat Diagn 2014;34(4):307–9.
[25] Bredaki FE, Sciorio C, Wright A, et al. Serum alpha-fetoprotein in the three trimesters of pregnancy: effects of maternal characteristics and medical history. Ultrasound Obstet Gynecol 2015;46(1):34–41.
[26] Dashe JS, McIntire DD, Twickler DM. Maternal obesity limits the ultrasound evaluation of fetal anatomy. J Ultrasound Med 2009;28(8):1025–30.
[27] Pasko DN, Wood SL, Jenkins SM, et al. Completion and sensitivity of the second-trimester fetal anatomic survey in obese gravidas. J Ultrasound Med 2016;35(11):2449–57.
[28] Adekola H, Soto E, Dai J, et al. Optimal visualization of the fetal four-chamber and outflow tract views with transabdominal ultrasound in the morbidly obese: are we there yet? J Clin Ultrasound 2015;43(9):548–55.
[29] Dashe JS. Effect of maternal obesity on the ultrasound detection of anomalous fetuses. Obstet Gynecol 2010;115(2, Part 1):385–6.

[30] Best KE, Tennant PWG, Bell R, et al. Impact of maternal body mass index on the antenatal detection of congenital anomalies. BJOG 2012;119(12):1503–11.
[31] Paladini D, Vassallo M, Tartaglione A, et al. The role of tissue harmonic imaging in fetal echocardiography. Ultrasound Obstet Gynecol 2004;23(2):159–64.
[32] Paladini D. Sonography in obese and overweight pregnant women: clinical, medicolegal and technical issues. Ultrasound Obstet Gynecol 2009;33(6):720–9.
[33] Benacerraf BR. How do we do it? Practical advice on imaging-based techniques and investigations: a technical tip on scanning obese gravidae. Ultrasound Obstet Gynecol 2010;35(5):615–6.
[34] Rosenberg JC, Guzman ER, Vintzileos AM, et al. Transumbilical placement of the vaginal probe in obese pregnant women. Obstet Gynecol 1995;85(1):132–4.
[35] Chung JH, Pelayo R, Hatfield TJ, et al. Limitations of the fetal anatomic survey via ultrasound in the obese obstetrical population. J Matern Fetal Neonatal Med 2012;25(10):1945–9.
[36] Schoenfeld A, Goverman J, Weiss DM, et al. Transducer user syndrome: an occupational hazard of the ultrasonographer. Eur J Ultrasound 1999;10(1):41–5.
[37] Janga D, Akinfenwa O. Work-related repetitive strain injuries amongst practitioners of obstetric and gynaecological ultrasound worldwide. Arch Gynecol Obstet 2012;286(2):353–6.
[38] Hendler I, Blackwell SC, Bujold E, et al. Suboptimal second-trimester ultrasonographic visualization of the fetal heart in obese women: should we repeat the examination? J Ultrasound Med 2005;24(9):1205-9-1.
[39] Lim J, Whittle W, Lee Y, et al. Early anatomy ultrasound in women at increased risk of fetal anomalies. Prenat Diagn 2013;33(9):1–6.
[40] Harper LM, Biggio JR, Wood SL, et al. The performance of first-trimester anatomy scan: a decision analysis. Am J Perinatol 2016;1(212).
[41] Gupta S, Timor-Tritsch IE, Oh C, et al. Early second-trimester sonography to improve the fetal anatomic survey in obese patients. J Ultrasound Med 2014;33(9):1579–83.
[42] Ray JG, Vermeulen MJ, Bharatha A, et al. Association between MRI exposure during pregnancy and fetal and childhood outcomes. JAMA 2016;316(9):952.
[43] Glanc P, O'Hayon BE, Singh DK, et al. Challenges of pelvic imaging in obese women. Radiographics 2012;32(6):1839–62.
[44] Harper LM, Cahill AG, Smith K, et al. Effect of maternal obesity on the risk of fetal loss after amniocentesis and chorionic villus sampling. Obstet Gynecol 2012;119(4):745–51.
[45] Adzick NS, Thom EA, Spong CY, et al. A randomized trial of prenatal versus postnatal repair of myelomeningocele. N Engl J Med 2011;364(11):993–1004.
[46] Johnson MP, Bennett KA, Rand L, et al. The Management of Myelomeningocele Study: obstetrical outcomes and risk factors for obstetrical complications following prenatal surgery. Am J Obstet Gynecol 2016.
[47] Guenot C, Robyr R, Jastrow N, et al. Fetal intra-peritoneal transfusion for the management of very early spontaneous twin anemia-polycythemia sequence in an obese patient with a whole anterior placenta. Twin Res Hum Genet 2016;19(2):154–7.
[48] Halvorsen CP, Ek S, Dellgren A, et al. Survival and neonatal outcome after fetoscopic guided laser occlusion (FLOC) of twin-to-twin transfusion syndrome (TTTS) in Sweden. J Perinat Med 2012;40(5):533–8.

Frank A. Chervenak and Laurence B. McCullough

14 The professional responsibility model of obstetrics ethics: implications for the management of obesity during pregnancy

14.1 Introduction

The management of obesity during pregnancy presents daunting challenges to obstetricians, as documented in the other chapters in this volume. Clinically, the most important objective is to mitigate the complications of obesity for pregnant, fetal, and neonatal patients during a current as well as future pregnancy. Modifying the pregnant patient's behavior is essential but often very difficult to achieve. Persuading pregnant patients is an obvious tool that has significant ethical dimensions. This chapter addresses these ethical dimensions by identifying the implications for the management of obesity during pregnancy of the professional responsibility model of obstetric ethics [1, 2].

We begin with an account of the professional responsibility model of obstetric ethics. We will then demonstrate its application to the management of obesity during pregnancy.

14.2 The professional responsibility model of obstetric ethics

14.2.1 Key concepts from medical ethics

The professional responsibility model of obstetric ethics draws on key concepts from medical ethics. Medical ethics is the disciplined study of morality in medicine. Medical ethics undertakes this study by asking specific questions: What does it mean to say that a physician is a professional? What obligations do physicians owe their patients, healthcare organizations, and society? What obligations do patients owe their physicians, healthcare organizations, and society? What obligations do healthcare organizations owe their patients, healthcare professionals, and society? What obligations do societies have to physicians, patients, and healthcare organizations?

Medical ethics should not be confused with the many sources of morality in a pluralistic society. These include, but are not limited to, law, the world's religions, ethnic and cultural traditions, families, and personal experience. Professional medical ethics seeks to bridge these differences and identify the obligations of physicians to their patients in all global cultures and national settings.

The first step in doing so is to recognize that professional medical ethics is secular. This recognition was achieved in the eighteenth century European and American

https://doi.org/10.1515/9783110487817-014

Enlightenments [3]. Secular professional medical ethics makes no reference to deity or deities or to revealed tradition, but to what reasoned, evidence-based discourse requires and its products. At the same time, secular professional medical ethics is not intrinsically hostile to but respectful of religious beliefs. Therefore, ethical principles and virtues should be understood to apply to all physicians, regardless of their personal religious and spiritual beliefs and regardless of their nationality or place of practice [4]. The advantage of secular medical ethics is that it is transreligious, transcultural, and transnational.

The traditions and practices of medicine constitute an obvious source of morality for physicians. These traditions provide an important reference point for professional medical ethics because they are based on the obligation to protect and promote the health-related interests of the patient. This obligation tells physicians what morality in medicine ought to be, but only in very general, abstract terms. Providing a clinically applicable account of that obligation is in clinical practice the central task of professional medical ethics, using ethical principles [2, 4]. We start with ethical principles that play a central role in professional medical ethics, beneficence and respect for autonomy.

In ethics, generally, the ethical principle of beneficence requires one to act in a way that is reliably expected to produce a greater balance of benefits over harms in the lives of others [2, 4]. In professional medical ethics, this principle requires the physician to seek a greater balance of clinical over clinical harms in the lives of patients [2]. The task of beneficence-based clinical judgment is to reach reasoned judgments about the appropriate balance of clinical goods and harms in a particular clinical situation, such as the decision to perform a cesarean delivery for the management of fetal macrosomia in an obese pregnant patient. On the basis of the best available evidence, beneficence-based clinical judgment identifies the clinical benefits that can be achieved for the patient based on the competencies of medicine. The clinical benefits that medicine is competent to seek for patients are the prevention and management of disease, injury, disability, loss of functional status, and unnecessary pain, distress, and suffering, and the prevention of premature or unnecessary death. Pain and suffering become unnecessary when they do not result in achieving the other goods of clinical care, e.g., allowing a woman to labor without effective analgesia [2].

In beneficence-based clinical judgment, pregnancy is not a disease. It is instead a clinical condition: a naturally occurring biological process that creates risks of disease, injury, disability, loss of functional status, and unnecessary pain, distress, and suffering. As a consequence, the clinical management of the clinical condition of pregnancy comes under beneficence-based clinical judgment.

The ethical principle of nonmaleficence requires the physician not to cause harm. This is sometimes treated as an absolute, allowing no exceptions. This is a common mistake; nonmaleficence is best understood as expressing the limits of beneficence-based clinical judgment. This ethical principle is also known as *Primum non nocere* or "first do no harm." This commonly invoked dogma is really a Latinized misinterpretation of the Hippocratic texts, which emphasized beneficence while avoiding harm when approaching the limits of medicine to maintain or improve the patient's condition or to alter the course of disease or injury [2, 4]. Nonmaleficence should be incorporated into beneficence-based clinical judgment: when the physician approaches the limits of beneficence-based clinical judgment, i.e., when the evidence for expected clinical benefit diminishes and the risks of clinical harm increases, then deliberative beneficence-based clinical ethical judgment requires the physician to proceed with great caution. The physician should be especially concerned in such clinical circumstances to prevent serious, far-reaching, and irreversible clinical harm to the patient.

This ethical principle requires the physician to empower the pregnant woman to make informed decisions about the management of her pregnancy. The most important way that physicians fulfill this obligation is to identify medically reasonable alternatives to the pregnant woman and to identify alternatives that, although technically possible, are not reliably judged to be medically reasonable. "Medically reasonable" means that there is a beneficence-based clinical judgment that a form of clinical management or intervention has a reliable evidence base for expected net clinical benefit. There is no ethical obligation to offer a technically possible alternative that does not meet this test for being medically reasonable.

14.2.2 The professional responsibility model

The professional responsibility model of obstetrics ethics is designed to guide obstetricians in responsibly managing ethical challenges in clinical practice and research [2]. For example, directive counseling for fetal benefit in the management of obesity during pregnancy must take account of obligations to the pregnant woman, which creates the possibility of conflict between the physician's recommendation and a pregnant woman's autonomous decision to the contrary. Such conflict is best managed preventively through the informed consent process as an ongoing dialogue throughout a woman's pregnancy, augmented as necessary by negotiation and respectful persuasion [2, 5]. Respectful persuasion is based on an appeal to the pregnant woman's values, such as achieving a good outcome for her pregnancy, make recommendations based on those values, and respond to refusal with engaged dialogue aiming at having the pregnant woman reconsider her refusal.

This approach to obstetric ethics is known as the professional responsibility model of obstetric ethics [1, 2]. The professional responsibility model provides a powerful antidote to the rights-based reductionism that characterizes much of the literature on obstetric ethics. This oversimplification of obstetric ethics occurs when the only or overriding ethical consideration is the rights of either the pregnant woman or the fetus.

Rights-based reductionism is best illustrated by the abortion controversy. One extreme asserts that fetal rights always override the rights of the pregnant woman. This is fetal-rights reductionism. Termination of pregnancy at any gestational age or for any reason is impermissible, regardless of whether the pregnancy is voluntary or not or viable [6]. The other extreme asserts that the pregnant woman's rights always override fetal rights. This is maternal-rights reductionism. Termination of pregnancy is therefore permissible at any gestational age and for any reason that is important to the pregnant woman [7, 8].

Rights-talk is initially appealing because of the simple dichotomy at its heart: one either has rights or one does not and, if one does, others must respect one's rights. This simple dichotomy is simplistic and does not withstand close clinical ethical scrutiny. There is unavoidable controversy about the nature and limits of both fetal and women's rights. Such rights are based on many factors, including cultural, political, and religious beliefs that do not lend themselves to compromise and are outside of the physician-patient relationship.

Consider the simplistic claim that a pregnant woman has unconditional rights to control what happens to her body. The claim ignores a fundamental question: should this right be understood to come with limits or with no exceptions throughout the entire pregnancy? Professional integrity sets justified limits on the preferences of patients [9, 10], pregnant patients included. For example, a distraught woman who is 34 weeks pregnant reports that her husband has deserted her and insists on induced abortion immediately. The professional responsibility model requires her obstetrician not to implement her request because feticide is ruled out by the obstetrician's beneficence-based obligation to protect the life of this fetal patient. The obstetrician should therefore recommend against feticide and explain that no conscientious obstetrician should implement her request. There are many such circumstances in which a pregnant woman's request for an induced abortion should not be implemented unquestioningly.

By contrast, consider the simplistic claim that the fetus has an unconditional right to life or to complete gestation. The presence of a fetal anomaly incompatible with life belies such claims as lacking scientific and clinical foundation because medicine has no capacity to correct such anomalies. Such claims lack an authoritative foundation in either religion or philosophy. There is no single authoritative perspective from which the incompatible differences of these diverse views on fetal rights can be resolved [2]. To insist on an unconditional right to life or to complete gestation therefore has no place in professional obstetric ethics.

The existence of maternal-rights reductionism approach in the literature is well documented in the context of intrapartum management. This approach asserts an unconditional right of the pregnant woman to control her body in all aspects of the management of pregnancy: "...the moral and legal primacy of the competent, informed pregnant woman in decision making is overwhelming" [11]. Another expression of this approach at first seems to be nonreductionist. Its authors acknowledge patient safety as a "first-order issue" [6] and support what they call "restrictive guidelines" based on protecting the life and health of pregnant women [6]. The proponents of this seemingly nuanced approach, however, abandoned it in favor of the maternal rights reductionism model when they asserted: "Crucially, even when restrictive guidelines are warranted, the rights of pregnant women to bodily integrity must be maintained" [7]. Some express this approach explicitly, e.g., that "women have fully endowed rights that do not diminish with conception, nor progressively degrade as pregnancy advances to viability and birth" [7]. The woman's rights reductionism approach has been used to claim the right of pregnant women to have a clinically non-indicated cesarean delivery [12, 13]. Another example is the assertion of the pregnant woman's autonomy as an "unrestricted negative right," i.e., an unconditional right to noninterference with refusal of cesarean delivery: "autonomy is an inter-relational right—ultimately, there is no circumstance in which someone should be brought to an operating room against their will" [14].

Rights-based reductionism has no place in professional obstetric ethics because it unacceptably distorts the professional nature of the relationship of an obstetrician to his or her patients. The professional obligations of the obstetrician originate in the ethical concept of medicine as a profession.

The concept of medicine as a profession was introduced into the history of medicine by Drs. John Gregory (1724–1773) of Scotland and Thomas Percival (1740–1804) of England. This concept requires the physician to make three commitments: (1) becoming and remaining scientifically and clinically competent; (2) protecting and promoting the health-related and other interests of the patient as the physician's primary concern and motivation; and (3) preserving and strengthening medicine as what Percival called a "public trust," a social institution that exists primarily for the benefit of society not its members (in contrast to the concept of medicine as a merchant guild) [15].

In the professional responsibility model of obstetric ethics, obstetricians have beneficence-based an autonomy-based obligations to the pregnant patient and beneficence-based obligations to the fetal patient [1, 2]. The beneficence-based obligation of the obstetrician is to make evidence-based clinical judgments about diagnostic and therapeutic measures that are medically reasonable because they are reliably expected to result in a greater balance of clinical goods over clinical harms for the pregnant or fetal patient. The obstetrician then empowers the pregnant woman's autonomy by offering or recommending medically reasonable alternatives in the informed consent process. When the condition for being medically reasonable is met, the alternative should be offered, along with the other medically reasonable alternatives. Sometimes, the evidence clearly supports one alternative as clinically superior to others or as the only medically reasonable alternative. In such clinical circumstances, the physician should recommend this alternative to the pregnant woman. Sometimes, the evidence clearly supports an alternative as not medically reasonable. In such clinical circumstances, the physician should not offer this alternative to the pregnant woman and should recommend against it should the pregnant woman ask about it.

Patients exercise their capacity for autonomous decision-making in response to alternatives that are offered or recommended by the physician in the informed consent process. The capacity for autonomous decision making has three components: (1) absorbing and retaining information about her condition and the medically reasonable diagnostic and therapeutic responses to it; (2) understanding that information, i.e., evaluating and rank-ordering those responses and appreciating that she could experience the risks of treatment; and (3) expressing a value-based preference [16]. The physician has a role to play in each of these. They are, respectively: (1) to recognize the capacity of each patient to deal with medical information and not to underestimate that capacity, provide information (i.e., disclose and explain all medically reasonable alternatives) and recognize the validity of the values and beliefs of the patient; (2) not to interfere with but, when necessary, to assist the patient in her evaluation and ranking of the medically reasonable diagnostic and therapeutic alternatives for managing her condition; and (3) to elicit and implement the patient's value-based preference [4].

14.3 Implications for the management of pregnancy complicated by obesity

From the perspective of the professional responsibility model of obstetric ethics, the informed consent process should be seen as one of the tools for modifying behavior before, during, and after pregnancy. This process begins with educating obese patients about the risks of pregnancy and how these risks might be reduced. Educating some patients may motivate them to change. For most patients, more than education will be needed. Respect for autonomy rules out interfering with patient's decisions as well as coercion, which is interference accompanied by a threat. Between these two poles are frank communication and persuasion.

Frank communication means being clear about the ill effects for pregnant, fetal, and neonatal patients of poor dietary control during pregnancy in an obese patient. These risks should not be sugarcoated. At the same time, communication about reducible risk should be respectful. The human central nervous system learns by repetition, which means that a single educational session is less likely to have durable effect than repeated educational sessions. This approach can try the patience and good nature of the obstetrician, especially when the patient is recalcitrant to behavior modification. The professional responsibility model reminds the obstetrician not to let these psychological challenges diminish a core commitment of the model, to keep the patient's interests systematically primary and self-interest systematically secondary.

Making evidence-based recommendations is obviously supported by the ethical principle of beneficence. Making evidence-based recommendations is also supported by the ethical principle of respect for autonomy because recommendations empower the pregnant patient by signaling to her the obstetrician's commitment to her health and that of her fetus and future child. It is therefore a mistake to think that directive counseling in the form of making recommendations is not compatible with the ethical principle of respect for autonomy. When the evidence is as it is in the case of dietary modification for obese patients, making recommendations is mandated by the professional responsibility model. It is therefore unprofessional to adhere to a nondirective approach in such clinical circumstances.

Directive counseling regarding intrapartum management for maternal or fetal benefit when the evidence is clear will be discussed in the other chapters in this volume. Given the evidence-based controversies that these chapters document, obstetricians should be especially careful in evaluating evidence and tempering the strength of recommendations accordingly. In beneficence-based clinical judgment, the stronger the evidence for maternal or fetal benefit, the stronger the professional responsibility to make recommendations and explain their evidence base. The weaker the evidence, the stronger the professional responsibility to present medically reasonable alternatives and respect the pregnant woman's informed decision. This approach balances beneficence-based obligations to the fetal patient against beneficence-based and autonomy-based obligations to the pregnant woman. Such balancing also recognizes that a pregnant woman is obligated only to take reasonable risks of medical interventions that are reliably expected to benefit the fetal and neonatal patient [2].

14.4 Conclusion

The professional responsibility model of obstetric ethics is an essential component of the management of obesity during pregnancy. This chapter helps the obstetrician to fulfill his or her professional responsibility to this at-risk patient population by identifying the clinical implications of beneficence-based obligations to pregnant, fetal, and neonatal patients and of autonomy-based obligations to the pregnant patient.

Bibliography

[1] Chervenak FA, McCullough LB, Brent RL. The professional responsibility model of obstetric ethics: avoiding the perils of clashing rights. Am J Obstet Gynecol 2011;205:315.e1–5.
[2] Chervenak FA, McCullough LB. The professional responsibility model of perinatal ethics. Berlin: Walter de Gruyter, 2014.
[3] Engelhardt HT, Jr. The foundations of bioethics. 2nd ed. New York, NY: Oxford University Press, 1995.
[4] Beauchamp TL, Childress JF. Principles of biomedical ethics. 7th ed. New York, NY: Oxford University Press, 2012.
[5] Chervenak FA, McCullough LB. Clinical guides to preventing ethical conflicts between pregnant women and their physicians. Am J Obstet Gynecol 1990;162:303–7.
[6] Johnson LSM. Abortion: II. Contemporary ethical and legal aspects: A. Ethical perspectives. In: Post SG (ed.), Encyclopedia of bioethics, pp. 7–18. New York: Macmillan References USA, 2004.
[7] Lyerly AD, Little MO. Toward an ethically responsible approach to vaginal birth after cesarean. Semin Perinatol 2010;34:337–44.
[8] Minkoff H, Paltrow L. Obstetricians and the rights of pregnant women. Womens Health (Lond) 2007;3:315–9.
[9] Brett AS, McCullough LB. When patients request specific interventions: defining the limits of the physician's obligation. N Engl J Med 1986;315:1347–51.
[10] Brett AS, McCullough LB. Addressing requests by patients for non-beneficial interventions. JAMA 2012;307:149–50.
[11] Annas GJ. Protecting the liberty of pregnant patient. N Engl J Med 1988;316:1213–4.

[12] Högberg U, Lynöe N, Wulff M. Cesarean by choice? Empirical study of public attitudes. Acta Obstet Gynecol Scand 2008;87:1301–8.
[13] Buckley S. Reclaiming every woman's birthright. Midwifery Today Int Midwife 2010;94:40–41.
[14] Minkoff H. NIH vaginal birth after cesarean: new insights. National Institutes of Health Consensus Development Conference, March 10–13, 2010. Page 6, Day 2 Discussion, available at http://videocast.nih.gov/summary.asp?Live=8408, accessed June 29, 2012.
[15] McCullough LB. The ethical concept of medicine as a profession: its origins in modern medical ethics and implications for physicians. In: Kenny N, Shelton W (eds.). Lost virtue: professional character development in medical education, pp. 17–27. New York: Elsevier, 2006.
[16] McCullough LB, Coverdale JH, Chervenak FA. Ethical challenges of decision making with pregnant patients who have schizophrenia. Am J Obstet Gynecol 2002;187:696–702.

Amir Aviram and Yariv Yogev

15 The obese patient: losing weight in pregnancy

15.1 Scope of the problem

Obesity has already been recognized as an epidemic. According to the World Health Organization, obesity has more than doubled in the last three decades, with more than 600 million obese adults worldwide, which translated into 13% of the entire adult population in 2014 [1]. Data recently published by the Organization of Economic Cooperation and Development reported that 24% of adult females were obese in 2014 [2]. According to Statistics Canada, since 2003, there has been an increase in female obesity from 14.5% to 18.7%, whereas the rate of overweight women remained stable at 27.5% [3]. In the United States, the prevalence of overweight and obesity is substantially greater, with more than a third of the adult population classified as obese, of which 34.4% are women of reproductive age [4]. It had been previously reported that maternal obesity is associated with pregnancy complications [5–11] such as gestational diabetes mellitus (GDM), hypertensive disorders, fetal overgrowth, and labor complications. The Institute of Medicine (IOM) issued recommendations regarding gestational weight gain (GWG) in 1990, which were revised almost two decades later, in 2009 [12]. These guidelines do not differentiate between classes of obesity, and recommend GWG of 11 to 20 lb. (5–9 kg) for women with a singleton gestation and body mass index (BMI) of 30 kg/m^2 and above (Tab. 15.1). These recommendations also do not advocate for gestational weight loss, although it is stated that further research is needed.

Tab. 15.1: Recommendations for total and rate of weight gain in pregnancy.

Prepregnancy BMI		Total weight gain (range in kg)	Total weight gain (range in lb.)	Rates of weight gain in second and third trimester (mean kg/week)	Rates of weight gain in second and third trimester (mean kg/week)
Underweight	<18.5 kg/m^2	12.5–18	28–40	0.51	1
Normal weight	18.5–24.9 kg/m^2	11.5–16	25–35	0.42	1
Overweight	25–29.9 kg/m^2	7–11.5	15–25	0.28	0.6
Obese	≥30 kg/m^2	5–9	11–20	0.22	0.5

Note: Adapted from Institute of Medicine [12] “Weight gain during pregnancy: reexamining the guidelines”.

https://doi.org/10.1515/9783110487817-015

15.2 Gestational weight loss among obese patients

The question remains whether gestational weight loss (GWL) may reduce maternal and neonatal complications among obese parturients. To answer this question, a causal relationship (rather than merely an association) between obesity and pregnancy complications must be demonstrated. If this is the case, losing weight to reduce complications would have a biological plausibility. The pivotal study of Villamor and Cnattingius [13] lends support to this claim, as they studied the effect of interpregnancy weight change on pregnancy complications in more than 150,000 women, in which each woman served as her own control during two consecutive pregnancies. They found that compared with women who had minimal BMI change, those who gained three BMI points or more had a higher prevalence of preeclampsia, gestational hypertension, GDM, cesarean deliveries (CD) and large-for-gestational age neonate (LGA, birth weight >90% centile). This study demonstrated that higher BMI underlies pregnancy complications, thus preconception weight reduction may be associated with decreased risk. However, will weight reduction during pregnancy be associated with the same risk reduction? Beyerlein et al. [14] performed a retrospective cohort study of more than 700,000 deliveries to evaluate the association between GWL and pregnancy outcomes stratified by BMI category. They found that the proportion of women with GWL increased with increasing BMI. They also found that GWL was associated with approximately 40% lower risk for preeclampsia and 25% to 35% lower risk for LGA among class 2 and 3 obese patients, and a 25% to 35% lower risk for nonscheduled CD among overweight and class 1 and 3 obese patients. Additionally, GWL was associated with preterm delivery (PTD) among normal-weight and overweight women (adjusted odds ratio (aOR) 2.7 and 1.4, respectively), and with small-for gestational age (SGA) infants among all but the class 3 obese patients. They concluded that the association of GWL with a decreased risk of pregnancy complications seems to be outweighed by increased risks of prematurity and SGA in all but obese class 3 mothers. Another retrospective cohort study published by Bogaerts and associates [15] investigated the effect of GWL on pregnancy outcomes. They included only live births at term, reaching a cohort of more than 510,000 women. They calculated the risk of adverse outcomes by GWL categories (e.g., greater GWL, 5 kg or more; lesser GWL, 0–5 kg) in each class of obesity, adjusted for parity, gestational age, and maternal age. In their cohort, 4.7% of women lost weight during pregnancy. Similar to the findings of Beyerlien et al. discussed previously, they too reported that the higher the BMI, the greater the proportion of women with GWL—3.2% in the obesity class 1 category, 7% in the obesity class 2 category, and 13.4% in the obesity class 3 category ($p = 0.003$). GWL was found to be associated with decreased incidence of gestational hypertension among obese class 1 patients (aOR 0.31 and 0.46 for greater than 5 kg GWL and 0–5 kg GWL, respectively), lower risk of emergency CD among obese class 2 patients (aOR 0.24 and 0.50 for greater than 5 kg GWL and 0–5 kg GWL, respectively), and a lower rate of macrosomia and LGA in all obese patients (ranging from aOR 0.15 to aOR 0.79). Contrary to Beyerlein's study, they did not find an association between GWL and SGA. Yet, because only term deliveries were included, they could not examine the prevalence of PTD among the GWL population.

A population-based cohort study by Marie Blomberg [16] aimed at estimating whether GWL or low GWG according to the 2009 IOM recommendations among obese patients was associated with adverse outcomes. She also found the same association between BMI and proportion of women with GWL: with 4.1%, 7.9%, and 14.6% experiencing GWL in the obesity classes 1, 2, and 3 categories, respectively. The results of this study demonstrated that GWL was associated with a decreased risk for CD (OR 0.76, 95% CI 0.65–0.89; OR 0.66, 95% CI 0.54–0.82; and OR 0.77, 95% CI 0.60–0.99 for obesity classes 1, 2, and 3, respectively) and LGA (OR 0.73, 95% CI 0.58–0.92;

Outcome	Number of studies	Adjusted OR (95% CI)	I^2(%)
Primary Outcomes			
SGA (<10th percentile)	5	1.76 (1.45, 2.14)	56
LGA (>90th percentile)	5	0.57 (0.52, 0.62)	0
Secondary Outcomes			
Macrosomia (>4000 g & >4500 g)	2	0.58 (0.38, 0.89)	0
LGA (>97th percentile)	1	0.64 (0.54, 0.76)	NA
Cesarean birth	3	0.73 (0.67, 0.80)	0
Shoulder dystocia	1	0.82 (0.49, 1.37)	NA
Preeclampsia	1	0.82 (0.66, 1.02)	NA
Gestational diabetes mellitus	1	0.88 (0.62, 1.25)	NA
Induction of labor	1	0.92 (0.73, 1.15)	NA
Postpartum hemorrhage	2	0.93 (0.78, 1.12)	0
NICU admission	2	0.98 (0.81, 1.19)	0
Operative vaginal delivery	2	1.06 (0.83, 1.37)	43
Apgar score (<7 at 5 minutes)	2	1.08 (0.81, 1.44)	0
Fetal distress	1	1.12 (0.63, 1.98)	NA
SGA (<3rd percentile)	2	1.62 (1.19, 2.20)	0
Low birth weight (<2500 g)	1	1.68 (1.10, 2.57)	NA

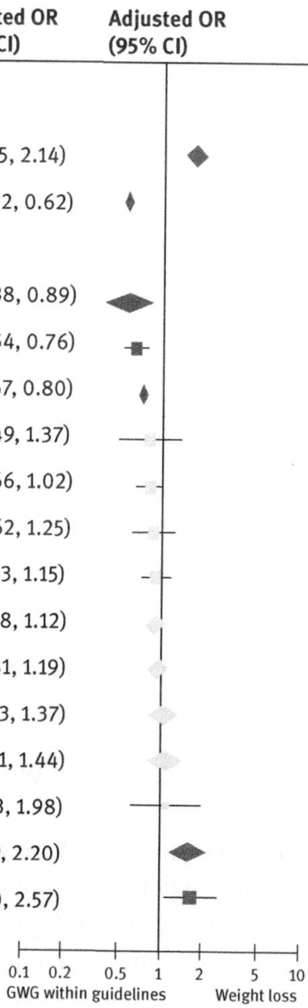

Fig. 15.1: Adapted from Kapadia et al. [18] "Weight loss instead of weight gain within the guidelines in obese women during pregnancy: a systematic review and meta-analyses of maternal and infant outcomes".

OR 0.54, 95% CI 0.40–0.72; and OR 0.64, 95% CI 0.46–0.90 for obesity classes 1, 2, and 3, respectively), with an increased risk for SGA (OR 2.14, 95% CI 1.56–2.95; and OR 2.34, 95% CI 1.15–4.76 for obesity classes 1 and 3, respectively). This study did not report gestational age at delivery.

Contrary to these findings, Durie et al. [17] studied the effect of GWG and GWL in a retrospective cohort study of approximately 74,000 women. In their cohort, 1.5% of women experienced weight loss. Net weight loss was not associated with a reduction in the risk of CD, LGA, or GDM, nor with SGA.

In 2015, Kapadia and associates [18] published a systematic review and meta-analysis regarding weight loss during pregnancy among obese women. Their meta-analysis included six trials, all of which were retrospective cohort studies. They concluded that GWL was associated with a lower risk of LGA (aOR 0.57, 95% CI 0.52–0.62), macrosomia (aOR 0.58, 95% CI 0.58–0.89), and CD (aOR 0.73, 95% CI 0.67–0.80). They also found that GWL translated to a higher of SGA (aOR 1.76, 95% CI 1.45–2.14) (Fig. 15.1).

15.3 Gestational weight loss in GDM patients

As for GDM and GWL, only limited data exist. Katon and colleagues [19] evaluated the effect of losing weight among overweight and obese individuals after the diagnosis of GDM. Their cohort included only 322 women, but almost 20% lost weight during their pregnancy. They reported that GWL was associated with lower birth weight among overweight but not obese mothers. A larger retrospective cohort study aimed to investigate the association of GWL among the overweight and obese patients diagnosed with GDM [20]. The study population consisted of more than 26,000 women with GDM with BMI of ≥25 kg/m^2, of which 5.2% experienced GWL. Overweight and obese patients with GWL experienced less CD (aOR 0.86, 95% CI 0.75–0.98), macrosomia (aOR 0.66, 95% CI 0.53–0.83), LGA (0.63, 95% CI 0.52–0.77), and NICU admissions (aOR 0.51, 95% CI 0.27–0.95) with the cost being a higher risk for PTD prior to 34 weeks of gestation (aOR 1.71, 95% CI 1.23–2.37) and SGA (aOR 1.69, 95% CI 1.32–2.17).

15.4 Risks of gestational weight loss

According to these studies, GWL is associated with a decreased risk for certain outcomes, with the cost of increasing the risk of SGA, and perhaps PTD. Yet, we need to ask ourselves two important questions: first, is GWL associated with a potential harm other than potential SGA and PTD? Second, are interventions aimed at reducing weight during pregnancy effective? The 2009 IOM guidelines summarized the risks of fasting in pregnancy [12]. Reviewing the evidence, a pregnant woman is more prone to develop ketonuria and ketonemia during prolonged fasting of 12 to 18 h as the result of physiological changes that occur during pregnancy, and this tendency increases among diabetic patients. Because most interventions and dietary plans consist of regular calories intake, usually with primary and secondary meals, the risk of prolonged fasting in this setting, resulting in ketonuria or ketonemia, is minimal.

15.5 Interventions aimed at reducing weight in pregnancy

As for the second question, Dodd and colleagues [21] performed a randomized trial aimed at determining the effect of dietary and lifestyle interventions during pregnancy on the outcomes of pregnancies among overweight and obese women. They recruited more than 2,000 patients between 10 and 20 weeks' gestation, with BMI of 25 kg/m^2 and above, half of whom received consultation regarding their lifestyle and dietary habits. Although no difference was detected in the rate of LGA infants, the risk of birth weight exceeding 4,000 g was significantly lower in the intervention group (adjusted relative risk 0.82, 95% CI 0.68–0.99). They calculated that 28 women needed to receive the intervention to prevent one case of macrosomia. Thangaratinam and associates [22] performed a systematic review regarding interventions to reduce or prevent obesity in pregnant women. In their review, they included 88 studies, of which 40 were randomized and 48 nonrandomized, regarding interventions aiming at weight reduction among overweight and obese gravidas. Interventions were demonstrated to result in approximately 1 kg less of GWG, less preeclampsia (RR 0.74, 95% CI 0.59–0.92) and shoulder dystocia (RR 0.39, 95% CI 0.22–0.70), with no differences in SGA or other adverse maternal, fetal, or neonatal outcomes. The authors concluded that dietary and lifestyle interventions result in less GWG and pregnancy complications, yet the included studies varied greatly in their design, interventions, compliance, and more. Additionally, this study did not specifically report the risks or benefits of GWL per se. Furber and colleagues [23] summarized the lack of evidence regarding GWL in obese women in the conclusion of their Cochrane review: "There are no trials designed to reduce weight in obese pregnant women. Until the safety of weight loss in obese pregnant women can be established, there can be no practice recommendations for these women to intentionally lose weight during the pregnancy period. Further study is required to explore the potential benefits, or harm, of weight loss in pregnancy when obese before weight loss interventions in pregnancy can be designed. Qualitative research is also required to explore dietary habits of obese pregnant women, especially those who are morbidly obese".

15.6 Conclusion

In conclusion, gestational weight loss is more frequent as maternal BMI increases. Gestational weight loss may have benefits such as lower rate of macrosomia, LGA, and the need for a cesarean delivery, yet it may also be associated with SGA and PTD.

It is not clear whether interventions specifically aimed at reducing weight in pregnancy will have a benefit concerning pregnancy outcomes. Additional research is needed to elucidate the exact association between gestational weight loss and pregnancy outcomes and the value of intervention programs.

Bibliography

[1] WHO. Obesity and overweight. http://www.who.int/mediacentre/factsheets/fs311/en/. Published 2016. Accessed November 11, 2016.

[2] OECD. OECD Health Statistics 2016. http://www.oecd.org/health/health-data.htm. Published 2016. Accessed November 11, 2016.

[3] Overweight and obese adults. Statistics Canada 82–625–X. http://www.statcan.gc.ca/pub/82–625–x/2015001/article/14185–eng.htm. Published 2016. Accessed November 11, 2016.

[4] Ogden CL, Carroll MD, Fryar CD, Flegal KM. Prevalence of obesity among adults and youth: United States, 2011–2014. NCHS Data Brief 2015;(219):1–8. http://www.ncbi.nlm.nih.gov/pubmed/26633046.

[5] Reece EA. Perspectives on obesity, pregnancy and birth outcomes in the United States: the scope of the problem. Am J Obstet Gynecol 2008;198(1):23–7. doi:10.1016/j.ajog.2007.06.076.

[6] Sebire NJ, Jolly M, Harris JP, Wadsworth J, Joffe M, Beard RW, Regan L, Robinson S. Maternal obesity and pregnancy outcome: a study of 287,213 pregnancies in London. Int J Obes Relat Metab Disord 2001;25(8):1175–82. doi:10.1038/sj.ijo.0801670.

[7] Aviram A, Yogev Y. The association between maternal obesity and hypertensive disease in pregnancy. In: Sheiner E, Yogev Y, eds. Controversies in preeclampsia. New York: Nova Science Publishers, Inc.; 2014:85–98.

[8] Aviram A, Yogev Y. Ask the experts: risks of obesity to pregnancy and fetal health. In: Sheiner E, Yogev Y, eds. Obesity & pregnancy. London: Future Medicine, Ltd.; 2014. http://www.futuremedicine.com/doi/pdf/10.2217/9781780843667#page=27. Accessed November 2, 2014.

[9] Aviram A, Hod M, Yogev Y. Maternal obesity: implications for pregnancy outcome and long-term risks-a link to maternal nutrition. Int J Gynaecol Obstet 2011;115 Suppl:S6–10. doi:10.1016/S0020–7292(11)60004–0.

[10] Yogev Y, Catalano PM. Pregnancy and obesity. Obstet Gynecol Clin North Am 2009;36(2):285–300, viii. doi:10.1016/j.ogc.2009.03.003.

[11] Doherty DA, Magann EF, Francis J, Morrison JC, Newnham JP. Pre-pregnancy body mass index and pregnancy outcomes. Int J Gynecol Obstet 2006;95(3):242–7. doi:10.1016/j.ijgo.2006.06.021.

[12] IOM (Institute of Medicine). Weight gain during pregnancy: reexamining the guidelines. Washington, DC: The National Academies Press, 2009.

[13] Villamor E, Cnattingius S. Interpregnancy weight change and risk of adverse pregnancy outcomes: a population-based study. Lancet 2006;368(9542):1164–70. doi: 10.1016/S0140–6736(06)69473–7.

[14] Beyerlein A, Schiessl B, Lack N, Von Kries R. Associations of gestational weight loss with birth-related outcome: a retrospective cohort study. BJOG 2011;118(1):55–61. doi:10.1111/j.1471–0528.2010.02761.x.

[15] Bogaerts A, Ameye L, Martens E, Devlieger R. Weight loss in obese pregnant women and risk for adverse perinatal outcomes. Obstet Gynecol 2015;125(3):566–75. doi:10.1097/AOG.0000000000000677.

[16] Blomberg M. Maternal and neonatal outcomes among obese women with weight gain below the new Institute of Medicine recommendations. Obstet Gynecol 2011;117(5):1065–70. doi:10.1097/AOG.0b013e318214f1d1.
[17] Durie DE, Thornburg LL, Glantz JC. Effect of second-trimester and third-trimester rate of gestational weight gain on maternal and neonatal outcomes. Obstet Gynecol 2011;118(3):569–75. doi:10.1097/AOG.0b013e3182289f42.
[18] Kapadia MZ, Park CK, Beyene J, Giglia L, Maxwell C, McDonald SD. Weight loss instead of weight gain within the guidelines in obese women during pregnancy: a systematic review and meta-analyses of maternal and infant outcomes. PLoS One 2015;10(7):1–22. doi:10.1371/journal.pone.0132650.
[19] Katon J, Reiber G, Williams MA, Yanez D, Miller E. Weight loss after diagnosis with gestational diabetes and birth weight among overweight and obese women. Matern Child Health J 2013;17(2):374–83. doi:10.1007/s10995-012-1044-5.
[20] Yee LM, Cheng YW, Inturrisi M, Caughey AB. Gestational weight loss and perinatal outcomes in overweight and obese women subsequent to diagnosis of gestational diabetes mellitus. Obesity (Silver Spring) 2013;21(12):E770–4. doi:10.1002/oby.20490.
[21] Dodd JM, Turnbull D, McPhee AJ, Deussen AR, Grivell RM, Yelland LN, Crowther C a, Wittert G, Owens JA, Robinson JS. Antenatal lifestyle advice for women who are overweight or obese: LIMIT randomised trial. Br Med J 2014;348(February):g1285. doi:10.1136/bmj.g1285.
[22] Thangaratinam S, Rogozińska E, Jolly K, Glinkowski S, Duda W, Borowiack E, Roseboom T, Tomlinson J, Walczak J, Kunz R, Mol BW, Coomarasamy A, Khan KS. Interventions to reduce or prevent obesity in pregnant women: a systematic review. Health Technol Assess 2012;16(31):iii–191. doi:10.3310/hta16310.
[23] Furber CM, McGowan L, Bower P, Kontopantelis E, Quenby S, Lavender T. Antenatal interventions for reducing weight in obese women for improving pregnancy outcome. Cochrane Database Syst Rev 2013;(1):CD009334. doi:10.1002/14651858.CD009334.pub2.

Sepand Alavifard, Minakshi Shukla and Rohan D'Souza

16 Obesity and hypertension

16.1 Introduction

Obesity and hypertension are two growing health concerns facing contemporary obstetric practice. The prevalence of obesity, defined as prepregnancy body mass index (BMI) of ≥30 kg/m^2, is increasing and now affects more than 30% of reproductive-aged women in the United States. The prevalence of preexisting hypertension among pregnant women is similarly increasing, and now affects up to 5% of pregnancies (of which 30%–35% are also complicated by obesity) [1]. Even in industrialized countries, hypertension is the leading cause of maternal mortality and accounts for 16% of maternal deaths [2]. With the increase in prevalence of both obesity and chronic hypertension, as well as the increase in other comorbidities such as pregestational diabetes and renal disease that is seen in this group of women, the management of the obese hypertensive pregnant patient has become one of the biggest challenges for an obstetrician [1, 3]. This chapter aims to outline the pathophysiology and mechanisms that could explain the relationship between obesity and hypertension in the obstetric setting, describe the maternal and fetal/neonatal concerns specific to the hypertensive obese patient, and suggest management strategies based on published evidence.

16.2 Epidemiology

When compared with men, premenopausal (nonobese) women are relatively protected against developing hypertension due to the effects of estrogen. However, this is not the case with obese premenopausal women who seem to be at a considerably higher risk of developing hypertension compared with age-matched obese men [4].

In addition, there is strong epidemiological evidence showing an association between prepregnancy obesity and the development of hypertensive disorders of pregnancy (HDPs) (Tab. 16.1) [3]. In a study of singleton pregnancies among women without prepregnancy chronic disease, the relative risk of HDP in women with Class I, Class II, and Class III obesity (Tab. 16.2) was 2.34 (95% confidence intervals (CI) 2.20–2.49), 2.78 (95% CI 2.56–3.01), and 3.55 (95% CI 3.26–3.86), respectively [5].

https://doi.org/10.1515/9783110487817-016

Tab. 16.1: Hypertensive disorders of pregnancy [37].

Type	Definition
Chronic hypertension	Hypertension[a] that predates pregnancy
Gestational hypertension	Hypertension after 20 weeks of gestation (in absence of preeclampsia)
Preeclampsia-eclampsia	Hypertension and proteinuria[b] or, in the absence of proteinuria, new-onset hypertension with the new onset of any of the following: thrombocytopenia (platelet ≤100,000/μL), impaired liver function (elevated blood levels of liver transaminases to twice the normal concentration), the new development of renal insufficiency (elevated serum creatinine >1.1 mg/dL or a doubling of serum creatinine in the absence of other renal disease), pulmonary edema, or new-onset cerebral or visual disturbances
Preeclampsia superimposed on chronic hypertension	Chronic hypertension in association with preeclampsia

[a] Systolic blood pressure ≥140 mmHg and diastolic blood pressure ≥90 mmHg.
[b] Defined as ≥300 mg per 24-h urine collection (or this amount extrapolated from a timed collection or protein/creatinine ratio (each measured as ≥0.3 mg/DL) and dipstick reading of 1+ (used only if other quantitative methods are not available).

Tab. 16.2: Classes of obesity [15].

Class	BMI (kg/m²)
Class I	30–34.9
Class II	35–39.9
Class III	≥40

Although obesity has been shown to be an independent risk factor for both gestational hypertension (adjusted odds ratio (aOR) 2.91; 95% CI 2.76–3.07) [6, 7] and preeclampsia (aOR 3.16; 95% CI 2.96–3.35) [8], a Norwegian cohort study suggests that obesity is a stronger predictor of gestational hypertension than of preeclampsia [9]. In addition, although the reasons remain unknown, there is evidence to suggest that obese multiparous women are at a higher risk for preeclampsia when compared with multiparous women of normal BMI, a relationship which is absent when comparing obese primigravida to their normal-weight counterparts [6].

16.3 Pathophysiology

The relationship between obesity and hypertension is multifactorial, with diet, genetics, epigenetics, and environmental factors described as contributors. For example, obesity-associated hypertension can develop due to lack of exercise, development of insulin residence, pathology of the sympathetic nervous system, dysfunction of the renin-angiotensin-aldosterone system, kidney damage, and inappropriate activation of immune and inflammatory pathways [4, 6].

Although there is strong epidemiological evidence associating obesity and HDPs, conclusive cellular and molecular mechanisms are yet to be proposed. A number of hypotheses have been proposed:

A. A proinflammatory state – There is evidence to suggest that the increase in the body's adipose content triggers a number of inflammatory pathways in the white adipose tissue, plasma, and the placenta. The proinflammatory state of obesity has been thought to be the underlying mechanism behind the association of obesity and gestational hypertension and preeclampsia [10].
B. Cytokines – Tumor necrosis factor-α (TNF-α) and interleukin 6 (IL-6): TNF-α is a vital contributor to trophoblast implantation as well as placental development. It is hypothesized that variation in the levels of TNF-α in obesity compromise placental vasculature, lead to shallow trophoblast implantation of spiral arteries, and jeopardize fetal-placental circulation and therefore may play a role in the development of preterm preeclampsia [11]. Adipose tissue is an important contributor to circulating levels of IL-6, another cytokine that may explain the increased risk of preeclampsia among the obese population. IL-6 is found at higher levels in both obese patients and those with preeclampsia. With IL-6 playing a role in inflammation-induced vascular damage, higher levels in obese patients may alter placental wall function leading to preeclampsia [12].
C. Fetal size – Obese women have higher numbers of large-for-gestational age (LGA) babies [11, 13]. Increased fetal size creates a mismatch between the fetal demand on the placenta and the placental supply thereby resulting in uteroplacental ischemia, which may contribute to the increased risk of preeclampsia [13]. Therefore, the association between obesity and preeclampsia may be mediated by the higher risk of carrying an LGA fetus.

16.4 The effect of obesity and hypertension on pregnant women and their offspring

In addition to the increased odds of developing gestational hypertension [7] and preeclampsia [14], and higher rates of cesarean deliveries [5], the obese hypertensive patient is at increased risk for short-term and long-term adverse outcomes in their offspring. The relationship between obesity, hypertension, and offspring health is complex. Prepregnancy obesity is commonly associated with an increased risk of high birth weight (>4,000 g; OR 2.00; 95% CI 1.94–2.18) and fetal macrosomia (>4,500 g; 3.23; 95% CI 2.39–4.37) [3]. Indeed, when compared with women with normal BMI, the relative risk of having an LGA baby increases from 1.52 (1.45–1.58) for overweight women to 2.32 (2.14–2.52) for those with Class III obesity [5]. Yet, obese women with hypertension exhibit varying degrees of placental insufficiency resulting in reduced placental vascularity and blood flow, putting them at an increased risk for developing superimposed preeclampsia, fetal growth restriction, preterm delivery, placental abruption, transient tachypnea of the newborn, sepsis, and intensive care unit admission [1, 5, 11]. These sometimes opposing signals regulating placental function may contribute to the diversity of short-term and long-term outcomes observed in offspring born to pregnant obese women.

Maternal adipokines such as IL-6, TNF-α, leptin, and adiponectin link maternal adipose tissue metabolism to placental function and along with metabolic hormones have a direct effect on placental function by modulating placental nutrient transport. Nutrient delivery to the fetus, which is regulated by a complex interaction including insulin signaling, cytokine profile and insulin responsiveness, modulated by adiponectin and IL-1β could explain, at least in part, some of the fetal growth effects seen in these pregnancies.

In addition to the development of pregnancy complications, changes in placental function seen in obese patients may also be involved in linking maternal obesity to long-term health risks in the infant, including obesity and metabolic disease and making them susceptible to neuropsychiatric and cognitive disorders in later life [11].

16.5 Management strategies

16.5.1 The prepregnancy period

Although weight-control interventions during pregnancy have some effect on reducing maternal and offspring complications, this effect is limited. It is therefore recommended that the focus for intervention should move to the preconception and postpartum periods [15]. Most of the health professionals surveyed in the United Kingdom thought the onus for prepregnancy management should be on primary health care providers; however, the primary care professionals felt they were seldom involved in preconception care. Given that most women do not actively seek the help of health care providers in this regard, while planning pregnancies, it has been suggested that prepregnancy management should involve a broader social movement that generates bottom-up mobilization of communities and individuals to create demand, coupled with a top-down approach from policy initiatives to provide supply of services. However, there are no current guidelines to suggest which preconception health programs and interventions are of benefit to women and their infants, and a Cochrane systematic review was not able to make any recommendations as no randomized trials were identified [16]. The implementation of preconception interventions in practice is challenging and constitutes the biggest gap in evidence with regard to the management of obesity and hypertension. In an attempt to address this gap, an integrated approach comprising pregnancy prevention, planning, and preparation, involving more than the primary health care sector and adopting an ecological approach to risk reduction that addresses personal, societal, and cultural influences has been suggested [15]. Based on behavioral theory that individual capacity to act and community empowerment have a reciprocal relation, with empowered communities creating empowered citizens and vice versa, the focus should move to mobilizing communities and individuals to create a demand for obesity prevention policies and better access to good food for women of childbearing age. A community that generates consensus puts pressure on politicians to respond to voters and on commercial organizations to cater to their customers. Community mobilization, identification of political opportunities, definition of common goals, followed by sustained collective action to generate popular demand for policies and political actions that support preconception health and address the challenge of obesity, has been suggested as the only true way of meeting the challenge of prepregnancy reduction of weight-control interventions.

Until this is achieved, the following interventions have been recommended in the prepregnancy period from a practical point of view:

A. Lifestyle interventions for weight control – These include interventions based on diet, physical activity, and a combination of both. Women with a BMI higher than 35 are recommended to obtain advice from a dietician. Compliance with diet and physical activity is better prior to pregnancy than during pregnancy and novel web-based platforms have shown high compliance and usability, with users showing improvements in dietary and lifestyle behaviors [17].
B. Medical interventions – Obese women enter pregnancy in a state of increased insulin resistance, which raises the possibility that drugs such as metformin could be used as adjunct therapy to improve insulin sensitivity and the pattern of fetal growth. However, randomized trials in obese women without preexisting diabetes have not shown a beneficial effect on the development of gestational diabetes, gestational weight gain, or adverse fetal/neonatal outcomes.
C. Invasive procedures – Bariatric surgery comprises surgical weight-loss methods, the most common of which include Roux-en-Y gastric bypass (malabsorptive), sleeve gastrectomy (restrictive), and adjustable gastric banding (restrictive) [18, 19].

Epidemiological evidence suggests that bariatric surgery reduces the risk of obese women developing HDPs, including preeclampsia, by as much as 75% after bariatric surgery [20–23]. A meta-analysis similarly showed that bariatric surgery could reduce the risk of preeclampsia by one half (OR 0.45; 95% CI 0.25–0.80). The relationship was maintained in subgroup analysis which compared (1) pregnancies with maternal obesity postbariatric surgery to those without bariatric surgery and (2) mothers who have had a pregnancy both before and after bariatric surgery (OR 0.20; 95% CI 0.08–0.51) [24].

Bariatric surgery has also been shown to reduce the risk of developing an LGA fetus (OR 0.40; 95% CI 0.2–0.8) [24, 25]. Due to the hypothesized relationship between LGA and preeclampsia described earlier, this may explain at least part of the reduction in the risk of developing preeclampsia among postbariatric pregnancies. On the other hand, however, there is evidence to suggest an increased risk for small-for-gestational age (SGA) fetuses after bariatric surgery (OR 1.93; 95% CI 1.52–2.44) [24]. Reduced rates of LGA and increased rates of SGA are thought to be associated with poor maternal nutrition status because of postbariatric surgery malabsorption issues, inadequate nutrition, and/or dietary restrictions. Therefore, for obstetrical patients that have previously undergone bariatric surgery, special attention has to be paid to maternal nutrition status as well as fetal growth.

16.5.2 Prepregnancy counseling

Health care providers should seize the opportunity to discuss the above strategies for weight loss prior to planning a conception. In addition, the following routine advice is extremely relevant in the context of obesity and hypertension:

A. Assessment of baseline renal and cardiac function – In women with long-standing chronic hypertension of five or more years, an echocardiogram should be performed to assess global heart function as well as left ventricular function [1]. It is also good practice to establish baseline renal function, including assessment for proteinuria and serum creatinine levels.
B. Optimization of blood pressure (BP) and antihypertensive medications – All medications should be reviewed and consideration should be given to discontinuing medications that are potentially teratogenic such as angiotensin-converting enzyme inhibitors, angiotensin receptor blockers, renin inhibitors, and mineralocorticoid receptor antagonists unless there is compelling reason such as the presence of proteinuric renal disease. Stopping these medications could result in the deterioration of renal function and a consultation with a nephrologist and a maternal-fetal specialist to discuss the pros and cons of continuing these medications versus using alternate medications such as labetalol, nifedipine, and methyldopa, should be encouraged. Time should be allowed for optimizing BP on the new medications prior to planning conception.
C. Folic acid supplementation – Given the higher rates of congenital malformations in obese patients and some suggestion that hypertension might increase the risk further, folic acid supplementation should be commenced at least 3 months prior to planning a conception.

16.5.3 The antepartum period

Management in the antepartum period involves the following:

16.5.3.1 Weight management in pregnancy

Although obese women have increased odds of developing gestational hypertension regardless of gestational weight gain [26], a prospective population-based cohort study of

245,526 singleton term pregnancies in Sweden showed that obese women with low gestational weight gain (<8 kg) had lower odds of developing preeclampsia (aOR 0.52; 95% CI 0.42–0.62), cesarean sections (0.81, 0.73–0.90), instrumental deliveries (0.75, 0.63–0.88), and LGA births (0.66, 0.59–0.75) [27]. Systematic reviews and meta-analyses have suggested that interventions in pregnancy are successful in reducing gestational weight gain (0.97 kg, 0.34–1.6 kg), the risk of preeclampsia (RR 0.74, 0.59–0.92), and shoulder dystocia (RR 0.39, 0.22–0.70) [28]. Dietary interventions are the most effective, also resulting in a reduction in the risk of gestational hypertension (RR 0.30, 0.10–0.88) and preterm birth (RR 0.68, 0.48–0.96). The effect of diet and physical activity in pregnancy on gestational weight gain is consistent irrespective of BMI category and has a positive effect on clinical outcomes including cesarean section rates and the outcomes of labor induction. There is no evidence of harm as a result of dietary and physical activity based interventions in pregnancy.

A substantial body of published work identifies the components of effective diet and lifestyle interventions, but the challenge is in engaging pregnant women to improve their diets and lifestyles. However, it must be remembered that the effect of interventions in pregnancy is still more limited than lifestyle interventions instituted in the preconceptual period [15]. Although highly motivated at this point of time, women cite physical inconvenience, the limitations of being pregnant, and the lack of time for noncompliance with interventions, especially physical activity during pregnancy [29]. The use of web-based platforms [17] to promote diet and lifestyle improvement could show promise in pregnancy too.

16.5.3.2 Pharmacology

(A) *Metformin* – As mentioned earlier, although metformin should theoretically improve insulin sensitivity and result in improved pregnancy outcomes, randomized trials in obese women without preexisting diabetes do not show a beneficial effect on the development of gestational diabetes, gestational weight gain, or fetal/neonatal outcomes [15].

(B) *Probiotics* – Probiotics have been suggested because of their potential beneficial effects on the gut microbiome, resulting in modification of lipopolysaccharides and insulin sensitivity. The results of a randomized trial suggested that probiotic administration from the first trimester until the end of breast-feeding alongside dietary intervention helped to reduce the development of gestational diabetes in these women [30]; however, these findings have not been replicated in other studies. A more recent randomized trial did not show any improvement in glycemic status following a 4-week course of probiotics [31].

(C) *Multivitamins* – A study conducted by Griffith University, Australia that included 2,261 lean, overweight, and obese women as part of the Environments for Healthy Living Project showed that first trimester multivitamin/mineral use was associated with a 62% (95% CI 16%–92%) reduced risk of developing preeclampsia among obese women [32]. The study concluded that multivitamins may be beneficial in reducing the incidence of preeclampsia in general, and especially in women that are overweight and obese. It must be noted, however, that these findings were specific to the Australian population studied and may not be generalizable in other settings.

(D) *Low-dose aspirin* – Chronic hypertension and BMI >30 are both independent risk factors for developing preeclampsia (Tab. 16.3) and warrant the initiation of low-dose aspirin prior to 16 weeks of gestation to prevent preeclampsia and other placentally mediated problems in pregnancy [33, 34].

Tab. 16.3: Screening for preeclampsia before 16 weeks of gestation based on clinical risk factors (from D'Souza and Kingdom [38]).

Major risk factors	Moderate risk factors
– Prior preeclampsia – Known antiphospholipid syndrome – Known type 1 or type 2 diabetes mellitus – Chronic hypertension – Assisted reproductive therapy in the current pregnancy – Prepregnancy or early first trimester BMI >30 kg/m^2	– Prior placental abruption – Prior stillbirth – Prior fetal intrauterine growth restriction – Maternal age >40 years – Nulliparity – Multifetal pregnancy – Known chronic kidney disease – Known systemic lupus erythematosus
Women should be considered at increased risk for developing preeclampsia if they have one major risk factor, or at least two moderate risk factors	

(E) *Antihypertensive therapy* – As mentioned earlier, consideration should be given to changing potentially teratogenic antihypertensive medications such as angiotensin-converting enzyme inhibitors, angiotensin receptor blockers, renin inhibitors, and mineralocorticoid receptor antagonists to medications such as labetalol, methyldopa, and nifedipine.

16.5.3.3 Maternal and fetal surveillance

This should follow the guidelines set by the American College of Obstetricians and Gynecologists' Hypertension in pregnancy guidelines [37]. A summary of these guidelines include:

(A) Home BP monitoring is suggested for those with chronic hypertension. BP should be maintained between 120 and 160 mmHg systolic and 80 and 105 mmHg diastolic. Antihypertensive medications should be administered if BP is greater than 160 mmHg systolic or 100 mmHg diastolic.

(B) Close monitoring for severe features of HDP (Tab. 16.4) is recommended, with serial assessment of maternal symptoms and daily fetal movement, twice-weekly BP measurement and weekly assessment of platelet counts and liver enzymes.

Tab. 16.4: Severe features of HDP (any of these findings) – from ACOG [37].

– Systolic BP of 160 mmHg or higher or diastolic BP of 110 mmHg or higher on two occasions at least 4 hours apart while the patient is on bed rest
– Thrombocytopenia (platelet count less than 100,000/mL)
– Impaired liver function as indicated by abnormally elevated blood concentrations of liver enzymes (to twice normal concentration), severe persistent right upper quadrant or epigastric pain unresponsive to medication and not accounted for by alternative diagnoses or both
– Progressive renal insufficiency (serum creatinine concentrations greater than 1.1 mg/dL or a doubling of the serum creatinine concentration in the presence of other renal disease)
– Pulmonary edema
– New-onset cerebral or visual disturbance

(C) In the absence of severe features, two to four weekly ultrasound scans to assess fetal growth and well-being should be undertaken. If there is evidence of fetal growth restriction, feto-placental assessment that includes umbilical artery Doppler velocimetry as an adjunct antenatal test is recommended.

(D) The decision to hospitalize for maternal and/or fetal indications should be individualized.

16.5.3.4 The decision to deliver

The decision to deliver should be based on the presence of features of severe hypertension, gestational age, stability of the mother and fetus, and whether or not antenatal corticosteroids have been administered. The amount or change in amount of proteinuria should not be a consideration while planning delivery. In summary,

A. In the presence of gestational hypertension or preeclampsia without severe features, expectant management until 37 weeks is suggested. Beyond 37 weeks, delivery rather than continued observation is suggested, even in the absence of severe features.
B. If the presence of severe features of HDP and those with unstable maternal or fetal condition, delivery is recommended beyond 34 weeks, soon after maternal stabilization.
C. Under 34 weeks, with stable maternal and fetal conditions, it is recommended that antenatal corticosteroids be administered for fetal lung maturation and continued pregnancy be undertaken only at facilities with adequate maternal and neonatal intensive care resources. In the event of unstable maternal or fetal condition, delivery should be expedited regardless of whether antenatal corticosteroids have been administered.
D. Presence of severe features of HDP prior to fetal viability warrants delivery after maternal stabilization with no attempt at expectant management.

16.5.4 Labor and delivery

The mode of delivery should be determined by fetal gestation, fetal presentation, cervical status, and maternal and fetal conditions. Intrapartum monitoring and anesthesia

– wherever the clinical condition permits, neuraxial analgesia and anesthesia (either spinal or epidural) are recommended. Even with severe features, invasive hemodynamic monitoring is not routinely recommended, and the decision should be individualized. Magnesium sulfate for seizure prophylaxis is only recommended if the BP is >160 mmHg systolic and 110 mmHg diastolic.

16.5.5 The postpartum period

16.5.5.1 Thromboprophylaxis

Both obesity and hypertension are risk factors for postpartum thromboembolism and consideration should be given to thromboprophylaxis after both vaginal and especially cesarean delivery.

16.5.5.2 Monitoring for postpartum preeclampsia

Discharge instructions should be exhaustive and include warning signs for the development of severe features of hypertension. In case of the development of severe features, magnesium sulfate is indicated [37].

16.5.5.3 Lifestyle modifications for weight loss

Contrary to the lack of evidence in the preconception period, there is some evidence to guide lifestyle modifications in the postpartum period. Systematic reviews [35, 36] of randomized trials concluded that postpartum interventions were successful with some suggestion that the combination of diet and physical activity with an element of supervision or professional support was the most effective intervention for weight loss. However, the most effective time during the postpartum period for intervention is unclear as is the point between pregnancies at which weight loss might be most beneficial for the mother and her future offspring.

16.5.5.4 Breast-feeding

Exclusive breast-feeding increases the probability of returning to prepregnancy weight and BMI in the postpartum period, but its effectiveness as a weight-loss strategy postpartum seems to depend on the timing of measurements and whether or not the mother breast-feeds exclusively.

16.5.5.5 Follow up

Given the eight-to-ninefold increased risk for cardiovascular disease in later life, these women should be followed by yearly assessment of BP, lipids, fasting blood sugar, and BMI assessment [37].

Bibliography

[1] Ankumah NE, Sibai BM. Chronic hypertension in pregnancy: diagnosis, management, and outcomes. Clin Obstet Gynecol 2017;60:206–14.
[2] Lozano R, Naghavi M, Foreman K, et al. Global and regional mortality from 235 causes of death for 20 age groups in 1990 and 2010: a systematic analysis for the Global Burden of Disease Study 2010. Lancet 2012;380:2095–128.
[3] Poston L, Caleyachetty R, Cnattingius S, et al. Preconceptional and maternal obesity: epidemiology and health consequences. Lancet Diabetes Endocrinol 2016;4:1025–36.
[4] DeMarco VG, Aroor AR, Sowers JR. The pathophysiology of hypertension in patients with obesity. Nat Rev Endocrinol 2014;10:364+.
[5] Kim SS, Zhu Y, Grantz KL, et al. Obstetric and neonatal risks among obese women without chronic disease. Obstet Gynecol 2016;128:104–12.
[6] Hogan JL, Anglim B, Dwyer VO, Farah N, Stuart B, Turner MJ. Body mass index and hypertensive disorders of pregnancy. Pregnancy Hypertens 2012;2:28.
[7] Shin D, Song WO. Prepregnancy body mass index is an independent risk factor for gestational hypertension, gestational diabetes, preterm labor, and small- and large-for-gestational-age infants. J Matern Fetal Neonatal Med 2015;28:1679–86.
[8] Jalal P, Ensiyeh J. The association between body mass index and preeclampsia: a meta-analysis. J Matern Fetal Neonatal Med 2016;29:3670.
[9] Egeland GM, Klungsøyr K, Øyen N, Tell GS, Næss Ø, Skjærven R. Preconception cardiovascular risk factor differences between gestational hypertension and preeclampsia: Cohort Norway Study. Hypertension 2016;67(6):1173–80.
[10] Stupin JH, Arabin B. Overweight and obesity before, during and after pregnancy. Part 1: Pathophysiology, molecular biology and epigenetic consequences. Geburtshilfe Frauenheilkd 2014;74:639.
[11] Howell KR, Powell TL. Effects of maternal obesity on placental function and fetal development. Reproduction 2017;153:R97–108.
[12] Roberts JM, Bodnar LM, Patrick TE, Powers RW. The role of obesity in preeclampsia. Pregnancy Hypertens 2011;1:6.
[13] Rasmussen S, Irgens LM, Espinoza J. Maternal obesity and excess of fetal growth in pre-eclampsia. BJOG 2014;121:1351–7.
[14] Poorolajal J, Jenabi E. The association between body mass index and preeclampsia: a meta-analysis. J Matern Fetal Neonatal Med 2016;29:3670–6.
[15] Hanson M, Barker M, Dodd JM, et al. Interventions to prevent maternal obesity before conception, during pregnancy, and post partum. Lancet Diabetes Endocrinol 2017;5:65–76.
[16] Opray N, Grivell RM, Deussen AR, Dodd JM. Directed preconception health programs and interventions for improving pregnancy outcomes for women who are overweight or obese. Cochrane Database Syst Rev 2015:CD010932.
[17] Van Dijk MR, Huijgen NA, Willemsen SP, Laven JS, Steegers EA, Steegers-Theunissen RP. Impact of an mHealth platform for pregnancy on nutrition and lifestyle of the reproductive population: a survey. JMIR Mhealth Uhealth 2016;4:e53.
[18] Chevrot A, Kayem G, Coupaye M, Lesage N, Msika S, Mandelbrot L. Impact of bariatric surgery on fetal growth restriction: experience of a perinatal and bariatric surgery center. Am J Obstet Gynecol 2016;214:655.e1–7.
[19] Parker MH, Berghella V, Nijjar JB. Bariatric surgery and associated adverse pregnancy outcomes among obese women. J Matern Fetal Neonatal Med 2016;29:1747–50.

[20] Abenhaim HA, Alrowaily N, Czuzoj-Shulman N, Spence AR, Klam SL. Pregnancy outcomes in women with bariatric surgery as compared with morbidly obese women. J Matern Fetal Neonatal Med 2016;29(22):3596–601.
[21] Badreldin N, Kuller J, Rhee E, Brown L, Laifer S. Pregnancy management after bariatric surgery. Obstet Gynecol Surv 2016;71(6):361–8.
[22] Yi XY, Li QF, Zhang J, Wang ZH. A meta-analysis of maternal and fetal outcomes of pregnancy after bariatric surgery. Int J Gynaecol Obstet 2015;130(1):3–9.
[23] Willis K, Lieberman N, Sheiner E. Pregnancy and neonatal outcome after bariatric surgery. Best Pract Res Clin Obstet Gynaecol 2015;29(1):133–44.
[24] Galazis N, Docheva N, Simillis C, Nicolaides KH. Maternal and neonatal outcomes in women undergoing bariatric surgery: a systematic review and meta-analysis. Eur J Obstet Gynecol Reprod Biol 2014;181:45–53.
[25] Weintraub AY, Levy A, Levi I, Mazor M, Wiznitzer A, Sheiner E. Effect of bariatric surgery on pregnancy outcome. Int J Gynaecol Obstet 2008;103(3):246–51.
[26] Liu Y, Dai W, Dai X, Li Z. Prepregnancy body mass index and gestational weight gain with the outcome of pregnancy: a 13-year study of 292,568 cases in China. Arch Gynecol Obstet 2012;286:905–11.
[27] Cedergren M. Effects of gestational weight gain and body mass index on obstetric outcome in Sweden. Int J Gynaecol Obstet 2006;93:269–74.
[28] Thangaratinam S, Rogozinska E, Jolly K, et al. Interventions to reduce or prevent obesity in pregnant women: a systematic review. Health Technol Assess 2012;16:iii–iv, 1–191.
[29] Oostdam N, van Poppel MN, Wouters MG, et al. No effect of the FitFor2 exercise programme on blood glucose, insulin sensitivity, and birthweight in pregnant women who were overweight and at risk for gestational diabetes: results of a randomised controlled trial. BJOG 2012;119:1098–107.
[30] Luoto R, Laitinen K, Nermes M, Isolauri E. Impact of maternal probiotic-supplemented dietary counselling on pregnancy outcome and prenatal and postnatal growth: a double-blind, placebo-controlled study. Br J Nutr 2010;103:1792–9.
[31] Lindsay KL, Kennelly M, Culliton M, et al. Probiotics in obese pregnancy do not reduce maternal fasting glucose: a double-blind, placebo-controlled, randomized trial (Probiotics in Pregnancy Study). Am J Clin Nutr 2014;99:1432–9.
[32] Vanderlelie J, Scott R, Shibl R, Lewkowicz J, Perkins A, Scuffham PA. First trimester multivitamin/mineral use is associated with reduced risk of pre-eclampsia among overweight and obese women. Matern Child Nutr 2016;12(2):339–48.
[33] Bartsch E, Medcalf K, Park AL, Ray JG, High Risk of Pre-eclampsia Identification Group. Clinical risk factors for pre-eclampsia determined in early pregnancy: systematic review and meta-analysis of large cohort studies. BMJ 2016;353:i1753.
[34] Roberge S, Giguère Y, Villa P, Nicolaides K, Vainio M, Forest JC, von Dadelszen P, Vaiman D, Tapp S, Bujold E. Early administration of low-dose aspirin for the prevention of severe and mild preeclampsia: a systematic review and meta-analysis. Am J Perinatol 2012;29(7):551–6.
[35] Choi J, Fukuoka Y, Lee JH. The effects of physical activity and physical activity plus diet interventions on body weight in overweight or obese women who are pregnant or in postpartum: a systematic review and meta-analysis of randomized controlled trials. Prev Med 2013;56:351–64.
[36] van der Pligt P, Willcox J, Hesketh KD, et al. Systematic review of lifestyle interventions to limit postpartum weight retention: implications for future opportunities to prevent maternal overweight and obesity following childbirth. Obes Rev 2013;14:792–805.
[37] ACOG. Hypertension in pregnancy. Washington, DC: ACOG, 2013
[38] D'Souza R, Kingdom J. Preeclampsia. CMAJ 2016;188:1178.

Ann Kinga Malinowski and Jacqueline Parrish

17 Venous thromboembolism in the obese pregnant patient

17.1 Background and epidemiology

Venous thromboembolism (VTE) remains among the leading causes of maternal mortality in the developed world [1, 2]. VTE can take the form of deep vein thrombosis (DVT), pulmonary embolism (PE) or more rarely, cerebral vein thrombosis (CVT) [2]. Although the third trimester and the first three weeks postpartum convey a higher risk of an event [3, 4], the risk of VTE in the first and second trimesters remains significant [5].

The incidence of VTE in pregnancy stands at 5.4 events/10,000 pregnancies antenatally, 7.2/10,000 peripartum, and 4.3/10,000 postnatally [6]. This converts to a fivefold higher risk of VTE antepartum compared with the nonpregnant state, and a fourfold higher risk of DVT and 15-fold higher risk of PE postpartum as compared with antepartum [7].

The reported mortality rate of pregnancy-related VTE ranges between 0.79 and 1.1 per 100,000 deliveries [2, 8], with the most recent report of the Confidential Enquiries into Maternal Deaths in the UK (CEMD-UK) registering 18 VTE-related deaths (16 following PE and two following CVT) [2], and a Canadian report linking 17% (55 of 324) of maternal deaths between 1981 and 2004 to pregnancy-related PE [9].

VTE in pregnancy is potentially preventable through timely institution of thromboprophylaxis [2], as it is often heralded by readily identifiable risk factors [2, 10]. VTE risk has been noted to be 38% higher after age 35 and 64% higher in the African American population (compared with other races) [8]. Medical conditions were also significantly associated with an increased risk of VTE as follows: hypertension, odds ratio (OR) 1.8; obesity, OR 4.4; sickle cell disease, OR 6.7; heart disease, OR 7.1; lupus, OR 8.7; antiphospholipid antibody syndrome, OR 15.8; previous thrombosis, OR 24.8; and thrombophilia, OR 51.8 (38.7–69.2) [8]. Pregnancy-related factors and complications of pregnancy were likewise shown to increase risk of VTE as follows: multiple gestation, OR 1.6; anemia, OR 2.6; hyperemesis, OR 2.6; disorders of fluid/electrolyte/acid-base balance, OR 4.9; antepartum hemorrhage, OR 2.3; postpartum infection, OR 4.1; postpartum hemorrhage, OR 1.3; transfusion, OR 7.6 [8].

Obesity in particular has been recognized by the most recent report of the CEMD-UK as the principal contributor to the risk of VTE in pregnancy, with 12 of 16 women who died as a result of VTE observed to have an elevated body mass index (BMI) [2]. In a national matched case-control study utilizing the UK Obstetric Surveillance System, 70% of women with antenatal PE had a recognizable risk factor for VTE, with a BMI in the obesity range (>30 kg/m^2) noted in 28% [11]. A recent systematic review found a doubling of risk for VTE in the obese patient (OR of 2.33;

https://doi.org/10.1515/9783110487817-017

95% CI 1.68–2.34) [12]. Additionally, a gradient response for the risk of VTE and obesity has been observed, with morbidly obese patients (BMI >40 kg/m^2) at greater risk than those with a BMI of 30 to 40 kg/m^2 [13]. Furthermore, risk factors seem to have an additive effect on the degree of risk [10].

These findings are all the more concerning given the continued increase in the rate of prepregnancy obesity (BMI >30 kg/m^2) from 13% in 1994 to 22% in 2003 [14], with predictions that as the worldwide prevalence of obesity increases, the incidence of VTE will also increase in parallel [15].

17.2 Pathogenesis of VTE

Virchow's triad (comprised of venous stasis, hypercoagulable blood, and vascular damage) as the evoking mechanism for VTE has been well accepted [16]. The normal, physiological changes of pregnancy have the capacity to affect all three of these domains. Venous stasis is exacerbated with advancing gestation through progesterone-mediated venodilation, venous compression of the pelvic veins by the gravid uterus, and anatomic compression of the left iliac vein by the right iliac artery that crosses it [17]. This latter element explains the preponderance of VTE for the left lower extremity [15, 18]. Additionally, a shift within the coagulation pathway in favor of hypercoagulability is induced in anticipation of blood loss during parturition; reflected by the increase in procoagulant factors (fibrinogen and factors V, IX, X, and VIII), decrease in anticoagulant activity (reduction in protein S and increase in activated protein C resistance), and decrease in fibrinolytic activity (increase in plasminogen activator inhibitor type 1 and 2 and reduction in tissue plasminogen activator), leading to enhanced thrombin generation and diminished clot dissolution [17]. The risk for VTE in light of the hypercoagulable state of pregnancy is further increased in those with congenital or acquired thrombophilia [8]. Finally, vascular damage of pelvic vessels is induced during vaginal delivery, and more so during assisted delivery or cesarean section [17].

In addition to these pregnancy-related alterations, the elements of the Virchow's triad are further affected by obesity. The increased abdominal fat content and chronically elevated intra-abdominal pressure may limit venous return [15] beyond the reduction already exerted by the gravid uterus. Difficulties with mobility and altered gait may result in relative immobility [15], compromising venous return and increasing VTE risk.

Furthermore, the recognition that adipose tissue is highly metabolically active, releasing substances such as interleukin-6, plasminogen activator inhibitor-1, tumor necrosis factor-α, and tissue factor [19], creating proinflammatory, prothrombotic, and hypofibrinolytic effects [10], as well as enhanced oxidative stress and endothelial dysfunction, compounding the risk of a thromboembolic event [20].

17.3 Prevention of VTE in obese pregnant women

Current guidelines recommend that patients at risk for VTE receive prophylactic anticoagulation when the estimated risk of VTE is considered to be greater than 1% [18]. Although obesity alone is not considered an indication for antenatal thromboprophylaxis [18, 21, 22], the compounding effect of multiple risk factors on the risk of VTE must be considered. In particular, the finding by Jacobsen et al. [23] that pregnant women with a BMI of >25 kg/m^2 who were immobilized antenatally had a markedly greater risk of VTE (aOR 62.3; 95% CI 11.5–338.0). Various professional organizations have developed recommendations for thromboprophylaxis against VTE in pregnancy that reflects these considerations [18, 21, 22, 24].

Low-molecular weight heparin (LMWH) has replaced unfractionated heparin (UFH) as the preferred anticoagulation agent in pregnancy [18, 21, 22, 24], as discussed under the section Choice of treatment agent. Table 17.1 delineates the proposed weight-based doses for LMWH prophylaxis. Initial or current pregnancy weight is used for calculation of the prophylactic dose [21]. Although some guidelines recommend absolute prophylactic doses [18], with a caveat that doses may need to be adjusted at extremes of body weight [22, 24], others suggest weight-based dosing [21], given the observation that some obese women who experienced a PE antenatally were receiving prophylactic doses of LMWH recommended for women of lower weight [11]; although these weight-based doses are not evidence-based [21].

Tab: 17.1: Weight-based dosing of LMWH.

Indication	Weight (kg)	Agent (administered subcutaneously)		
		Enoxaparin (mg)	Dalteparin (units)	Tinzaparin (units)
Prophylactic [21]	<50	20 mg daily	2,500 units daily	3,500 units daily
	50–90	40 mg daily	5,000 units daily	4,500 units daily
	91–130	60 mg daily	7,500 units daily	7,000 units daily
	131–170	80 mg daily	10,000 units daily	9,000 units daily
	>170	0.6 mg/kg	75 units/kg daily	75 units/kg daily
Therapeutic [18, 24]		1 mg/kg bid or 1.5 mg/kg daily	200 units/kg daily or 100 units/kg bid	175 units/kg daily

17.4 Clinical manifestations of VTE

A raised index of suspicion for the signs and symptoms of VTE is vital for prompt investigation and management, which may in turn diminish mortality [25]. This aim, however, is hampered by the overlap of the typical symptoms of VTE (particularly leg swelling, dyspnea, tachypnea, and tachycardia), with the nonspecific complaints often reported by individuals experiencing an uncomplicated pregnancy [26], and even more frequently by pregnant obese patients [25], at times resulting in a delay of diagnosis [27].

Unilateral leg swelling and pain (particularly in the left leg) are more suggestive of DVT [28], and may be accompanied by local tenderness and warmth, and sometimes leukocytosis [25]. More specific features, such as recent immobilization, calf asymmetry of ≥3 cm (with calf circumference measured 10 cm below the tibial tuberosity), or swelling of one entire leg [29] should prompt investigation. Likewise, atypical symptoms, including abdominal pain, or isolated pain in the groin, flank, or buttock may also be seen and should not be dismissed, given the higher frequency of isolated iliac vein thrombosis in pregnancy [30]. The most common symptoms of PE include shortness of breath and chest pain, followed by cough, syncope, and hemoptysis [29, 31]. Increased jugular venous pressure and cardiovascular collapse have also been noted [29]. The symptoms of PE may be present in the absence of or in addition to symptoms of DVT [29].

In the absence of a specific contraindication, once suspicion of VTE exists, therapeutic anticoagulation should be initiated pending confirmatory investigations [17].

17.5 Diagnostic modalities

Diagnosis of VTE in pregnancy requires a modification of standard VTE testing, as prediction rules and algorithms are extrapolated from the nonpregnant population and remain unvalidated in pregnancy [17, 18]. Diagnostic VTE algorithms for nonpregnant patients often call for inclusion of a D-dimer level, a marker with high sensitivity, but low specificity [32]. Interestingly, D-dimer levels do not seem to be affected by BMI [33]. However, in the context of pregnancy, the interpretation of D-dimer is hindered by its normal, physiologic increase [34]. Although some suggest the D-dimer may have a role in the evaluation of VTE in pregnancy given its high negative predictive value [35], others caution that further validation is necessary before its incorporation [30]. Current guidelines discourage the use of clinical prediction rules or sole reliance on negative D-dimer results (without objective investigations/imaging) for exclusion of VTE in pregnancy [18].

17.6 Deep vein thrombosis

The approach for the diagnosis of VTE in pregnancy is shown in Fig. 17.1. Compression ultrasound (CUS) of the proximal venous system is the imaging modality of choice for the diagnosis of DVT in pregnancy [30], particularly given its noninvasive nature and the absence of radiation exposure [36]. Ultrasound examination targeted to visualize areas from the iliac vein to the popliteal vein [18, 25, 37], including Doppler assessment of blood flow in the iliac vein (which is noncompressible), is vital given the higher incidence of iliac vein DVT [38]. Although a single CUS negative for DVT has been shown to have a negative predictive value of 98.9% (95% CI 95.5–99.8) in pregnant and postpartum women [36], current recommendations suggest a repeat CUS within 7 days [18]. Where absence of flow is noted in the iliac vein, suggesting obstruction, an MRI could be considered to further delineate the findings [18].

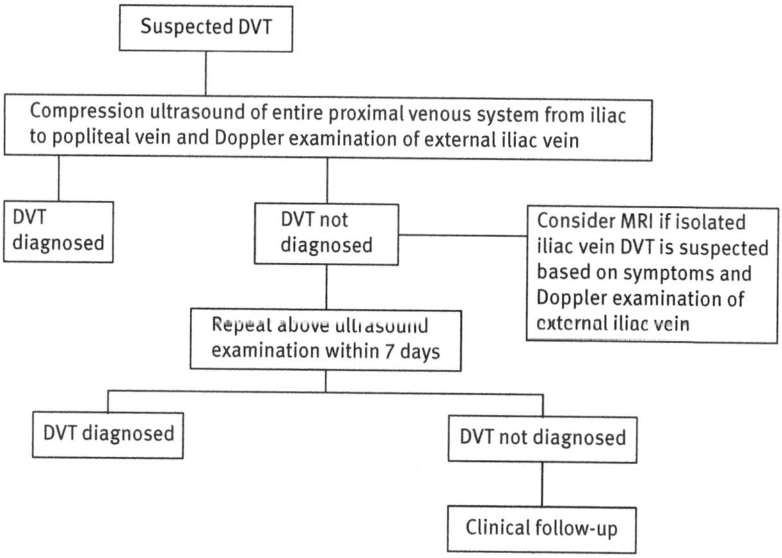

Fig. 17.1: Proposed algorithm for the diagnosis of DVT in pregnant women (from Chan et al. J Obstet Gynaecol Can 2014;36(6):527–53) [18].

17.7 Pulmonary embolism

The approach for the diagnosis of PE in pregnancy is shown in Fig. 17.2. When a PE is suspected based on respiratory symptomatology, evaluation for a DVT should still be carried out [18, 30, 39]. When a DVT is confirmed, therapeutic anticoagulation is indicated as it would be for a PE, and confirmation of a PE may not be necessary, permitting the avoidance of radiation exposure inherent to imaging modalities for the diagnosis of PE [30, 39]. When CUS is negative for DVT or is unavailable, diagnostic imaging in the form of ventilation/perfusion (V/Q) scan or computer tomographic pulmonary angiography (CT-PA) will be required for the diagnosis of PE [18, 39].

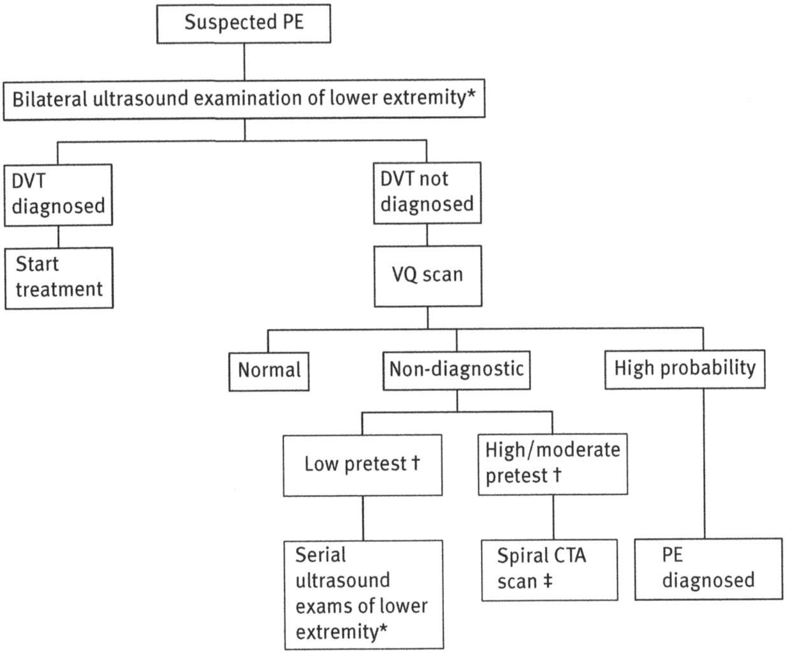

* Bilateral US should include examination of the iliac veins with Doppler manoeuvers
† Pretest determined by clinician's subjective assessment
‡ Modification in spiral CT protocol should be considered for pregnant patients

Fig. 17.2: Proposed algorithm for the diagnosis of PE in pregnant women (from Chan et al. J Obstet Gynaecol Can 2014;36(6):527–53) [18].

The fetal dose of radiation has been reported as 0.01 mGy for CT-PA and 0.12 mGy for the perfusion portion of the V/Q scan; corresponding with estimates of fatal malignancy to 15 years of age of <1/1,000,000 and 1/280,000, respectively [40]. Although CT-PA is advantageous to the fetus, it is worth considering that the levels of fetal radiation for both modalities are well below the accepted safety thresholds, reflect extremely low absolute risks, and are not associated with teratogenicity [41]. In contrast, the radiation dose to the maternal breast has been reported at 10 mGy for CT-PA versus 0.28 mGy for the perfusion part of a V/Q scan, translating to 40 times the dose at a sensitive time of breast tissue proliferation [40], raising concerns of increased lifetime risk of breast cancer [30, 39].

Considering that significantly fewer pregnant women with suspected PE will have nondiagnostic V/Q scans in comparison to the nonpregnant population (likely owing to less concomitant respiratory disease) [42], V/Q scans provide an attractive option for imaging of pregnant women suspected of PE, particularly when only the perfusion portion of the V/Q scan is performed. Indeed, preferential utilization of V/Q over CT-PA in these circumstances has been endorsed and imbedded in current guidelines

[18, 39]. However, when lung pathology is present (increasing the risk of a nondiagnostic V/Q scan), proceeding straight to CT-PA may be prudent. The most appropriate modality can be clarified by first requesting a chest X-ray (CXR), with subsequent perfusion portion of a V/Q scan if CXR is negative, or CT-PA instead if CXR is positive [39].

17.8 Cerebral vein thrombosis

Although CVT is encountered more rarely than DVT and PE, with a documented incidence of 0.01% to 0.04% [18]. In a case-control study, obesity (BMI >30 kg/m^2) in women was found to be associated with CVT (with an adjusted odds ratio (aOR) of 3.50; 95% CI, 2.00–6.14), whereby oral contraceptive use increased the risk even further (aOR 29.26; 95% CI, 13.47–63.60) [43]. Pregnancy, particularly the third trimester and the puerperium, has likewise been found to be a risk factor for CVT [44]. Characteristic symptoms include diffuse, increasingly more severe headache, and occasionally "thunderclap" headache, which may be the sole manifestation [45]. Headache may be accompanied by papilledema and sometimes diplopia, as a result of sixth nerve palsy [44]. Seizures, altered level of mentation, and focal deficits are also commonly seen [46]. Computed tomography (CT) without contrast will often be normal despite the presence of CVT [44]. Time-of-flight magnetic resonance venography is the imaging modality of choice for the diagnosis of CVT [47], particularly in pregnancy, as it does not require contrast and eliminates concerns with respect to exposure to ionizing radiation used in CT venography. Once diagnosed, therapeutic anticoagulation, as described below for VTE in pregnancy should be initiated [18].

17.9 Management of acute VTE

17.9.1 Choice of treatment agent

LMWH is currently considered to be the first-line treatment for VTE in pregnancy, with UFH remaining an option if LMWH is unavailable or contraindicated [18, 22, 24, 39]. Both agents enhance antithrombin's activity (including anti-factor Xa and anti-factor IIa activity), decrease continued thrombus formation, and permit fibrinolysis of the existing thrombus [17]. Neither LMWH nor UFH cross the placenta [48, 49]. The safety and efficacy of LMWH for treatment of VTE in pregnancy has been demonstrated in a systematic review [50], particularly in relation to the lower risk of heparin-induced thrombocytopenia (HIT), osteoporosis, and bleeding, favoring LMWH as compared with UFH [50–52]. Although no cases of HIT have thus far been reported in pregnant patients receiving LMWH [50], in the setting of HIT or allergy to UFH/LMWH, heparanoids (i.e., danaparoid and fondaparinux), which do not cross-react with HIT antibodies, may be administered in pregnancy in consultation with a hematologist [53, 54].

Warfarin, a vitamin K antagonist, crosses the placenta and given the risks of embryopathy, fetal loss, and fetal bleeding [55–57], it should not be used for the treatment of VTE in pregnancy, except under exceptional circumstances [18, 22]. Avoidance of novel anticoagulation agents such as oral direct thrombin inhibitors (i.e., dabigatran) and anti-Xa inhibitors (i.e., rivaroxaban, apixaban) is likewise recommended, as there is no data on their use in pregnancy [18, 22, 24].

In view of the potential hemorrhagic complications, thrombolytic therapy (streptokinase, r-tPA, urokinase) in pregnancy should be reserved strictly for cases of massive, life- or limb-threatening VTE, or ones characterized by hemodynamic instability [18, 24, 39, 58, 59].

The role of vena cava filters in pregnancy is likewise limited. These can be considered in the setting of acute VTE where labor is imminent or where anticoagulation is contraindicated by significant bleeding [18, 60–62].

17.9.2 Anticoagulation dosage and duration

Therapeutic LMWH is weight-based and the recommended treatment doses in pregnancy for the most commonly used formulations are presented in Tab. 17.1.

Physiologic changes in pregnancy, including expansion of maternal blood volume nearing 50% by the third trimester, enhancement of glomerular filtration with consequently higher renal excretion, and intensification of protein-binding, affect the pharmacokinetics of UFH and LMWH [63]. Twice-daily dosing has been suggested by some to maintain therapeutic anticoagulation levels [18, 39]. Yet uncertainty with respect to the need for twice daily dosing remains, as some studies have questioned its lack of superiority to once-daily dosing [64], and a population study of the pharmacokinetics of LMWH in pregnancy demonstrated that the half-life of enoxaparin is prolonged as pregnancy advances, supporting the use of once-daily dosing [63]. Although some current guidelines suggest twice-daily dosing [18, 39], others mention the possible utility of twice-daily dosing but leave open the option of once-daily LMWH administration [22, 24].

Similarly, the need for anti-FXa monitoring in pregnancy has been questioned, as adjustment of LWMH to maintain specific anti-FXa targets has not been shown to affect outcomes in pregnant women with VTE [65]. Given the costs of the assay, inconsistency between assays, and lack of correlation of laboratory levels with clinical events, one guideline labels anti-FXa monitoring controversial [18], another suggests it is hard to justify [5], and a third does not recommend it except at extremes of weight or in complex circumstances such as renal impairment [39].

Anticoagulation treatment for acute VTE in pregnancy should continue for the length of the pregnancy and for at least 6 weeks postpartum, and for a total duration of at least 3 months [18, 24, 39]. Either LMWH or warfarin may be used postpartum and both are compatible with breast-feeding [18, 24, 39].

17.9.3 Peripartum management of anticoagulation

Prophylaxis should be halted at the onset of labor, or in the case of planned induction of labor or cesarean section, the last dose should be taken the day before [15, 18, 39]. It is recommended that patients being managed with therapeutic anticoagulation have a planned delivery [15, 18]. Neuraxial anesthesia may be administered safely 12 hours following a prophylactic dose of LMWH and 24 hours after a therapeutic dose [66].

If the VTE was diagnosed 2 to 4 weeks prior to delivery, LMWH should be transitioned to intravenous UFH during labor, as this minimizes the length of time anticoagulation is interrupted [18, 24]. Neuraxial anesthesia may be placed 4 hours after discontinuation of IV UFH, when aPTT returns to normal [18].

17.9.4 Re-initiation of anticoagulation postpartum

LMWH should be re-initiated 4 to 6 hours following vaginal delivery and 6 to 12 hours following cesarean section [22], and at least 4 hours following removal of the epidural catheter [66]. A prophylactic dose of LMWH may be given at that time once hemostasis is satisfactory, and followed by a therapeutic dose 24 hours later, as indicated [18].

Bibliography

[1] Lisonkova S, Bartholomew S, Rouleau J, et al. Temporal trends in maternal mortality in Canada I: estimates based on vital statistics data. J Obstet Gynaecol Can 2011;33(10):1011–9.

[2] Cantwell R, Clutton-Brock T, Cooper G, et al. Saving mothers' lives: reviewing maternal deaths to make motherhood safer: 2006–2008. The Eighth Report of the Confidential Enquiries into Maternal Deaths in the United Kingdom. BJOG 2011;118 Suppl 1:1–203.

[3] Sultan AA, West J, Tata LJ, Fleming KM, Nelson-Piercy C, Grainge MJ. Risk of first venous thromboembolism in and around pregnancy: a population-based cohort study. Br J Haematol 2012;156(3):366–73.

[4] Virkus RA, Lokkegaard EC, Bergholt T, Mogensen U, Langhoff-Roos J, Lidegaard O. Venous thromboembolism in pregnant and puerperal women in Denmark 1995–2005. A national cohort study. Thromb Haemost 2011;106(2):304–9.

[5] Blanco-Molina A, Trujillo-Santos J, Criado J, et al. Venous thromboembolism during pregnancy or postpartum: findings from the RIETE Registry. Thromb Haemost 2007;97(2):186–90.

[6] Liu S, Rouleau J, Joseph KS, et al. Epidemiology of pregnancy-associated venous thromboembolism: a population-based study in Canada. J Obstet Gynaecol Can 2009;31(7):611–20.

[7] Heit JA, Kobbervig CE, James AH, Petterson TM, Bailey KR, Melton LJ, 3rd. Trends in the incidence of venous thromboembolism during pregnancy or postpartum: a 30-year population-based study. Ann Intern Med 2005;143(10):697–706.

[8] James AH, Jamison MG, Brancazio LR, Myers ER. Venous thromboembolism during pregnancy and the postpartum period: incidence, risk factors, and mortality. Am J Obstet Gynecol 2006;194(5):1311–5.

[9] Public Health Agency of Canada. Canadian Perinatal Health Report, 2008 Edition. Ottawa; 2008:1–168.

[10] Braekkan SK, Siegerink B, Lijfering WM, Hansen JB, Cannegieter SC, Rosendaal FR. Role of obesity in the etiology of deep vein thrombosis and pulmonary embolism: current epidemiological insights. Semin Thromb Hemost 2013;39(5):533–40.
[11] Knight M, UKOSS. Antenatal pulmonary embolism: risk factors, management and outcomes. BJOG 2008;115(4):453–61.
[12] Ageno W, Becattini C, Brighton T, Selby R, Kamphuisen PW. Cardiovascular risk factors and venous thromboembolism: a meta-analysis. Circulation 2008;117(1):93–102.
[13] Cushman M. Epidemiology and risk factors for venous thrombosis. Semin Hematol 2007;44(2):62–9.
[14] Kim SY, Dietz PM, England L, Morrow B, Callaghan WM. Trends in pre-pregnancy obesity in nine states, 1993–2003. Obesity (Silver Spring) 2007;15(4):986–93.
[15] Allman-Farinelli MA. Obesity and venous thrombosis: a review. Semin Thromb Hemost 2011;37(8):903–7.
[16] Esmon CT. Basic mechanisms and pathogenesis of venous thrombosis. Blood Rev 2009;23(5):225–9.
[17] Bourjeily G, Paidas M, Khalil H, Rosene-Montella K, Rodger M. Pulmonary embolism in pregnancy. Lancet 2010;375(9713):500–12.
[18] Chan WS, Rey E, Kent NE, et al. Venous thromboembolism and antithrombotic therapy in pregnancy. J Obstet Gynaecol Can 2014;36(6):527–53.
[19] Despres JP, Lemieux I. Abdominal obesity and metabolic syndrome. Nature 2006;444(7121):881–7.
[20] Darvall KA, Sam RC, Silverman SH, Bradbury AW, Adam DJ. Obesity and thrombosis. Eur J Vasc Endovasc Surg 2007;33(2):223–33.
[21] Royal College of Obstetricians and Gynaecologists. Reducing the risk of thrombosis and embolism during pregnancy and the puerperium. Green-top Guideline No 37a; 2015:1–40.
[22] James A, Committee on Practice B-O. Practice bulletin no. 123: thromboembolism in pregnancy. Obstet Gynecol 2011;118(3):718–29.
[23] Jacobsen AF, Skjeldestad FE, Sandset PM. Ante- and postnatal risk factors of venous thrombosis: a hospital-based case-control study. J Thromb Haemost 2008;6(6):905–12.
[24] Bates SM, Greer IA, Middeldorp S, et al. VTE, thrombophilia, antithrombotic therapy, and pregnancy: antithrombotic therapy and prevention of thrombosis, 9th ed: American College of Chest Physicians Evidence-Based Clinical Practice Guidelines. Chest 2012;141(2 Suppl):e691S–736S.
[25] Drife J. Deep venous thrombosis and pulmonary embolism in obese women. Best Pract Res Clin Obstet Gynaecol 2015;29(3):365–76.
[26] Marik PE, Plante LA. Venous thromboembolic disease and pregnancy. N Engl J Med 2008;359(19):2025–33.
[27] Smith SB, Geske JB, Morgenthaler TI. Risk factors associated with delayed diagnosis of acute pulmonary embolism. J Emerg Med 2012;42(1):1–6.
[28] Dresang LT, Fontaine P, Leeman L, King VJ. Venous thromboembolism during pregnancy. Am Fam Physician 2008;77(12):1709–16.
[29] Drife J. Thromboembolism. Br Med Bull 2003;67:177–90.
[30] Rodger M. Evidence base for the management of venous thromboembolism in pregnancy. Hematology Am Soc Hematol Educ Program 2010;2010:173–180.
[31] Goldhaber SZ, Visani L, De Rosa M. Acute pulmonary embolism: clinical outcomes in the International Cooperative Pulmonary Embolism Registry (ICOPER). Lancet 1999; 353(9162):1386–9.
[32] Bates SM, Takach Lapner S, Douketis JD, et al. Rapid quantitative D-dimer to exclude pulmonary embolism: a prospective cohort management study. J Thromb Haemost 2016;14(3):504–9.
[33] Kabrhel C, Mark Courtney D, Camargo CA, Jr., et al. Factors associated with positive D-dimer results in patients evaluated for pulmonary embolism. Acad Emerg Med 2010;17(6):589–97.

[34] Kjellberg U, Andersson NE, Rosen S, Tengborn L, Hellgren M. APC resistance and other haemostatic variables during pregnancy and puerperium. Thromb Haemost 1999;81(4):527–531.
[35] Chan WS, Chunilal S, Lee A, Crowther M, Rodger M, Ginsberg JS. A red blood cell agglutination D-dimer test to exclude deep venous thrombosis in pregnancy. Ann Intern Med 2007;147(3):165–70.
[36] Le Gal G, Kercret G, Ben Yahmed K, et al. Diagnostic value of single complete compression ultrasonography in pregnant and postpartum women with suspected deep vein thrombosis: prospective study. BMJ 2012;344:e2635.
[37] Le Gal G, Righini M. Controversies in the diagnosis of venous thromboembolism. J Thromb Haemost 2015;13 Suppl 1:S259–65.
[38] Chan WS, Spencer FA, Ginsberg JS. Anatomic distribution of deep vein thrombosis in pregnancy. CMAJ 2010;182(7):657–660.
[39] Royal College of Obstetricians and Gynaecologists. The acute management of thrombosis and embolism during pregnancy and the puerperium. Green-top Guideline No 37b; 2015.
[40] Cook JV, Kyriou J. Radiation from CT and perfusion scanning in pregnancy. BMJ 2005;331(7512):350.
[41] Tan M, Huisman MV. The diagnostic management of acute venous thromboembolism during pregnancy: recent advancements and unresolved issues. Thromb Res 2011;127 Suppl 3:S13–16.
[42] Chan WS, Ray JG, Murray S, Coady GE, Coates G, Ginsberg JS. Suspected pulmonary embolism in pregnancy. Arch Intern Med 2002;162(10):1170.
[43] Zuurbier SM, Arnold M, Middeldorp S, et al. Risk of cerebral venous thrombosis in obese women. JAMA Neurol 2016;73(5):579–84.
[44] Saposnik G, Barinagarrementeria F, Brown RD, Jr., et al. Diagnosis and management of cerebral venous thrombosis: a statement for healthcare professionals from the American Heart Association/American Stroke Association. Stroke 2011;42(4):1158–92.
[45] Cumurciuc R, Crassard I, Sarov M, Valade D, Bousser MG. Headache as the only neurological sign of cerebral venous thrombosis: a series of 17 cases. J Neurol Neurosurg Psychiatry 2005;76(8):1084–7.
[46] Sidhom Y, Mansour M, Messelmani M, et al. Cerebral venous thrombosis: clinical features, risk factors, and long-term outcome in a Tunisian cohort. J Stroke Cerebrovasc Dis 2014;23(6):1291–5.
[47] Leach JL, Fortuna RB, Jones BV, Gaskill-Shipley MF. Imaging of cerebral venous thrombosis: current techniques, spectrum of findings, and diagnostic pitfalls. Radiographics 2006;26 Suppl 1:S19–41; discussion S42–13.
[48] Harenberg J, Schneider D, Heilmann L, Wolf H. Lack of anti-factor Xa activity in umbilical cord vein samples after subcutaneous administration of heparin or low molecular mass heparin in pregnant women. Haemostasis 1993;23(6):314–20.
[49] Flessa HC, Kapstrom AB, Glueck HI, Will JJ. Placental transport of heparin. Am J Obstet Gynecol 1965;93(4):570–3.
[50] Greer IA, Nelson-Piercy C. Low-molecular-weight heparins for thromboprophylaxis and treatment of venous thromboembolism in pregnancy: a systematic review of safety and efficacy. Blood 2005;106(2):401–7.
[51] Sanson BJ, Lensing AW, Prins MH, et al. Safety of low-molecular-weight heparin in pregnancy: a systematic review. Thromb Haemost 1999;81(5):668–72.
[52] Pettila V, Leinonen P, Markkola A, Hiilesmaa V, Kaaja R. Postpartum bone mineral density in women treated for thromboprophylaxis with unfractionated heparin or LMW heparin. Thromb Haemost 2002;87(2):182–6.
[53] Schindewolf M, Mosch G, Bauersachs RM, Lindhoff-Last E. Safe anticoagulation with danaparoid in pregnancy and lactation. Thromb Haemost 2004;92(1):211.
[54] Mazzolai L, Hohlfeld P, Spertini F, Hayoz D, Schapira M, Duchosal MA. Fondaparinux is a safe alternative in case of heparin intolerance during pregnancy. Blood 2006;108(5):1569–70.

[55] Blickstein D, Blickstein I. The risk of fetal loss associated with warfarin anticoagulation. Int J Gynaecol Obstet 2002;78(3):221–5.
[56] Della Corte A, De Feo M, Romano G, et al. Risk of warfarin anticoagulation in pregnant patients with mechanical heart valve prostheses. J Heart Valve Dis 2004;13 Suppl 1:S90.
[57] Walfisch A, Koren G. The "warfarin window" in pregnancy: the importance of half-life. J Obstet Gynaecol Can 2010;32(10):988–9.
[58] Turrentine MA, Braems G, Ramirez MM. Use of thrombolytics for the treatment of thromboembolic disease during pregnancy. Obstet Gynecol Surv 1995;50(7):534–41.
[59] Leonhardt G, Gaul C, Nietsch HH, Buerke M, Schleussner E. Thrombolytic therapy in pregnancy. J Thromb Thrombolysis 2006;21(3):271–6.
[60] Kawamata K, Chiba Y, Tanaka R, Higashi M, Nishigami K. Experience of temporary inferior vena cava filters inserted in the perinatal period to prevent pulmonary embolism in pregnant women with deep vein thrombosis. J Vasc Surg 2005;41(4):652–6.
[61] Decousus H, Leizorovicz A, Parent F, et al. A clinical trial of vena caval filters in the prevention of pulmonary embolism in patients with proximal deep-vein thrombosis. Prevention du Risque d'Embolie Pulmonaire par Interruption Cave Study Group. N Engl J Med 1998;338(7):409–15.
[62] Miyahara T, Miyata T, Shigematsu K, et al. Clinical outcome and complications of temporary inferior vena cava filter placement. J Vasc Surg 2006;44(3):620–4.
[63] Patel JP, Green B, Patel RK, Marsh MS, Davies JG, Arya R. Population pharmacokinetics of enoxaparin during the antenatal period. Circulation 2013;128(13):1462–9.
[64] Voke J, Keidan J, Pavord S, Spencer NH, Hunt BJ, British Society for Haematology Obstetric Haematology Group. The management of antenatal venous thromboembolism in the UK and Ireland: a prospective multicentre observational survey. Br J Haematol 2007;139(4):545–58.
[65] McDonnell BP, Glennon K, McTiernan A, et al. Adjustment of therapeutic LMWH to achieve specific target anti-FXa activity does not affect outcomes in pregnant patients with venous thromboembolism. J Thromb Thrombolysis 2017;43(1):105–111.
[66] Horlocker TT, Wedel DJ, Rowlingson JC, et al. Regional anesthesia in the patient receiving antithrombotic or thrombolytic therapy: American Society of Regional Anesthesia and Pain Medicine Evidence-Based Guidelines (3rd ed.). Reg Anesth Pain Med 2010;35(1):64–101.

Kristin L. Connor

18 MicrObesity in pregnancy: the inside story

18.1 Introduction

Despite the alarming prevalence of obesity worldwide, current efforts to mitigate the adverse effects of obesity and its comorbidities by behavior modification or dietary restriction have produced mixed results [1–3]. Importantly, these treatment challenges extend to women of reproductive age, a population in which overweight and obesity are increasing [4]. In countries such as Canada and America, more than 30% of women of reproductive age are estimated to be obese [4–6]. Prepregnancy overweight and obesity, and increasingly even normal weight, are also associated with excessive gestational weight gain and postpartum weight retention [7, 8]. Left unresolved, maternal obesity and postpartum weight retention have long-term implications for the health of the mother and that of her child [9]. The lack of progress in reducing the incidence and burden of obesity suggests that the mechanisms driving its pathogenesis have yet to be fully elucidated. Furthermore, it is likely that a new approach is needed for early identification of girls and women at-risk for metabolic compromise, and for the development of new therapies that target modifiable factors on the causal pathway to obesity and its comorbidities. Emerging evidence suggests that the gut may be a potential mediator of obesity and provide new insights into the pathogenesis and treatment of the disease.

18.2 The gut as a gatekeeper of health

Obesity is a complex disease and there are many factors that are associated with weight. These include (epi)genetics, nutrition, environment, behavior, and physiology (including normal physiologic adaptations permissive of increased adipose deposition, such as pregnancy). Gut bacteria (microbiota) may be another factor underlying obesity onset and additionally explain relationships between host genetics, the environment, and the obese phenotype.

It should not be surprising that there is renewed interest in the gut and its role in health and disease states. The gastrointestinal system and its resident microbes are critical for nutrient production, metabolism, and uptake [10, 11]; development and function of gut epithelial cells [12]; metabolism of drugs [13, 14]; and development and activity of the immune system [12]. Recent evidence has linked microbiota in the gut and their collective genomes/gene products (the microbiome) to human health, where shifts in microbial community structure and function (dysbiosis) are associated with diseases such as obesity and type 2 diabetes (T2D) [15–19]. Changes in diet can also affect the host's gut microbiome [20, 21], and an individual's nutritional history

https://doi.org/10.1515/9783110487817-018

likely has a profound effect on establishing the community of gut bacteria that reside and persist there [22, 23]. Collectively, these observations have led to the development of a new concept "MicrObesity", which aims to understand the contributions of the gut microbiome to host metabolism and energy storage [24].

18.2.1 Contributions of the gut microbiome to obesity onset in the nonpregnant state

The precise contributions of gut microbiota to the regulation of weight and metabolic function of the host are not well understood. This may in part be due to the vast number and diversity of bacteria that inhabit the gut. New estimates place the number of bacterial cells in the human gut to be only slightly more than our total number of human cells, and reveal that gut bacterial concentrations are similar in obese and nonobese individuals [25]. Yet, to fully appreciate the influence of gut microbes on health, one must look beyond bacterial types and numbers and assess what these microbes are in fact doing by studying their function at the genetic and metabolic levels. This is a daunting task, for there are more than 3 million microbial genes in the human gut microbiome [26] (compared with the ~20,000 genes in the human genome), and we do not yet know the extent to which functional redundancy is built in to the gut microbiome. The result is a complex ecosystem that behaves like an organ and whose dynamic nature can affect not only the local environment in which these microbes reside (and thus, the function of the microbes themselves) but also distal tissues and organs in the host. In fact, gut microbes may modify the permeability of key tissue barriers [27–29], and it has been estimated that up to one-third of blood metabolites have bacterial origin [30, 31], highlighting the expansive reach microbes can have throughout the body.

Despite the complexity of the gut microbiome and its interactions with the host, research over the last decade has begun to reveal that gut microbes participate in key pathways linked to metabolic dysfunction and obesity onset: inflammation, fat storage, and insulin resistance. It is recognized that bacteria are critical for immune system regulation and that inflammation in the gut may influence that in the periphery [32]. Obesity [33, 34] and T2D [35, 36] are associated with chronic systemic low-grade inflammation. Bacterial endotoxins (lipid components of the cell wall of Gram-negative bacteria) are considered key activators of inflammatory pathways in these diseases. Endotoxin levels have been shown to increase with a high-fat diet, and they initiate inflammation and weight gain in animals [37]. In obese humans, altered composition of the gut microbiome, characterized by reduced bacterial diversity and increased abundance of proinflammatory bacteria, is associated with increased inflammation in the gut and periphery compared with nonobese subjects [38]. It has thus been proposed that the gut microbiome should be thought of as an immune system [39], functioning to maintain physiologic homeostasis in the host, but at times, activating immune pathways that underlie many noncommunicable diseases.

Gut microbes also permit fat deposition in the host and have increased capacity to utilize energy [16, 40]. The mechanism through which this occurs is being investigated in detail and broadly involves altered communication between the gut and peripheral sites critical for maintaining host energy balance. In brief (reviewed by Geurts et al. [41] and Musso et al. [42]), the gut and its resident microbes sense signals from the environment, including nutrients, metabolites, hormones, and inflammatory factors. In response, the gut signals, through the circulation and afferent nerves, to organs that regulate food intake and energy expenditure, namely, the brain, liver, adipose tissue, and muscle [41, 42]. Crucially important to energy balance may be the ability of gut bacteria to metabolize complex carbohydrates indigestible by human intestinal enzymes. Bacteria that can ferment these carbohydrates produce simple sugars and short-chain fatty acids (SCFAs; namely, acetate, propionate, and butyrate), the latter of which are readily available for intestinal absorption and serve as substrates for different metabolic processes [43]. Butyrate is a source of energy for epithelial cells in the colon, whereas acetate and propionate are taken up by the portal circulation and are used in cholesterol synthesis or hepatic gluconeogenesis and lipogenesis, respectively [43]. SCFAs provide excess energy to the host, and can regulate fat storage and further nutrient absorption [40, 44, 45]. In humans and animals, obesity is associated with a microbiome enriched in bacteria that enhance these fermentation processes, in part, rendering the microbiome more effective in producing SCFAs and harvesting energy, which may underlie adipose tissue expansion and obesity onset [15, 16]. Therefore, dietary substrates consumed by the host are important not only for determining host nutritional status but also for feeding the resident microbes that influence host nutrient availability and metabolism.

Another factor that may be critical to energy balance regulation and link these processes with immune and microbial systems is the adipokine leptin [46]. Independent of obesity, leptin concentrations increase following acute phase cytokine stimulation, endotoxin challenge, and bacterial infection [37]. Additionally, experimental models have shown that leptin deficiency [15], or the absence of the leptin receptor [47], result in an obese phenotype, low-grade inflammation, and gut microbial dysbiosis. Leptin resistance in the brain [48] or at peripheral sites [49], key features of obesity, may be regulated in part by gut microbes, and changing the types of microbes present in the gut can reduce inflammation, which may improve leptin sensitivity [49, 50]. Importantly, new evidence has revealed that leptin plays a direct role in regulating the composition of the gut microbiome independent of food intake by the host [51]. Whether gut microbes can directly influence inflammatory signals in the brain that regulate central leptin resistance [52] remains to be determined. Thus, interactions between leptin and the gut microbiome may offer new insights into the etiology of obesity.

Although it is difficult to isolate the effects of gut microbes on host glucose metabolism and insulin sensitivity independent of changes in adiposity, a growing body of evidence indicates that the microbiome does play a role in glucose control [42].

Impaired glucose tolerance and insulin sensitivity and T2D have all been associated with higher bacterial endotoxin levels [37, 53, 54]. More specifically, gut microbial dysbiosis, including a decrease in the abundance of bacteria that produce butyrate, has been observed in human and animal models of insulin resistance and diabetes [17, 18, 55]. One small intervention study has even shown that fecal transfer from lean donors to insulin-resistant men with metabolic syndrome improves muscle insulin resistance in recipient men, associated with increased gut microbial diversity and abundance of butyrate-producing bacteria [56]. The mechanisms through which gut microbes may confer an insulin-resistant phenotype in the host are slowly being uncovered (reviewed in detail by Musso et al. [42] and Caricilli and Saad [57]). These include microbial interactions with the environment (namely, dietary substrates consumed by the host) and with the intestinal barrier (including factors that govern intestinal permeability, hormone production, and gene expression) to activate inflammatory and stress pathways that contribute to the onset of insulin resistance.

18.3 Expanding the pregnancy narrative to include the microbiome

Major physiologic adaptations that occur with normal pregnancy resemble phenotypes associated with metabolic dysfunction in the nonpregnant state. For example, inflammation in the maternal peripheral circulation and in the local environments of the uterus and placenta is altered with advancing gestation in normal pregnancy [58, 59]. Pregnancy is also characterized by an increase in maternal fat deposition [60], and as gestation advances, the increased fat stores are distributed at visceral rather than subcutaneous sites [61]. This parallels the increases seen in peripheral leptin [62] and lipid [63] concentrations with advancing gestation in normal pregnancy. Furthermore, early pregnancy is associated with maternal insulin sensitivity, whereas late pregnancy is characterized by insulin resistance [64, 65]. Collectively, these physiologic shifts are required to provide more resources to the rapidly developing fetus and placenta, and to provide the mother with energy and nutrients essential for parturition and lactation [66]. In contrast, elevated maternal BMI is associated with an increase in proinflammatory biomarkers in the maternal circulation and an activation of proinflammatory pathways in the placenta [67]. Throughout pregnancy, overweight and obese women have greater fat stores in all anatomic sites compared with normal weight women, but gestational measures of the abdominal fat index (a surrogate for visceral fat) indicate that it increases to a lesser degree across pregnancy in overweight and obese than in normal weight women [61]. This may in part be explained by the common observation that overweight and obese women gain weight more slowly during pregnancy than women with a normal prepregnancy BMI. Consistent with this, in overweight and obese women, leptin levels are higher, but increase to a lesser degree (as do peripheral lipid levels [63]), over the course of pregnancy than in normal weight women [62].

Interestingly, the concentration of leptin per kilogram of maternal body weight has been observed to decrease in overweight and obese women, but increase in normal weight women, with advancing gestation [62], suggesting that although leptin generally circulates in the body at levels proportional to body fat, there may be additional mechanisms that regulate leptin levels in the overweight or obese woman during pregnancy. Beyond the fact that prepregnancy overweight and obesity can situate mothers on a path towards increased inflammation and decreased insulin sensitivity [33, 68], and put these women at increased risk for gestational diabetes [69], these metabolic conditions also have consequences for the developing fetus, including earlier and greater delivery of nutrient substrates and proinflammatory factors through the placenta [70].

18.3.1 The gut microbiome and maternal adaptation to pregnancy

If gut microbes modify blood metabolites, these, and other signals originating from the gut, can thus target not only maternal tissues but also the placenta and fetus. We therefore must consider that the maternal gut microbiome represents a third genome, actively participating in the adaptation to pregnancy and the programming of fetal development. Although limited evidence points to a role for gut microbes in pregnancy-associated physiologic changes, it is likely that the interactions that occur between the environment, host physiology, and the microbiome in the nonpregnant state also exist in pregnancy. It has been shown that normal pregnancy alters the gut microbiome, where the abundance and diversity of microbes in the maternal gut change with advancing gestation, including a reduction in the abundance of butyrate-producing bacteria [71]. The maternal gut microbiome in the first trimester of pregnancy more closely resembles that of a nonpregnant individual than that of a woman in the third trimester [71]. The third trimester microbiome is characterized by reduced bacterial diversity compared with the first trimester microbiome [71], similar to the microbial dysbiosis seen in overweight, obese, and inflammatory phenotypes [55, 72, 73], and the composition of this late pregnancy gut microbiome seems to be maintained at least until 1 month postpartum [71, 74]. Elegant experiments using germ-free mice (mice that do not have a microbiome of their own) have aimed to determine what these microbial changes mean for normal pregnancy. In these studies, stool (and hence, the microbiome) from pregnant women collected either in the first or third trimester was transferred to germ-free mice [71]. Mice that received the third trimester stool showed increased adiposity and insulin insensitivity compared with first trimester recipients [71]. Collectively, these data suggest that gut microbes may be permissive of the normal metabolic changes that occur in pregnancy, namely, increased adipose deposition and insulin resistance with advancing gestation, and may therefore aid the mother in meeting the increased energy requirements for pregnancy, parturition, and lactation.

Late pregnancy is also a time of increased inflammation [58, 59], and gut microbes may be active participants in these proinflammatory processes. Biomarkers of intestinal inflammation are present in stool from third trimester pregnant women [74], and induce a small inflammatory response in germ-free mice [71]. Experimental models that influence maternal weight have found significant relationships between the abundance of specific bacteria in the maternal gut microbiome at the end of pregnancy and circulating, or small intestinal, proinflammatory cytokine and chemokine concentrations [75]. These relationships are similar to those seen in nonpregnant obese individuals where increased inflammation has been observed locally and peripherally, and is associated with changes in levels of potentially proinflammatory gut bacteria [38].

Therefore, as in the nonpregnant state, immune, endocrine, and metabolic signals of pregnancy may converge at the gut. Resident microbes may be necessary for the physiologic changes that occur with normal pregnancy, and consequently represent a new entity that must be considered to comprehensively understand maternal adaptation to pregnancy.

18.4 MicrObesity in pregnancy

Given the established links between gut microbial dysbiosis and metabolic diseases in the host, and that the gut microbiome likely plays a role in normal physiologic adaptations to pregnancy, it is natural to wonder what effect prepregnancy overweight or obesity have on the maternal gut microbiome. Studies are under way to answer this question. One of the earliest (that did not benefit from next generation sequencing that is commonplace today) found that as in normal weight women, the composition of the gut microbiome changed from the first to third trimester in women who were obese before pregnancy [76]. Furthermore, the abundance of bacteria representative of the Firmicutes phyla was higher in overweight stool, as were *Staphylococcus* and *Bacteroides*, and although there were no differences in gestational weight gain between normal weight and obese women in this cohort, women with excessive gestational weight gain had altered composition of their gut microbiomes [76]. These data are consistent with reports of changes in specific types of bacteria in the nonpregnant obese individual [16, 19], and also suggest a role for these obesogenic maternal gut microbes in energy balance and inflammatory processes in pregnancy.

More recent data have shown direct relationships between metabolic biomarkers in overweight and obese women in early pregnancy and abundance and types of their gut microbes. In this cohort, compared with overweight women, obese women had higher fasting glucose, HOMA-IR, insulin, C-peptide, leptin, gastroinhibitory polypeptide, and resistin concentrations in early pregnancy (<16 weeks gestation) [77]. Obese women also had reduced microbial richness in early pregnancy compared with overweight counterparts, and abundance levels of key bacterial phyla and families were found to be different between overweight and obese women [77]. Importantly, there was no difference in the composition of the maternal gut microbiome in early pregnancy in women who developed gestational diabetes compared with those who did not [77]. There were, however, significant associations between abundance of specific gut microbes and levels of hormones involved in glucose metabolism (including insulin, C-peptide, and HOMA-IR), energy metabolism (including leptin, ghrelin, and resistin) and lipid metabolism (including triglycerides, VLDL and HDL cholesterol) [77]. Early assessment of the composition (and function) of the maternal gut microbiome may thus prove a valuable prognostic tool for adverse outcomes in later pregnancy.

It is important to reiterate that host diet, rather than adiposity or weight, may be the principal driver of gut microbial dynamics. This is also true in pregnancy, evidenced by studies that have begun to disentangle the effects of diet and weight on the composition and function of the maternal gut microbiome [78, 79]. Female mice fed a high-fat diet before and during pregnancy, but not females that were calorically restricted and exhibited weight faltering in pregnancy, were observed to have reduced microbial richness and altered microbial abundance levels in late pregnancy compared with control-fed and calorically restricted mothers [79]. These changes were independent of maternal weight, as high-fat fed mothers did not weigh more than controls, but may be related to leptin, as the abundance of specific bacterial taxa was associated with peripheral leptin concentrations at the end of pregnancy [79]. Collectively, these data are consistent with structural and functional changes in the maternal gut microbiome seen in other high-fat feeding experimental models [80]. In a primate model of maternal high-fat nutrition, females fed a high-fat diet became either sensitive to its effects, and developed obesity and insulin resistance, or were resistant to its effects, and remained lean [78]. The composition of the gut microbiomes of the high-fat diet–resistant and lean females were essentially indistinguishable from each other, but both were different from the microbiome composition (microbial abundance and diversity) of control-fed females [78]. Sustained high-fat diet intake over multiple pregnancies further confirmed the strength of the effect that diet, rather than weight, had in restructuring the maternal gut microbiome, and suggests that long-term changes in maternal dietary intakes may be a mechanism through which permanent shifts in the microbial community can occur [22]. There is also increasing interest in the role of dietary probiotics and prebiotics on human health. For example, one study in normal weight pregnant women revealed that perinatal probiotic supplementation reduced the incidence of gestational diabetes [81]. Although there are limited data on microbiome-targeted interventions to improve adverse pregnancy outcomes associated with maternal overweight and obesity, two ongoing clinical trials aim to determine whether maternal probiotic consumption in obese women during pregnancy can improve the health of the pregnancy, including measures of excessive gestational weight gain, glucose homeostasis and birth weight, through effects on the maternal gut microbiome [82, 83]. Therefore, nutrition counseling, including attention paid to the consumption of prebiotics or probiotics, may be beneficial for overweight and obese women before conception and in the perinatal periods beyond helping them adhere to gestational weight gain guidelines.

18.4.1 Implications of maternal obesity and gut microbial dysbiosis

The reduced microbial richness seen in obese, nonpregnant individuals has been associated with greater weight gain over time [55]. This may be important to bear in mind when considering prepregnancy BMI, as a woman entering pregnancy overweight or obese may have a gut microbiome that predisposes to greater gestational weight gain. Although such putative relationships in pregnancy require further study, the observation that many overweight women gain more than the recommended amount of weight during pregnancy [7] suggests that interventions that can modify the gut microbiome could be a target for weight management not only before but during pregnancy. Furthermore, given that the postpartum maternal gut microbiome seems to reflect that in late pregnancy, and proinflammatory markers have been measured in late pregnancy stool, a pro-obese or proinflammatory microbiome in the antenatal period (a consequence or driver of maternal obesity) may persist postnatally, exaggerating the postpartum inflammatory state [58] and contributing to the increased risk of postpartum weight retention [84] and T2D [85] seen with maternal overweight and obesity.

Although outside the scope of this chapter, mounting evidence reveals that a bidirectional communication system exists between microbes in the gut and the brain, establishing a brain-gut-microbiota axis [86, 87]. The mechanisms regulating this communication are complex and include the host's metabolic, immune, and (neuro)endocrine systems [86, 87]. The brain-gut-microbiota axis is likely to play a role in pregnancy, including neuroendocrine processes such as hypothalamic-pituitary-adrenal axis function [86], and may also have implications for maternal mental health, as it does in nonpregnant individuals [87]. Obese mothers are at increased risk for depressive symptoms in the antenatal and postpartum periods [88]. It is therefore intriguing to speculate that obesity-associated changes in the maternal gut microbiome could contribute to altered maternal hypothalamic-pituitary-adrenal axis function and the pathogenesis of maternal depression and anxiety. Interventions that target the gut microbiome to prevent or manage maternal obesity may also have positive effects on maternal mental health.

It should also be noted that restructuring of microbial niches with normal pregnancy is not limited to the gut, but also occurs in the vagina [89] and in breast milk postpartum [90, 91]. Furthermore, spatially distinct microbial communities have been shown to be similar, suggesting that microbiota can spread through the circulation [92–94]. The composition of the maternal gut and vaginal (and possibly placental [94]) microbiomes in late pregnancy will have implications for the types of microbes seeded in the newborn during delivery and the infant during breastfeeding [95, 96]. Changes in these maternal microbial niches, a result of maternal obesity, metabolic dysfunction, and/or inflammation, may influence the initial colonizers in the infant gut, and the microbes that persist there [87]. As such, these early microbial cues can have a profound effect on the infant, shaping its own immune and metabolic systems. It is well documented that maternal obesity is a risk factor for suboptimal fetal and infant development, including earlier and greater weight gain in fetuses and infants, and increased risk for obesity and T2D from childhood to adulthood [66, 97, 98]. An obesogenic maternal gut microbiome may establish a suboptimal gut microbiome in the infant [78, 99, 100] that is also primed for increased energy harvest and permissive of increased adipose tissue deposition. Additionally, maternal obesity and endocrine status at delivery have been associated with reduced microbial diversity and altered composition of the breast milk microbiome [91], thereby influencing the community of microbes the infant is exposed to through breastfeeding. Therefore, the early life infant gut microbiome, established through interactions with the mother and the perinatal nutritional environment, may represent an underexplored link between maternal obesity, postnatal catch-up growth, and later obesity risk in children [98].

18.5 Conclusions and future perspectives

Research over the last decade has confirmed a role for the gut microbiome in the pathogenesis of obesity and its comorbidities in the nonpregnant state. However, the extent to which changes in the gut microbiome precede obesity, are a result of it, or both, is not definitively known. More recent studies have provided insight into the contributions of gut microbes to physiologic adaptations that occur with normal pregnancy. The mechanisms through which the gut microbiome is permissive of obese and pregnant phenotypes seem to be similar. Although the data are more limited, maternal obesity is also associated with gut microbial dysbiosis, which may extend to other microbial niches including the vagina, placenta and breast milk. This will have implications for maternal perinatal health, pregnancy outcomes, and development of the fetus and infant.

Although more work needs to be done to clarify the role of diet and metabolic status before and during pregnancy in shaping the gut microbiome, the development of new therapies that harness the modifiable nature of the gut microbiome may hold great promise for obesity prevention and management before pregnancy and in the perinatal periods. Furthermore, early assessment of the structure and function of the maternal (or prepregnancy) gut microbiome may allow us to predict which women are at risk for undesirable pregnancy outcomes including excessive gestational weight gain, postpartum weight retention, and risk for gestational and type 2 diabetes, and intervene early to correct these adverse health trajectories. Recognizing the importance of the gut to the pathogenesis of obesity and pregnancy adaptations provides a window of opportunity to reduce the incidence and burden of obesity in pregnancy and affect the life-long health of mothers and their babies.

Bibliography

[1] Kalupahana NS, Voy BH, Saxton AM, Moustaid-Moussa N. Energy-restricted high-fat diets only partially improve markers of systemic and adipose tissue inflammation. Obesity (Silver Spring) 2011;19:245–54.

[2] Sumithran P, Prendergast LA, Delbridge E, et al. Long-term persistence of hormonal adaptations to weight loss. N Engl J Med 2011;365:1597–604.
[3] Garner DM. Confronting the failure of behavioral and dietary treatments for obesity. Clin Psychol Rev 1991;6:729–80.
[4] Institute for Health Metrics and Evaluation (IHME). GBD cause patterns. Seattle: IHME, University of Washington;2013.
[5] Gotay CC, Katzmarzyk PT, Janssen I, Dawson MY, Aminoltejari A, Bartley NL. Updating the Canadian obesity maps: an epidemic in progress. Can J Publ Health 2013;104:e64–e8.
[6] National Center for Health Statistics. Health, United States, 2015: with special feature on racial and ethnic health disparities. In: Services UDoHaH, ed. Hyattsville, MD: National Center for Health Statistics, Centers for Disease Control and Prevention;2016.
[7] Lowell H, Miller DC. Weight gain during pregnancy: adherence to Health Canada's guidelines. Health Rep 2010;21:31–6.
[8] Jarman M, Yuan Y, Pakseresht M, Shi Q, Robson PJ, Bell RC. Patterns and trajectories of gestational weight gain: a prospective cohort study. CMAJ Open 2016;4:E338–45.
[9] Poston L, Harthoorn LF, Van Der Beek EM. Obesity in pregnancy: implications for the mother and lifelong health of the child. A consensus statement. Pediatr Res 2011;69:175–80.
[10] Kau AL, Ahern PP, Griffin NW, Goodman AL, Gordon JI. Human nutrition, the gut microbiome and the immune system. Nature 2011;474:327–36.
[11] LeBlanc JG, Milani C, de Giori GS, Sesma F, van Sinderen D, Ventura M. Bacteria as vitamin suppliers to their host: a gut microbiota perspective. Curr Opin Biotechnol 2013;24:160–8.
[12] Hooper LV, Littman DR, Macpherson AJ. Interactions between the microbiota and the immune system. Science 2012;336:1268–73.
[13] Swanson HI. Drug metabolism by the host and gut microbiota: a partnership or rivalry? Drug Metab Dispos 2015;43:1499–504.
[14] Yip LY, Chan EC. Investigation of host-gut microbiota modulation of therapeutic outcome. Drug Metab Dispos 2015;43:1619–31.
[15] Ley RE, Backhed F, Turnbaugh P, Lozupone CA, Knight RD, Gordon JI. Obesity alters gut microbial ecology. Proc Natl Acad Sci U S A 2005;102:11070–5.
[16] Turnbaugh PJ, Ley RE, Mahowald MA, Magrini V, Mardis ER, Gordon JI. An obesity-associated gut microbiome with increased capacity for energy harvest. Nature 2006;444:1027–31.
[17] Qin J, Li Y, Cai Z, et al. A metagenome-wide association study of gut microbiota in type 2 diabetes. Nature 2012;490:55–60.
[18] Karlsson FH, Tremaroli V, Nookaew I, et al. Gut metagenome in European women with normal, impaired and diabetic glucose control. Nature 2013;498:99–103.
[19] Ley RE, Turnbaugh PJ, Klein S, Gordon JI. Microbial ecology: human gut microbes associated with obesity. Nature 2006;444:1022–3.
[20] Turnbaugh PJ, Ridaura VK, Faith JJ, Rey FE, Knight R, Gordon JI. The effect of diet on the human gut microbiome: a metagenomic analysis in humanized gnotobiotic mice. Sci Transl Med 2009;1:6ra14.
[21] David LA, Maurice CF, Carmody RN, et al. Diet rapidly and reproducibly alters the human gut microbiome. Nature 2014;505:559–63.
[22] Wu GD, Chen J, Hoffmann C, et al. Linking long-term dietary patterns with gut microbial enterotypes. Science 2011;334:105–8.
[23] Yatsunenko T, Rey FE, Manary MJ, et al. Human gut microbiome viewed across age and geography. Nature 2012;486:222–7.
[24] Cani PD, Delzenne NM. The gut microbiome as therapeutic target. Pharmacol Ther 2011;130:202–12.
[25] Sender R, Fuchs S, Milo R. Revised estimates for the number of human and bacteria cells in the body. PLoS Biol 2016;14:e1002533.

[26] Qin J, Li R, Raes J, et al. A human gut microbial gene catalogue established by metagenomic sequencing. Nature 2010;464:59–65.
[27] Cani PD, Possemiers S, Van de Wiele T, et al. Changes in gut microbiota control inflammation in obese mice through a mechanism involving GLP-2-driven improvement of gut permeability. Gut 2009;58:1091–103.
[28] Braniste V, Al-Asmakh M, Kowal C, et al. The gut microbiota influences blood-brain barrier permeability in mice. Sci Transl Med 2014;6:263ra158.
[29] Suzuki T, Yoshida S, Hara H. Physiological concentrations of short-chain fatty acids immediately suppress colonic epithelial permeability. Br J Nutr 2008;100:297–305.
[30] Wikoff WR, Anfora AT, Liu J, et al. Metabolomics analysis reveals large effects of gut microflora on mammalian blood metabolites. Proc Natl Acad Sci U S A 2009;106:3698–703.
[31] Swann JR, Want EJ, Geier FM, et al. Systemic gut microbial modulation of bile acid metabolism in host tissue compartments. Proc Natl Acad Sci U S A 2011;108 Suppl 1:4523–30.
[32] Lathrop SK, Bloom SM, Rao SM, et al. Peripheral education of the immune system by colonic commensal microbiota. Nature 2011;478:250–4.
[33] Lumeng CN, Saltiel AR. Inflammatory links between obesity and metabolic disease. J Clin Invest 2011;121:2111–7.
[34] Makki K, Froguel P, Wolowczuk I. Adipose tissue in obesity-related inflammation and insulin resistance: cells, cytokines, and chemokines. ISRN Inflamm 2013;2013:139239.
[35] Pickup JC, Crook MA. Is type II diabetes mellitus a disease of the innate immune system? Diabetologia 1998;41:1241–8.
[36] Grimble RF. Inflammatory status and insulin resistance. Curr Opin Clin Nutr Metab Care 2002;5:551–9.
[37] Cani PD, Amar J, Iglesias MA, et al. Metabolic endotoxemia initiates obesity and insulin resistance. Diabetes 2007;56:1761–72.
[38] Verdam FJ, Fuentes S, de Jonge C, et al. Human intestinal microbiota composition is associated with local and systemic inflammation in obesity. Obesity (Silver Spring) 2013;21:E607–15.
[39] Marchesi JR, Adams DH, Fava F, et al. The gut microbiota and host health: a new clinical frontier. Gut 2016;65:330–9.
[40] Samuel BS, Shaito A, Motoike T, et al. Effects of the gut microbiota on host adiposity are modulated by the short-chain fatty-acid binding G protein-coupled receptor, Gpr41. Proc Natl Acad Sci U S A 2008;105:16767–72.
[41] Geurts L, Neyrinck AM, Delzenne NM, Knauf C, Cani PD. Gut microbiota controls adipose tissue expansion, gut barrier and glucose metabolism: novel insights into molecular targets and interventions using prebiotics. Benef Microbes 2014;5:3–17.
[42] Musso G, Gambino R, Cassader M. Interactions between gut microbiota and host metabolism predisposing to obesity and diabetes. Annu Rev Med 2011;62:361–80.
[43] Arora T, Sharma R. Fermentation potential of the gut microbiome: implications for energy homeostasis and weight management. Nutr Rev 2011;69:99–106.
[44] El Kaoutari A, Armougom F, Gordon JI, Raoult D, Henrissat B. The abundance and variety of carbohydrate-active enzymes in the human gut microbiota. Nat Rev Microbiol 2013;11:497–504.
[45] Backhed F, Ding H, Wang T, et al. The gut microbiota as an environmental factor that regulates fat storage. Proc Natl Acad Sci U S A 2004;101:15718–23.
[46] Lord GM, Matarese G, Howard JK, Baker RJ, Bloom SR, Lechler RI. Leptin modulates the T-cell immune response and reverses starvation-induced immunosuppression. Nature 1998;394:897–901.
[47] Geurts L, Lazarevic V, Derrien M, et al. Altered gut microbiota and endocannabinoid system tone in obese and diabetic leptin-resistant mice: impact on apelin regulation in adipose tissue. Front Microbiol 2011;2:149.

[48] Schele E, Grahnemo L, Anesten F, Hallen A, Backhed F, Jansson JO. The gut microbiota reduces leptin sensitivity and the expression of the obesity-suppressing neuropeptides proglucagon (GCG) and brain-derived neurotrophic factor (BDNF) in the central nervous system. Endocrinology 2013;154:3643–51.
[49] Everard A, Lazarevic V, Derrien M, et al. Responses of gut microbiota and glucose and lipid metabolism to prebiotics in genetic obese and diet-induced leptin-resistant mice. Diabetes 2011;60:2775–86.
[50] Cani PD, Bibiloni R, Knauf C, et al. Changes in gut microbiota control metabolic endotoxemia-induced inflammation in high-fat diet-induced obesity and diabetes in mice. Diabetes 2008;57:1470–81.
[51] Rajala MW, Patterson CM, Opp JS, Foltin SK, Young VB, Myers MG, Jr. Leptin acts independently of food intake to modulate gut microbial composition in male mice. Endocrinology 2014;155:748–57.
[52] Milanski M, Arruda AP, Coope A, et al. Inhibition of hypothalamic inflammation reverses diet-induced insulin resistance in the liver. Diabetes 2012;61:1455–62.
[53] Mehta NN, McGillicuddy FC, Anderson PD, et al. Experimental endotoxemia induces adipose inflammation and insulin resistance in humans. Diabetes 2010;59:172–81.
[54] Harte AL, Varma MC, Tripathi G, et al. High fat intake leads to acute postprandial exposure to circulating endotoxin in type 2 diabetic subjects. Diabetes Care 2012;35:375–82.
[55] Le Chatelier E, Nielsen T, Qin J, et al. Richness of human gut microbiome correlates with metabolic markers. Nature 2013;500:541–6.
[56] Vrieze A, Van Nood E, Holleman F, et al. Transfer of intestinal microbiota from lean donors increases insulin sensitivity in individuals with metabolic syndrome. Gastroenterology 2012;143:913–6 e7.
[57] Caricilli AM, Saad MJ. The role of gut microbiota on insulin resistance. Nutrients 2013;5:829–51.
[58] Christian LM, Porter K. Longitudinal changes in serum proinflammatory markers across pregnancy and postpartum: effects of maternal body mass index. Cytokine 2014;70:134–40.
[59] Mor G, Cardenas I, Abrahams V, Guller S. Inflammation and pregnancy: the role of the immune system at the implantation site. Ann N Y Acad Sci 2011;1221:80–7.
[60] Catalano PM, Roman-Drago NM, Amini SB, Sims EA. Longitudinal changes in body composition and energy balance in lean women with normal and abnormal glucose tolerance during pregnancy. Am J Obstet Gynecol 1998;179:156–65.
[61] Straughen JK, Trudeau S, Misra VK. Changes in adipose tissue distribution during pregnancy in overweight and obese compared with normal weight women. Nutr Diabetes 2013;3:e84.
[62] Misra VK, Trudeau S. The influence of overweight and obesity on longitudinal trends in maternal serum leptin levels during pregnancy. Obesity (Silver Spring) 2011;19:416–21.
[63] Vahratian A, Misra VK, Trudeau S, Misra DP. Prepregnancy body mass index and gestational age-dependent changes in lipid levels during pregnancy. Obstet Gynecol 2010;116:107–13.
[64] Catalano PM, Huston L, Amini SB, Kalhan SC. Longitudinal changes in glucose metabolism during pregnancy in obese women with normal glucose tolerance and gestational diabetes mellitus. Am J Obstet Gynecol 1999;180:903–16.
[65] Lain KY, Catalano PM. Metabolic changes in pregnancy. Clin Obstet Gynecol 2007;50:938–48.
[66] O'Reilly JR, Reynolds RM. The risk of maternal obesity to the long-term health of the offspring. Clin Endocrinol (Oxf) 2013;78:9–16.
[67] Aye IL, Lager S, Ramirez VI, et al. Increasing maternal body mass index is associated with systemic inflammation in the mother and the activation of distinct placental inflammatory pathways. Biol Reprod 2014;90:129.
[68] Kahn BB, Flier JS. Obesity and insulin resistance. J Clin Invest 2000;106:473–81.
[69] Chu SY, Callaghan WM, Kim SY, et al. Maternal obesity and risk of gestational diabetes mellitus. Diabetes Care 2007;30:2070–6.

[70] Tenenbaum-Gavish K, Hod M. Impact of maternal obesity on fetal health. Fetal Diagn Ther 2013;34:1–7.
[71] Koren O, Goodrich JK, Cullender TC, et al. Host remodeling of the gut microbiome and metabolic changes during pregnancy. Cell 2012;150:470–80.
[72] Turnbaugh PJ, Hamady M, Yatsunenko T, et al. A core gut microbiome in obese and lean twins. Nature 2009;457:480–4.
[73] Greenblum S, Turnbaugh PJ, Borenstein E. Metagenomic systems biology of the human gut microbiome reveals topological shifts associated with obesity and inflammatory bowel disease. Proc Natl Acad Sci U S A 2012;109:594–9.
[74] Jost T, Lacroix C, Braegger C, Chassard C. Stability of the maternal gut microbiota during late pregnancy and early lactation. Curr Microbiol 2014;68:419–27.
[75] Connor KL, Chehoud C, Chan L, DiStefano P, DeSantis T, Lye SJ. Maternal diet shapes the gut microbiome, impacting immune status in pregnancy. Reprod Sci 2014:137A Abstract T-025.
[76] Collado MC, Isolauri E, Laitinen K, Salminen S. Distinct composition of gut microbiota during pregnancy in overweight and normal-weight women. Am J Clin Nutr 2008;88:894–9.
[77] Gomez-Arango LF, Barrett HL, McIntyre HD, et al. Connections between the gut microbiome and metabolic hormones in early pregnancy in overweight and obese women. Diabetes 2016;65:2214–23.
[78] Ma J, Prince AL, Bader D, et al. High-fat maternal diet during pregnancy persistently alters the offspring microbiome in a primate model. Nat Commun 2014;5:3889.
[79] Connor KL, Chehoud C, Chan L, DiStefano P, DeSantis T, Lye SJ. Weight gain and leptin impact the gut microbiome in pregnancy. Reprod Sci 2014:137A Abstract T-024.
[80] Gohir W, Whelan FJ, Surette MG, Moore C, Schertzer JD, Sloboda DM. Pregnancy-related changes in the maternal gut microbiota are dependent upon the mother's periconceptional diet. Gut Microbes 2015;6:310–20.
[81] Luoto R, Laitinen K, Nermes M, Isolauri E. Impact of maternal probiotic-supplemented dietary counselling on pregnancy outcome and prenatal and postnatal growth: a double-blind, placebo-controlled study. Br J Nutr 2010;103:1792–9.
[82] Halkjaer SI, Nilas L, Carlsen EM, et al. Effects of probiotics (Vivomixx(R)) in obese pregnant women and their newborn: study protocol for a randomized controlled trial. Trials 2016;17:491.
[83] Okesene-Gafa K, Li M, Taylor RS, et al. A randomised controlled demonstration trial of multifaceted nutritional intervention and or probiotics: the Healthy Mums and Babies (HUMBA) trial. BMC Pregnancy Childbirth 2016;16:373.
[84] Endres LK, Straub H, McKinney C, et al. Postpartum weight retention risk factors and relationship to obesity at 1 year. Obstet Gynecol 2015;125:144–52.
[85] Chescheir NC. Global obesity and the effect on women's health. Obstet Gynecol 2011;117:1213–22.
[86] Rea K, Dinan TG, Cryan JF. The microbiome: a key regulator of stress and neuroinflammation. Neurobiol Stress 2016;4:23–33.
[87] Dinan TG, Cryan JF. Gut instincts: microbiota as a key regulator of brain development, ageing and neurodegeneration. J Physiol 2016.[Q1]
[88] Molyneaux E, Poston L, Ashurst-Williams S, Howard LM. Obesity and mental disorders during pregnancy and postpartum: a systematic review and meta-analysis. Obstet Gynecol 2014;123:857–67.
[89] Aagaard K, Riehle K, Ma J, et al. A metagenomic approach to characterization of the vaginal microbiome signature in pregnancy. PLoS One 2012;7:e36466.
[90] Hunt KM, Foster JA, Forney LJ, et al. Characterization of the diversity and temporal stability of bacterial communities in human milk. PLoS One 2011;6:e21313.
[91] Cabrera-Rubio R, Collado MC, Laitinen K, Salminen S, Isolauri E, Mira A. The human milk microbiome changes over lactation and is shaped by maternal weight and mode of delivery. Am J Clin Nutr 2012;96:544–51.

[92] Han YW, Fardini Y, Chen C, et al. Term stillbirth caused by oral Fusobacterium nucleatum. Obstet Gynecol 2010;115:442–5.
[93] Fardini Y, Chung P, Dumm R, Joshi N, Han YW. Transmission of diverse oral bacteria to murine placenta: evidence for the oral microbiome as a potential source of intrauterine infection. Infect Immun 2010;78:1789–96.
[94] Aagaard K, Ma J, Antony KM, Ganu R, Petrosino J, Versalovic J. The placenta harbors a unique microbiome. Sci Transl Med 2014;6:237ra65.
[95] Backhed F, Roswall J, Peng Y, et al. Dynamics and stabilization of the human gut microbiome during the first year of life. Cell Host Microbe 2015;17:690–703.
[96] Koenig JE, Spor A, Scalfone N, et al. Succession of microbial consortia in the developing infant gut microbiome. Proc Natl Acad Sci U S A 2011;108 Suppl 1:4578–85.
[97] Poston L. Developmental programming and diabetes—The human experience and insight from animal models. Best Pract Res Clin Endocrinol Metab 2010;24:541–52.
[98] Ong KK, Loos RJ. Rapid infancy weight gain and subsequent obesity: systematic reviews and hopeful suggestions. Acta Paediatr 2006;95:904–8.
[99] Chu DM, Antony KM, Ma J, et al. The early infant gut microbiome varies in association with a maternal high-fat diet. Genome Med 2016;8:77.
[100] Galley JD, Bailey M, Kamp Dush C, Schoppe-Sullivan S, Christian LM. Maternal obesity is associated with alterations in the gut microbiome in toddlers. PLoS One 2014;9:e113026.

Shimrit Yaniv-Salem and Gustaaf Dekker

19 Obesity and the risk of stillbirth

19.1 Introduction

Stillbirths are a devastating event, affecting the physical, emotional, and social integrity of a family and their community [1]. The terminologies regarding fetal deaths and stillbirths are a source of great confusion leading to a great lack of uniformity in publications and reports on perinatal death in various countries.

There are more than 35 classification systems for perinatal mortality [2–4], and there is no international consensus on which one to use. The Stockholm Classification of stillbirth, which is exclusive for stillbirths, consists of 17 groups of causes of death and allows for one primary and several associated causes if needed. There is also a probability level (definite, probable, or possible) assigned to the diagnoses in this classification system [3].

The World Health Organization (WHO) defines "fetal death" as death of a fetus prior to complete expulsion from the mother, irrespective of the duration of pregnancy [5]. Although many Western countries including Canada, the United States, the United Kingdom, and Australia [6, 7] use a cutoff of ≥20 weeks to define stillbirth, the WHO uses the definition of a demised fetus of 1,000 g or more at birth, or after 28 completed weeks of gestation, or attainment of at least 35 cm crown-heel length to allow international comparability.

Although in recent years, there has been a growing body of literature regarding stillbirths, it is clear that there is still a substantial gap in knowledge [8, 9]. The WHO reported 2.6 million stillbirths worldwide in 2015, a daily rate of 7800 stillbirths per day. Rates of stillbirth range from as high as 42 per 1,000 deliveries in Nigeria, to as low as 2.1 per 1,000 deliveries in Japan [9]. The Every Newborn Action Plan has the stillbirth target at 12 per 1,000 births or less by 2030 [10].

A recent *Lancet* series, although demonstrating a constant annual rate reduction of 2%, compared with a previous *Lancet* series [11], also emphasized that this annual rate reduction is much lower than the one demonstrated in maternal and pediatric mortalities.

Numerous studies attempting to identify risk factors, and more so modifiable risk factors, have pointed toward an increased body mass index (BMI) as an important risk factor for stillbirths [11–21]. This is true for both developed and developing countries, as it is across the spectrum of socioeconomic and ethnic groups within these countries [22–24].

Although some studies recognized a BMI of 30 as the cutoff for associated risk of stillbirth, others show a more complex and continuous association. In a systemic review and meta-analysis of more than 16,274 stillbirths, Aune et al. [25] found that for every five-unit increase in maternal BMI, there was a 1.24 relative risk for stillbirth. Yao et al. [26] have shown, in a cohort of more than 2.6 million women, a dose-dependent relationship between overweight, obesity, and stillbirth throughout gestation and more so at term. In that study, BMI and stillbirth followed a linear

https://doi.org/10.1515/9783110487817-019

association throughout the gestation for all BMI groups, but for category III and BMI of 50 or more, an exponential one at term (see Fig. 19.1).

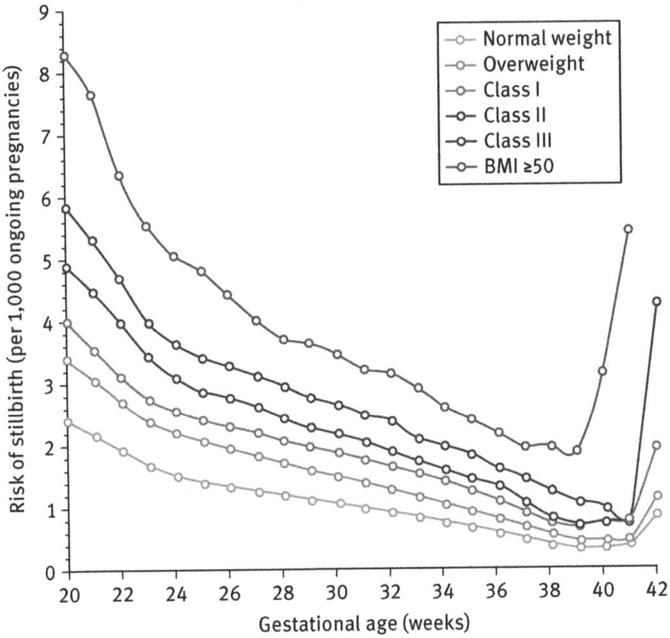

Fig. 19.1: Risk of stillbirth and BMI Class.

The big question is of course – will timely induction of labor result in a better outcome? Although there are no guidelines, many obstetricians do implement specific protocols for induction of labor for pregnant women with obesity (covered elsewhere in this text).

19.2 Pathophysiology of stillbirth in pregnancies affected by obesity

The mechanisms underlying the cause of stillbirth are likely numerous and a number of key risk factors associated with obesity may play an important role, including hypertension in pregnancy, gestational diabetes, and increased rate of congenital anomalies.

19.2.1 Increased risk for preeclampsia

Obesity increased the risk for hypertensive morbidity and preeclampsia in multiple reports [27–32]. Increased inflammatory stress and dyslipidemia are likely to be two main causes [33] O'Brien et al. [34], in a systematic review, found this to be a dose-dependent association. In this review of 13 cohort studies including nearly 1.4 million women, the risk of preeclampsia doubled with each 5 to 7 kg/m^2 increase in prepregnancy BMI. Increased BMI is a risk for both preterm and term preeclampsia [35]. Preeclampsia, in its severe form, has been long shown to have a causal relationship with stillbirths [12, 36–38]. In an 11-year cohort study of 1,089 stillbirths, from singleton pregnancies at gestational age ≥22 + 0 in the Stockholm population, Stormdal Bring et al. [39] found that preeclampsia is more prevalent in the preterm stillbirth group than in the term/post term group, implying that the association may correlate with severity of preeclampsia.

19.2.2 Increased risk for gestational diabetes mellitus

The prevalence of gestational diabetes mellitus (GDM) is significantly higher in obese women than in the general obstetrical population [40–42], and the risk increases with increasing maternal weight and BMI [43–46]. This correlation of increasing weight with increased risk of type 2 diabetes and GDM is related to the increase in insulin resistance in the obese state [47], superimposed on the endocrine effects of the placenta. Insulin-resistant states in pregnancy are associated with a higher risk of intrauterine fetal demise [48–53].

Although the increased risk for preeclampsia and GDM definitely contributes to the increased risk for stillbirth, changes in contemporary obstetrics, in particular, timely induction of labor, have probably mitigated their effect.

19.2.3 Increased risk of congenital anomalies

Research regarding maternal obesity and fetal anomalies is complex, both due to the heterogeneity of the birth defects studied, and the inconsistency in BMI categories [54, 55]. Block et al. [56] found an increased risk of birth defects with increased BMI. In their retrospective study from the Florida Birth Defect register, they reviewed more than one million births, from which 44,629 had at least one of 27 birth defects, including one composite outcome of any birth defect. Newborns affected with trisomies were excluded from analysis. Patients were divided into six BMI categories. In this large data set, overweight women were more likely to have delivered an infant diagnosed with "any birth defect." Compared with normal-weight women, obese women experienced increased odds of giving birth to a child with a number of birth defect outcomes: cleft lip with and without cleft palate, cleft palate without cleft lip, diaphragmatic hernia, endocardial cushion defect, obstructive genitourinary defect, pulmonary valve atresia and stenosis, pyloric stenosis, rectal and large intestinal atresia/stenosis, and spina bifida without anencephaly, tetralogy of Fallot (TOF), transposition of the great arteries, ventricular septal defect (VSD), and "any birth defect." Dose dependent relationship we observed between prepregnancy BMI and five congenital heart defects: hypoplastic left heart syndrome, pulmonary valve atresia/stenosis, TOF, transposition of the great arteries, and VSD. A similar dose-response association was also observed for cleft palate without cleft lip, diaphragmatic hernia, hydrocephalus without spina bifida, pyloric stenosis, and rectal and large intestinal atresia/stenosis.

The complexity of these associations was highlighted in the findings of Carmichael et al. [57]. This study examined the independent and combined effects of overweight or obese maternal BMI and low diet quality on risks of 32 types of structural birth defects. Twenty thousand cases were reviewed with 8,617 controls. Results indicated an association of elevated (overweight or obese) BMI alone, or lower diet quality alone, with 16 of the studied birth defects, with the authors stating that prepregnancy obesity and low diet quality are both important but complex factors that are associated with risks of several birth defects.

An anomaly-based approach yielded an association between increased BMI and specific cardiac anomalies [58], hydrocephalus [54, 59], recto-anal anomalies [60], renal anomalies [61], and neural tube defects [62].

19.3 Underdetection of congenital anomalies

Although it has been shown that obesity is associated with an increased risk of congenital anomalies, the technical difficulties in imaging this patient population cannot be ignored as a contributor to the underdetection of anomalies. The absorption of sound beam by subcutaneous tissue leads to signal attenuation and decreased image clarity [63, 64].

The effect of the decreased quality of imaging on detection rate has been subject to numerous studies [65–70]. Best et al. [71] reviewed 132,885 live births, with 3,096 cases of congenital anomalies from the Northern Congenital Abnormality Survey. This study found cardiovascular anomalies to be the most common postnatal finding, but the least likely to be detected prenatally. Detection rates decreased significantly with increasing BMI category for all anomalies.

The higher incidence and lower detection rates of congenital anomalies with higher BMI may both affect the increased risk of stillbirths in this population due to lack of identification of the fetus at risk.

19.4 Limitations of aneuploidy screening

Routine screening methods including first trimester screening and Integrated Prenatal Screening are based on the combination of a nuchal translucency scan and serum screening, both limited by increased BMI. The failure rate of nuchal translucency has been shown to be as high as 23% in the class III BMI group [72], and though not part of the formal risk calculation, nasal bone detection studies have shown that maternal obesity increases the chance of inadequate assessment [73]. Serum screening, although adjusted to BMI [74, 75], may be highly affected by small changes in reported maternal weight, further limiting the accuracy of aneuploidy screening [76].

High BMI also affects noninvasive prenatal testing, both by increasing the failure rate [77–79] and by increasing the false negative rates [79]. Higher failure rates have been found in all gestational ages, as reported by Yared et al. [80]. In this retrospective cohort study, 565 patients undergoing noninvasive prenatal testing were included. Maternal weight at initial screening was used, and obesity was defined as a BMI of >30 kg/m^2. Although maternal age, race, ethnicity, and gestational age at the time of screening were comparable between those women who had successful tests and those who had test failures, the failure rate increased dramatically as BMI increased, with a failure rate of 7.1% at a BMI of 28 to 29.9 kg/m^2 increasing to 50.0% at a BMI of >40 kg/m^2.

19.5 Fetal growth restriction

Another pathway linking obesity with of the increased risk of stillbirth is the incidence and difficulty in diagnosis of growth restriction. Maternal obesity has been found to be associated with a higher incidence of small-for-gestational age newborns [81, 82], whereas contrary to findings regarding limitations of ultrasound in anomaly detection, some studies reported that BMI did not affect the accuracy of growth estimation both in singleton and twin pregnancies [83, 84].

This impaired growth is most likely mediated by placental dysfunction. In addition to the aforementioned pathways linking obesity with preeclampsia, insulin resistance and the associated hyperinsulinemia may interfere with early placental growth and development [83, 85].

Furthermore, changes in glucose uptake and utilization, in lipid transport and metabolism, and in amino acid transport have been studied extensively in numerous animal models, and to a lesser extent in human studies [86]. These diverse changes share a common pathway; the proinflammatory milieu found with increased BMI.

These changes are not yet well understood but may be considered immediate factors in the processes leading to the increased risk of stillbirth associated with obesity.

19.6 Summary

Obesity is clearly a major contributor to stillbirth, particularly in countries with a "Western" lifestyle and diet, but also in large Asian populations currently facing an increasing diabetes epidemic. Obesity affects the inflammatory status, metabolism, placental function, and embryogenesis. Future research is urgently needed to better define the exact pathophysiologic pathways and, where possible, preventative strategies.

Obesity is theoretically both a preventable and curable condition. Prepregnancy counseling of obese women contemplating pregnancy, with appropriate involvement of allied health staff, is of pivotal importance if we hope to decrease the disease burden and pregnancy risks. Obesity must therefore be recognized as a real disorder for which prepregnancy counseling is indicated. Education of the patients and the general practitioners is a key ingredient of this strategy.

Bibliography

[1] Heazell AE, Siassakos D, Blencowe H, Burden C, Bhutta ZA, Cacciatore J, Dang N, Das J, Flenady V, Gold KJ, Mensah OK, Millum J, Nuzum D, O'Donoghue K, Redshaw M, Rizvi A, Roberts T, Saraki HET, Storey C, Wojcieszek AM, Downe S, Ending Preventable Stillbirths 3. Stillbirths: economic and psychosocial consequences. Lancet 2016;387:604–16.

[2] Gordijn SJ, Korteweg FJ, Erwich JJHM, Holm JP, Van Diem MT, Bergman KA, et al. A multilayered approach for the analysis of perinatal mortality using different classification systems. Eur J Obstet Gynecol Reprod Biol 2009;144:99–104.

[3] Varli IH, Petersson K, Bottinga R, Bremme K, Hofs OA, Holm M, et al. The Stockholm classification of stillbirth. Acta Obstet Gynecol Scand 2008;87:1202–12.

[4] Dudley DJ, Goldenberg R, Conway D, Silver RM, Saade GR, Varner MW, et al. A new system for determining the causes of stillbirth. Obstet Gynecol 2010;116:254–60.

[5] World Health Organization. International Statistical Classification of Diseases and Related Health Problems, 10th ed., World Health Organization, Geneva, 2004.

[6] Smith GCS, Fretts RC. Stillbirth. Lancet 2007;370:1715–25.

[7] www.stillbirthalliance.org. Accessed on February 28, 2007.

[8] Flenady V, Koopmans L, Middleton P, et al. Major risk factors for stillbirth in high income countries: a systematic review and meta-analysis. Lancet 2011;377(9774):1331–40.

[9] Lawn JE, Blencowe H, Waiswa P, Amouzou A, Mathers C, Hogan D, Flenady VJ, J Frøen F, Qureshi ZU, Calderwood C, Shiekh S, Jassir FB, You D, McClure EM, Mathai M, Cousens S, Ending Preventable Stillbirths 2. Stillbirths: rates, risk factors and acceleration towards 2030. Lancet 2016:587–603.

[10] WHO Every Newborn: An Action Plan to end preventable deaths, World Health Organization, Geneva, 2014. http://www.healthynewbornnetwork.org/issue/every-newborn/.

[11] Man J, Hutchinson JC, Ashworth M, Heazell AE, Jeffrey I, Sebire NJ, Stillbirth and intrauterine fetal death: contemporary demographic features of >1000 cases from an urban population. Ultrasound Obstet Gynecol 2016;48(5):591–595.

[12] Poston L, Caleyachetty R, Cnattingius S, Corvalán C, Uauy R, Herring S, Gillman MW. Preconceptional and maternal obesity: epidemiology and health consequences. Lancet Diabetes Endocrinol 2016;4:1025–36.

[13] Aminu M, Unkels R, Mdegela M, Utz B, Adaji S, van den Broek N. Causes of and factors associated with stillbirth in low- and middle-income countries: a systematic literature review. BJOG 2014;12:141–53.

[14] McClure EM, Saleem S, Pasha O, Goldenberg RL. Stillbirth in developing countries: a review of causes, risk factors and prevention strategies. J Matern Fetal Neonatal Med 2009;22:183–90.

[15] Di Mario S, Say L, Lincetto O. Risk factors for stillbirth in developing countries: a systematic review of the literature. Sex Transm Dis 2007;34:S11–21.
[16] Salihu HM, Dunlop AL, Hedayatzadeh M, et al. Extreme obesity and risk of stillbirth among black and white gravidas. Obstet Gynecol 2007;110:552.
[17] Johansson S, Villamor E, Altman M, et al. Maternal overweight and obesity in early pregnancy and risk of infant mortality: a population based cohort study in Sweden. BMJ 2014;349:g6572.
[18] Cnattingius S, Bergström R, Lipworth L, et al. Prepregnancy weight and the risk of adverse pregnancy outcomes. N Engl J Med 1998;338:147–52.
[19] Chen A, Feresu SA, Fernandez C, et al. Maternal obesity and the risk of infant death in the United States. Epidemiology 2009;20:74–81.
[20] Tennant PW, Rankin J, Bell R. Maternal body mass index and the risk of fetal and infant death: a cohort study from the North of England. Hum Reprod 2011;26:1501–11.
[21] Kristensen J, Vestergaard M, Wisborg K, et al. Pre-pregnancy weight and the risk of stillbirth and neonatal death. BJOG 2005;112:403–8.
[22] Gardosi J, Madurasinghe V, Williams M, Malik A, Francis A. Maternal and fetal risk factors for stillbirth: population based study. BMJ 2013;346:f108–21.
[23] Schumers L, Hutcheon JA, Bodnar LM, Lieberman E, Himes KP. Risk of adverse pregnancy outcomes by prepregnancy body mass index: a population-based study to inform prepregnancy weight loss counseling. Obstet Gynecol 2015;125(1):133–43.
[24] de Graaff EC, Wijs LA, Leemaqz S, Dekker GA. Risk factors for stillbirth in a socio-economically disadvantaged urban Australian population. J Matern Fetal Neonatal Med 2017;30:17–22.
[25] Aune D, Saugstad OD, Henriksen T, et al. Maternal body mass index and the risk of fetal death, stillbirth, and infant death: a systematic review and meta-analysis. JAMA 2014;311(15): 1536–46.
[26] Yao R, Ananth CV, Park BY, et al. Obesity and the risk of stillbirth: a population-based cohort study. Am J Obstet Gynecol 2014;210:457.e1–9.
[27] Robinson HE, O'Connell CM, Joseph KS, McLeod NL. Maternal outcomes in pregnancies complicated by obesity. Obstet Gynecol 2005;106:1357.
[28] Sibai BM, Gordon T, Thom E, et al. Risk factors for preeclampsia in healthy nulliparous women: a prospective multicenter study. The National Institute of Child Health and Human Development Network of Maternal-Fetal Medicine Units. Am J Obstet Gynecol 1995;172:642.
[29] Sibai BM, Ewell M, Levine RJ, et al. Risk factors associated with preeclampsia in healthy nulliparous women. The Calcium for Preeclampsia Prevention (CPEP) Study Group. Am J Obstet Gynecol 1997;177:1003.
[30] Weiss JL, Malone FD, Emig D, et al. Obesity, obstetric complications and cesarean delivery rate—a population-based screening study. Am J Obstet Gynecol 2004;190:1091.
[31] Gaillard R, Steegers EA, Hofman A, Jaddoe VW. Associations of maternal obesity with blood pressure and the risks of gestational hypertensive disorders. The Generation R Study. J Hypertens 2011; 29:937.
[32] Stuebe AM, Landon MB, Lai Y, et al. Maternal BMI, glucose tolerance, and adverse pregnancy outcomes. Am J Obstet Gynecol 2012;207:62.e1.
[33] Redman CW, Staff AC. Preeclampsia, biomarkers, syncytiotrophoblast stress, and placental capacity. Am J Obstet Gynecol 2015;213:S9.e1, S9–11.
[34] O'Brien TE, Ray JG, Chan WS. Maternal body mass index and the risk of preeclampsia: a systematic overview. Epidemiology 2003;14:368.
[35] Anderson NH, McCowan LM, Fyfe EM, Chan EH, Taylor RS, Stewart AW, Dekker GA, North RA, SCOPE Consortium. The impact of maternal body mass index on the phenotype of pre-eclampsia: a prospective cohort study. BJOG 2012;119(5):589–95.
[36] Ananth CV, Peltier MR, Chavez MR, et al. Recurrence of ischemic placental disease. Obstet Gynecol 2007;110:128.

[37] Ananth CV, Vintzileos AM. Ischemic placental disease: epidemiology and risk factors. Eur J Obstet Gynecol Reprod Biol. 2011;159(1):77–82.
[38] Abalos E, Cuesta C, Carroli G, Qureshi Z, Widmer M, Vogel JP, Souza JP, on behalf of the WHO Multicountry Survey on Maternal and Newborn Health Research Network. Pre-eclampsia, eclampsia and adverse maternal and perinatal outcomes: a secondary analysis of the World Health Organization Multicountry Survey on Maternal and Newborn Health. BJOG 2014;121(Suppl. 1):14–24.
[39] Stormdal Bring H, Hulth en Varli IA, Kublickas M, Papadogiannakis N, Peterson K. Causes of stillbirth at different gestational ages in singleton pregnancies. Acta Obstet Gynecol Scand 2014;93:86–92.
[40] Ehrenberg HM, Dierker L, Milluzzi C, Mercer BM. Prevalence of maternal obesity in an urban center. Am J Obstet Gynecol 2002;187:1189.
[41] Gross T, Sokol RJ, King KC. Obesity in pregnancy: risks and outcome. Obstet Gynecol 1980;56:446.
[42] HAPO Study Cooperative Research Group. Hyperglycaemia and Adverse Pregnancy Outcome (HAPO) study: associations with maternal body mass index. BJOG 2010;117:575.
[43] Sebire NJ, Jolly M, Harris JP, et al. Maternal obesity and pregnancy outcome: a study of 287,213 pregnancies in London. Int J Obes Relat Metab Disord 2001;25:1175.
[44] Chu SY, Callaghan WM, Kim SY, et al. Maternal obesity and risk of gestational diabetes mellitus. Diabetes Care 2007;30:2070.
[45] Catalano PM, Kirwan JP, Haugel-de Mouzon S, King J. Gestational diabetes and insulin resistance: role in short- and long-term implications for mother and fetus. J Nutr 2003;133:1674S.
[46] Torloni MR, Betrán AP, Horta BL, et al. Prepregnancy BMI and the risk of gestational diabetes: a systematic review of the literature with meta-analysis. Obes Rev 2009;10:194.
[47] Handwerger S, Freemark M. The roles of placental growth hormone and placental lactogen in the regulation of human fetal growth and development. J Pediatr Endocrinol Metab 2000;13:343.
[48] Girz BA, Divon MY, Merkatz IR. Sudden fetal death in women with well-controlled, intensively monitored gestational diabetes. J Perinatol 1992;12:229.
[49] Aberg A, Rydhström H, Källén B, Källén K. Impaired glucose tolerance during pregnancy is associated with increased fetal mortality in preceding sibs. Acta Obstet Gynecol Scand 1997;76:212.
[50] Dudley DJ. Diabetic-associated stillbirth: incidence, pathophysiology, and prevention. Obstet Gynecol Clin North Am 2007;34:293.
[51] Little SE, Zera CA, Clapp MA, et al. A multi-state analysis of early-term delivery trends and the association with term stillbirth. Obstet Gynecol 2015;126:1138.
[52] Starikov R, Dudley D, Reddy UM. Stillbirth in the pregnancy complicated by diabetes. Curr Diab Rep 2015;15:11.
[53] Melamed N, Hod M. Perinatal mortality in pregestational diabetes. Int J Gynaecol Obstet 2009;104 Suppl 1:S20–4.
[54] Stothard KJ, Tennant PW, Bell R, Rankin J. Maternal overweight and obesity and the risk of congenital anomalies: a systematic review and meta-analysis. JAMA 2009;301:636–50.
[55] Marengo L, Farag NH, Canfield M. Body mass index and birth defects: Texas, 2005–2008, Matern Child Health J 2013;17:1898–1907.
[56] Block SR, Watkins SM, Salemi JL, Rutkowski R, Tanner JP, Correia JA, Kirby RS. Maternal pre-pregnancy body mass index and risk of selected birth defects: evidence of a dose–response relationship. Paediatr Perinat Epidemiol 2013;27:521–31.
[57] Carmichael SL, Yang W, Gilboa SM, Ailes E, Correa A, Both LD, Feldkamp ML, Shaw GM. Elevated body mass index and decreased diet quality among women and risk of birth defects in their offspring. Birth Defects Res A Clin Mol Teratol 2016;106(3):164–71.

[58] Gilboa SM, Correa A, Botto LD, et al. Association between prepregnancy body mass index and congenital heart defects. Am J Obstet Gynecol 2010;202:51.e1–10.

[59] Kalyvas AV, Kalamatianos T, Pantazi M, Lianos GD, Stranjalis G, Alexiou GA. Maternal environmental risk factors for congenital hydrocephalus: a systematic review. Neurosurg Focus 2016;41(5):E3.

[60] Zwink N, Jenetzky Et, Brenner H. Parental risk factors and anorectal malformations: systematic review and meta-analysis. Orphanet J Rare Dis 2011;6:25–41.

[61] Macumber I, Schwartz S, Leca N. Maternal obesity is associated with congenital anomalies of the kidney and urinary tract in offspring. Pediatr Nephrol 2016;32(4):635–642.

[62] Huang HY, Chen HL, Feng LP. Maternal obesity and the risk of neural tube defects in offspring: a meta-analysis. Obes Res Clin Pract 2016: S1871–403X.

[63] Benacerraf BR. A technical tip on scanning obese gravidae. Ultrasound Obstet Gynecol. 2010;35:615–6.

[64] Weichert J, Hartge DR. Obstetrical sonography in obese women: a review. J Clin Ultrasound 2011, 39, 209–16.

[65] Zozzaro-Smith P, Gray LM, Bacak SJ, Thornburg LL. Limitations of aneuploidy and anomaly detection in the obese patient. J Clin Med 2014;3:795–808.

[66] Tabor A, Zdravkovic M, Perslev A, Møller LK, Pedersen BL. Screening for congenital malformations by ultrasonography in the general population of pregnant women: factors affecting the efficacy. Acta Obstet Gynecol Scand 2003;82:1092–8.

[67] Dashe JS, McIntire DD, Twickler DM. Effect of maternal obesity on the ultrasound detection of anomalous fetuses. Obstet Gynecol 2009;113:1001–7.

[68] Dashe JS, McIntire DD, Twickler DM. Maternal obesity limits the ultrasound evaluation of fetal anatomy. J Ultrasound Med 2009;28(8):1025–30.

[69] Benacerraf B. The use of obstetrical ultrasound in the obese gravida. Semin Perinatol 2013;37:345–7.

[70] Aagaard-Tillery KM, Flint Porter T, Malone FD, Nyberg DA, Collins J, Comstock CH, Hankins G, Eddleman K, Dugoff L, Wolfe HM, et al. Influence of maternal BMI on genetic sonography in the FaSTER trial. Prenat Diagn 2010;30:14–22.

[71] Best K, Tennant P, Bell R, Rankin J. Impact of maternal body mass index on the antenatal detection of congenital anomalies. BJOG 2012;119:1503–11.

[72] Thornburg LL, Mulconry M, Post A, Carpenter A, Grace D, Pressman EK. Fetal nuchal translucency thickness evaluation in the overweight and obese gravida. Ultrasound Obstet Gynecol 2009;33:665–9.

[73] Gandhi M, Fox NS, Russo-Stieglitz K, Hanley ME, Matthews G, Rebarber A. Effect of increased body mass index on first-trimester ultrasound examination for aneuploidy risk assessment. Obstet Gynecol 2009;114:856–9.

[74] Krantz DA, Hallahan TW, Macri VJ, Macri JN. Maternal weight and ethnic adjustment within a first-trimester Down syndrome and trisomy 18 screening program. Prenat Diagn 2005;25:635–40.

[75] Neveux LM, Palomaki GE, Larrivee DA, Knight GJ, Haddow JE. Refinements in managing maternal weight adjustment for interpreting prenatal screening results. Prenat Diagn 1996;16:1115–9.

[76] Huang T, Moschino WS, Okun N, Dennis A, Hoffman B, Lepage N, Rashid S, Au R, Farrell SA. The impact of maternal weight discrepancies on prenatal screening results for Down syndrome. Prenat Diagn 2013;33:471–6.

[77] Wang E, Batey A, Storable C, Musci T, Song K, Oliphant A. Gestational age and maternal weight effects on fetal cell-free DNA in maternal plasma. Prenat Diagn 2013;33:662–6.

[78] Ashoor G, Syngelaki A, Poon LC, Rezende JC, Nicolaides KH. Fetal fraction in maternal plasma cell-free DNA at 11–13 weeks' gestation: relation to maternal and fetal characteristics. Ultrasound Obstet Gynecol 2013;41:26–32.

[79] Canick JA, Palomaki GE, Khoza EM, Lambert-Messerlian GM, Haddow JE. The impact of maternal plasma DNA fetal fraction on next generation sequencing tests for common fetal aneuploidies. Prenat Diagn 2013;33:667–74.
[80] Yared E, Dinsmoor MJ, Endres LK, et al. Obesity increases the risk of failure of noninvasive prenatal screening regardless of gestational age. Am J Obstet Gynecol 2016;215:370.e1–6.
[81] Scott-Pillai R, Spence D, Cardwell C, Hunter A, Holmes V. The impact of body mass index on maternal and neonatal outcomes: a retrospective study in a UK obstetric population, 2004–2011. BJOG 2013;120:932–9.
[82] Leung T, Leung T, Sahota D, Chan O, Chan L, Fung T, Lau T. Trends in maternal obesity and associated risks of adverse pregnancy outcomes in a population of Chinese women. BJOG 2008;115:1529–37.
[83] Ahmadzia HK, Thomas SM, Dude AM, et al. Prediction of birthweight from third-trimester ultrasound in morbidly obese women. Am J Obstet Gynecol 2014;211:431.e1–7.
[84] Ryan HM, Morrison JJ, Breathnach FM, et al. The influence of maternal body mass index on fetal weight estimation in twin pregnancy. Am J Obstet Gynecol 2014;210:350.e1–6.
[85] Sferruzzi-Perri AN, Owens JA, Pringle KG, Roberts CT. The neglected role of insulin-like growth factors in the maternal circulation regulating fetal growth. J Physiol 2011;5891:7–20.
[86] Gallo LA, et al. Review: placental transport and metabolism of energy substrates in maternal obesity and diabetes. Placenta 2017;54:59–67.

Section III: **Intrapartum management**

Stefania Ronzoni and Gian Carlo Di Renzo

20 Induction of labor in the obese patient

20.1 Induction of labor in obese women

In developed countries, obesity represents one of the major challenges of modern medicine. Obesity prevalence has dramatically increased in the last decades showing a significant effect on women of reproductive age as well as on perinatal outcomes. In the Unites States, the incidence of obesity among pregnant women is estimated to be between 18.5% and 38.3% [1] and the recent Canadian Guidelines of Obesity in Pregnancy report an estimated obesity rate between 11% and 21% [2]. An increased body mass index (BMI) is associated with a significant greater likelihood of developing gestational diabetes, hypertensive disorders, postdates pregnancy, and fetal macrosomia as well as twice the rate of cesarean section compared with women with normal BMI [1, 2]. As a consequence, higher rates of induction of labor are required as women with gestational diabetes are often offered to be delivered at 38 to 39 weeks and women with hypertensive complications in pregnancy deliver by induction of labor between 34 and 37 weeks according to the severity of the disease [3]. Wolfe et al. [4] observed a progressively increased rate of induction of labor in association with the class of obesity; the rate of induction of labor results were 30.4%, 32.5%, and 34% in obese patients who belonged to class I (BMI = 30–34.9 kg/m^2), II (BMI = 35–39.9 kg/m^2), and III (BMI ≥ 40 (BMI > 40 kg/m^2), respectively, compared with an average induction of labor rate of approximately 23% of the general population.

20.2 Higher rate of failure of induction of labor in obese women

A large-scale study addressing the effect BMI has on induction of labor reported that in a cohort of more than 80,000 women, obesity was associated with induction failure rates twice as high as compared with normal weight controls (40.0% vs. 25.9%, respectively, $p < 0.022$) [4]. The rate of cesarean section followed by an induction of labor was found to be progressively higher according to the obesity class: 20.2% and 24.2% for women with obesity class I and II, respectively, and 31.6% for women with BMI from 40 to 50 kg/m^2. Obese patients with BMI >60 kg/m^2 presented a rate of cesarean section once induced of 63.2% and of 77.8% if nulliparous [4, 5]. Induction of labor failure rate observed in obese women was associated with lower starting Bishop score and was compounded by higher failure rates in obese women with Bishop score <3 [6]. However, in a multivariate logistic regression analysis, BMI was found to independently affect the rate of cesarean section after induction of labor when adjusted for other well-known factors such as advanced maternal age, fetal macrosomia, parity, gestational age, gestational weight gains, and cervical dilatation

https://doi.org/10.1515/9783110487817-020

at admission [7]. The same study showed that even for a population considered as ideal candidates for an induction of labor such as multiparae with a favorable cervix at admission, BMI represented a crucial factor in determining the success of trial of labor (Tab. 20.1) [7].

Tab. 20.1: Rate of failure of induction (CS) according to BMI class, parity, and admission cervical dilatation. Adapted from Ronzoni et al. [7].

Parity	Dilatation (cm)	BMI, underweight	BMI, normal weight	BMI, overweight	BMI, overweight
P = 0	≤1	35.5% (44/124)	38.7% (734/1,894)	51.4% (330/642)	61.4% (237/386)
	>1	16.1 (10/62)	27.6% (217/787)	30.4% (75/247)	36.0% (49/136)
P > 0	≤1	12.2% (7/57)	9.2% (73/792)	15.4% (46/299)	16.3% (36/220)
	>1	0% (0/69)	4.2% (38/902)	5.2% (17/329)	9.9% (17/171)

20.3 Different labor patterns in obese women

The onset of parturition in obese woman is frequently delayed compared with normal weight women. Obese women are, in fact, almost twice as likely as normal weight woman to have a prolonged pregnancy especially when there is a BMI of >35 kg/m^2 or higher [8]. Even after the spontaneous onset of labor, obese women present a prolonged and altered labor curve requiring a longer time period to achieve 6 cm cervical dilatation compared with normal weight women [9]. An impairment in the myometrial contractility with less Ca^{2+} flux in obese women compared with normal-weight women has been hypothesized as a possible mechanism involved in a prolonged first stage of labor and excessive blood loss in obese women [10]. Despite a decreased myometrial contractility, myometrial oxytocin receptor gene expression seems to be independent of BMI at the time of delivery [11]. It has been hypothesized that the normal parturition pathway is mainly altered by the characteristic metabolic dysregulation with changes in circulating hormones and free fatty acids [12]. Both leptin and cholesterol, which are significantly increased in obese women compared with normal weight pregnant women, have been proposed for the mechanisms behind the impaired contractility of the obese myometrium. In obese individuals and in pregnant women, in fact, there is an excess of adipose tissue resulting in altered expression patterns of leptin [13].

Leptin has been shown to decrease the influx of calcium ions into uterine smooth muscle [14]. Similarly, elevated levels of cholesterol have also been associated with decreased calcium influx in the myometrium [15]. The inhibition of calcium influx by both elevated leptin and cholesterol results in an antagonist effect against oxytocin, which normally causes myometrial contractions by releasing calcium from intracellular stores [10, 15]. Moreover, leptin stimulates prostaglandin E2 (PGE2) release from the placenta and adipose tissue through inflammatory signaling pathways [16]. Chronically elevated PGE2 in late pregnancy among obese women has been shown to decrease the sensitivity of maternal tissues to PGE2 during labor activation, a finding that has been documented clinically [17] and is supported by the known elevated PGE2 in obesity [18]. Thus, the chronic inflammatory state of obese women could negatively affect functional progesterone withdrawal and PGE2 activation. Leptin is also thought to play a role in inhibiting the cervical ripening by disrupting in vitro collagen degradation by matrix metalloproteinases and cervical cell apoptosis [19, 20] as well as stimulating the cervical collagen synthesis [19, 21]. Furthermore, high levels of circulating leptin in the second trimester have been demonstrated to inhibit fetal membrane weakening through decreased membrane apoptosis [20], leading to the inhibition of spontaneous rupture of membranes in obese women [22].

The clinical manifestations of this antagonistic effect include increased rates of postdates pregnancies, dysfunctional and prolonged labor patterns, and an increased rate of cesarean delivery in obese pregnant women.

20.4 Different responses to induction agents in obese women

Despite a well demonstrated different labor pattern in obese women compared with normal weight women, the consequences of obesity on cervical ripening have not been extensively studied and no guidelines about the dosage and duration of cervical ripening are known in the case of obesity. Only a few studies have specifically investigated the different responses of obese women to different medical induction methods. However, no studies have addressed the effect of mechanical induction methods on successful vaginal delivery in obese women.

Gauthier et al. [23] found that the failure rate of the first attempt at cervical ripening with the dinoprostone tampon was 1.6 times higher among obese patients compared with normal weight patients and the rate of cesarean section was two times higher in obese patients even after the administration of a second induction agent. Moreover, the length of labor in obese women who received the dinoprostone tampon was 5 hours longer compared with normal weight woman [23].

In another study, BMI >25 kg/m^2, nulliparity, low Bishop score, cervical length and the onset of uterine contractions were found to be independent predictors of failure of response to PGE2 when used for the induction of labor [24].

Suidan et al. [25] compared labor outcomes in obese women who underwent induction of labor with vaginal dinoprostone (10 mg) or misoprostol (either 25 µg vaginally or 50 µg orally). Obese women induced with misoprostol achieved a more successful cervical ripening, resulting in a lower cesarean section rate compared with obese women who underwent induction of labor with dinoprostone. This result was confirmed when adjusted for gestational age, parity, birth weight, and indication for induction and no differences in the rates of complications at delivery, such as necessity of emergent cesarean delivery, infection, or NICU admission, were found comparing the two groups. In addition, when the administration mode was considered for misoprostol, no differences were found between the group who received oral versus vaginal misoprostol in achieving a successful cervical ripening and vaginal delivery [25].

Lassiter et al. [26] found that women with higher BMIs required more doses of misoprostol during induction of labor compared with normal weight women. Pevzner et al. [27], in a secondary analysis during a multicenter double-blind, randomized trial (Misoprostol Vaginal Insert Trial), evaluated the duration, characteristics, and outcomes of labor for different BMI categories. Obese women who achieved a successful vaginal delivery had a longer labor compared with lean women, with a difference of more than 4 hours found when severely obese women (BMI >40 kg/m^2) were compared with normal weight women [27]. This is despite the fact that an obese BMI makes a woman more likely to not achieve active labor and have a higher rate of cesarean delivery for a failed induction that resulted in 29.8% and 36.5% in obese class I–II (BMI 30–39.5 kg/m^2) and obese class III (BMI >40 kg/m^2) women compared with a cesarean section rate of 21.3% in normal weight women [27]. Interestingly, women with elevated BMI required higher maximum doses of oxytocin and for longer time periods compared with nonobese women in the case of vaginal delivery or eventual cesarean delivery for induction failure [26–29].

20.5 Induction of labor in specific maternal medical conditions in obese women

Obesity is associated with a threefold increased risk of maternal preeclampsia and an increased risk of cesarean delivery [30]. Robinson et al. [31] evaluated the effect of maternal obesity on the mode of delivery among women undergoing an induction of labor for the diagnosis of preeclampsia. Based on multivariable logistic regression modeling, for every 5-unit increase in maternal BMI, a 16% increase in the odds of cesarean delivery was found in obese women with preeclampsia [31].

In a cohort of twin pregnancies requiring induction of labor, Park et al. [32] analyzed the predictive value of BMI, Bishop score, and sonographic measurement of cervical length for predicting successful labor induction. Only elevated BMI was associated with failure to achieve active labor after 24 hours of induction of labor. Obese women carrying a twin pregnancy showed an 82% rate of failure of induction within 24 hours.

Given the higher rate of failed labor induction resulting in a cesarean delivery, obese women are more likely to be potential candidates for a trial of labor after a cesarean section. It is well known that both obesity and induction of labor negatively affect a successful trial of labor after cesarean delivery [33, 34]. Chauhan et al. found that less than 15% of morbidly obese women with a prior cesarean delivery had a successful vaginal delivery. However, among the women who underwent induction of labor, none of them achieved a vaginal birth and more than half of them had infectious morbidity [35].

20.6 Excessive gestational weight gain in obese women requiring induction of labor

Excessive gestational weight gain (GWG) represents an additional negative predictive factor affecting a successful induction of labor and achieving vaginal delivery [36, 37]. In a population of women undergoing induction of labor for post dates, women gaining more than 12 kg showed an 8% increase in unsuccessful induction of labor by not achieving a vaginal delivery within 24 hours of beginning the induction [37]. Moreover, in case of induction of labor, an increased risk of cesarean section of 13% and 8% was found for every 5 kg in maternal weight gained and for every 1-unit increase in maternal BMI, respectively [36].

20.7 Conclusion

Considering the significant effect of elevated BMI on failed induction of labor rate, in particular in morbidly obese women, the management of obese women during pregnancy should be focused on minimizing the development of medical complications such as gestational hypertension and gestational diabetes in an attempt to reduce the indications for an induction of labor.

Furthermore, appropriate counseling, ideally preconceptionally and at the start of pregnancy regarding appropriate weight gain, nutrition, food choices, and physical activity, is necessary [2]. When an induction of labor is indicated, obstetric providers should make every attempt to increase the success of a labor induction in obese women, including being cognizant of the prolonged labor course and elevated required doses of oxytocin, and consider induction with misoprostol rather than dinoprostone [38]. Finally, in women with obesity well beyond class III and multiple risk factors for failing a trial of labor, there may be a role for individualized counseling and discussion of a planned cesarean delivery.

Bibliography

[1] Yogev Y, Catalano PM. Pregnancy and obesity. Obstet Gynecol Clin N Am 2009;36:285–300.
[2] Davies GAL, Maxwell C, McLeod L. SOGC clinical practice guidelines: obesity in pregnancy. J Obstet Gynaecol Can 2010;32(2):165–73.
[3] American College of Obstetricians and Gynecologists & Task Force on Hypertension in Pregnancy. Hypertension in pregnancy. Report of the American College of Obstetricians and Gynecologists' Task Force on Hypertension in Pregnancy. Obstet Gynecol 2013;122(5):1122–31.

[4] Wolfe KB, Rossi RA, Warshak CR. The effect of maternal obesity on the rate of failed induction of labor. Am J Obstet Gynecol 2011;205:128.e1–7.
[5] Gunatilake RP, Smrtka MP, Harris B, et al. Predictors of failed trial of labor among women with an extremely obese body mass index. Am J Obstet Gynecol 2013;209(6):562.e1–5.
[6] Zelig CM, Nichols SF, Dolinsky BM, Hecht MW, Napolitano PG. Interaction between maternal obesity and Bishop score in predicting successful induction of labor in term, nulliparous patients. Am J Perinatol 2013;30(1):75–80.
[7] Ronzoni S, Rosen H, Melamed N, Porat S, Farine D, Maxwell C. Maternal obesity class as a predictor of induction of failure: a practical risk assessment. Am J Perinatol 2015;32(14):1298–304.
[8] Arrowsmith S, Wray S, Quenby S. Maternal obesity and labor complications following induction of labor in prolonged pregnancy. BJOG 2011;118(5):578–88.
[9] Normal SM, Tuuli MG, Odibo AO, Caughey AB, Roehl KA, Cahill AG. The effects of obesity on the first stage of labor. Obstet Gynecol 2012;120(1):130–5.
[10] Zhang J, Bricker L, Wray S, Quenby S. Poor uterine contractility in obese women. BJOG 2007;114(3):343–8. Epub 2007 Jan 22.
[11] Grotegut CA, Gunatilake RP, Feng L, Heine RP, Murtha AP. The influence of maternal body mass index on myometrial oxytocin receptor expression in pregnancy. Reprod Sci 2013;20(12):1471–7.
[12] Karelis AD, St-Pierre DH, Conus F, Rabasa-Lhoret R, Poehlman ET. Metabolic and body composition factors in subgroups of obesity: what do we know? J Clin Endocrinol Metab 2004;89(6):2569–75.
[13] Hamed EA, Zakary MM, Ahmed NS, Gamal RM Circulating leptin and insulin in obese patients with and without type 2 diabetes mellitus: relation to ghrelin and oxidative stress. Diabetes Res Clin Pract 2011;94(3):434–41.
[14] Wuntakal R, Kaler M, Hollingworth T. Women with high BMI: should they be managed differently due to antagonising action of leptin in labour? Med Hypotheses 2013;80(6):767–8.
[15] Jie Z, Kendrick A, Quenby S, Wray S. Contractility and calcium signaling of human myometrium are profoundly affected by cholesterol manipulation: implications for labor? Reprod Sci 2007;14(5):456–66.
[16] Lappas M, Permezel M, Rice GE. Leptin and adiponectin stimulate the release of proinflammatory cytokines and prostaglandins from human placenta and maternal adipose tissue via nuclear factor-kappaB, peroxisomal proliferator-activated receptor-gamma and extracellularly regulated kinase 1/2. Endocrinology 2005;146:3334–42.
[17] Suidan RS, Rondon KC, Apuzzio JJ, Williams SF. Labor outcomes of obese patients undergoing induction of labor with misoprostol compared to dinoprostone. Am J Perinatol 2015;30:187–92.
[18] Subbaramaiah K, Morris PG, Zhou XK, Morrow M, Du B, Giri D, et al. Increased levels of COX-2 and prostaglandin E2 contribute to elevated aromatase expression in inflamed breast tissue of obese women. Cancer Discov 2012;2:356–65.
[19] Wendremaire M, Goirand F, Barrichon M, Lirussi F, Peyronel C, Dumas M, et al. Leptin prevents MMP activation in an in vitro model of myometrial inflammation. Fundam Clin Pharmacol 2012;26:83.
[20] Wendremaire M, Bardou M, Peyronel C, Hadi T, Sagot P, Morrison JJ, et al. Effects of leptin on lipopolysaccharide-induced myometrial apoptosis in an in vitro human model of chorioamnionitis. Am J Obstet Gynecol 2011;205:363.e1–9.
[21] Wendremaire M, Mourtialon P, Goirand F, Lirussi F, Barrichon M, Hadi T, et al. Effects of leptin on lipopolysaccharide-induced remodeling in an in vitro model of human myometrial inflammation. Biol Reprod 2013;88:45.
[22] Reti NG, Lappas M, Riley C, Wlodek ME, Permezel M, Walker S, et al. Why do membranes rupture at term? Evidence of increased cellular apoptosis in the supracervical fetal membranes. Am J Obstet Gynecol 2007;196:484.e1–10.

[23] Gauthier T, Mazeau S, Dalmay F, Eyraud JL, Catalan C, Marin B, Aubard Y. Obesity and cervical ripening failure risk. Matern Fetal Neonatal Med 2012;25(3):304–7.
[24] Melamed N, Yariv O, Hiersch L, Wiznitzer A, Meizner I, Yogev Y. Labor induction with prostaglandin E2: characteristics of response and prediction of failure. J Matern Fetal Neonatal Med 2013;26(2):132–6.
[25] Suidan RS, Rondon KC, Apuzzio JJ, Williams SF. Labor outcomes of obese patients undergoing induction of labor with misoprostol compared to dinoprostone. Am J Perinatol 2015;30(2):187–92.
[26] Lassiter JR, Holliday N, Lewis DF, Mulekar M, Abshire J, Brocato B. Induction of labor with an unfavorable cervix: how does BMI affect success? J Matern Fetal Neonatal Med 2016;29(18):3000–2.
[27] Pevzner L, Powers BL, Rayburn WF, Rumney P, Wing DA. Effects of maternal obesity on duration and outcomes of prostaglandin cervical ripening and labor induction. Obstet Gynecol 2009;114(6):1315–21.
[28] Hill M, Reed KL, Cohen WR. Oxytocin utilization for labor induction in obese and lean women. J Perinat Med 2015;43(6):703–6.
[29] Roloff K, Peng S, Sanchez-Ramos L, Valenzuela GJ. Cumulative oxytocin dose during induction of labor according to maternal body mass index. Int J Gynaecol Obstet 2015;131(1):54–8.
[30] Bodnar LM, Catov JM, Klebanoff MA, Ness RB, Roberts JM. Pre-pregnancy body mass index and the occurrence of severe hypertensive disorders of pregnancy. Epidemiology 2007;18:234–9.
[31] Robinson CJ, Hill EG, Alanis MC, Chang EY, Johnson DD, Almeida JS. Examining the effect of maternal obesity on outcome of labor induction in patients with preeclampsia. Hypertens Pregnancy 2010;29(4):446–56.
[32] Park KH, Hong JS, Kang WS, Shin DM, Kim SN. Body mass index, Bishop score, and sonographic measurement of the cervical length as predictors of successful labor induction in twin gestations. Perinat Med 2009;37(5):519–23.
[33] Durnwald CP, Ehrenberg HM, Mercer BM. The impact of maternal obesity and weight gain on vaginal birth after cesarean section success. Am J Obstet Gynecol 2004;191(3):954–7.
[34] American College of Obstetricians and Gynecologists. ACOG practice bulletin no. 115: vaginal birth after previous caesarean delivery. Obstet Gynecol 2010;116(2 Pt. 1):450–63.
[35] Chauhan SP, Magann EF, Carroll CS, Barrilleaux PS, Scardo JA, Martin JN, Jr. Mode of delivery for the morbidly obese with prior cesarean delivery: vaginal versus repeat cesarean section. Am J Obstet Gynecol 2001;185(2):349–54.
[36] Gawade P, Markenson G, Bsat F, Healy A, Pekow P, Plevyak M. Association of gestational weight gain with caesarean delivery rate after labor induction. J Reprod Med 2011;56(3–4):95–102.
[37] Torricelli M, Voltolini C, Conti N, Bocchi C, Severi FM, Petraglia F. Weight gain regardless of pre-pregnancy BMI and influence of fetal gender in response to labor induction in postdate pregnancy. J Matern Fetal Neonatal Med 2013;26(10):1016–9.
[38] Ruhstaller K. Induction of labor in the obese patient. Semin Perinatol 2015;39:437–40.

Aidan Sharkey and Mrinalini Balki

21 Analgesia and anesthesia for the obese parturient

21.1 Introduction

Obesity in pregnancy is of particular concern to the obstetric anesthesiologist owing to its potential for significant maternal morbidity and mortality. In a recent nationwide study, the prevalence of obesity was found to be five times higher among women who sustained cardiac arrest during hospitalization for delivery in Canada when compared with those who did not have a cardiac arrest [1]. Data from the Confidential Enquiries into Maternal Deaths in the UK and Ireland between 2012 and 2014 showed obesity to be associated with high odds of maternal deaths, with 33% of women who died being classified as obese and 18% being classified as overweight [2].

Despite the use of various efforts to combat obesity, its prevalence among women of child-bearing age is steadily increasing. Recent data from the National Centre for Health Statistics, United States, found that among women who delivered in 2014, 25.6% were overweight and 24.8% were obese [3]. With an increasing number of obese parturients in our labor wards, there is a proportional increase in demand on health care systems and health care practitioners alike.

Obesity during pregnancy carries with it an increased risk of both maternal and fetal complications (Tab. 21.1). An in-depth knowledge of the physiological changes and comorbidities associated with the obese pregnant woman is essential to the obstetric anesthesiologist looking after these high-risk patients to minimize morbidity and mortality.

Tab. 21.1: Maternal and fetal complications associated with obesity.

Maternal complications	Fetal complications
Hypertension	Miscarriage
Preeclampsia	Shoulder dystocia
Gestational diabetes	Macrosomia
Thromboembolic events	Congenital abnormalities
Obstructive sleep apnea	Stillbirth
Postpartum hemorrhage	Birth trauma
Assisted vaginal delivery	Neonatal death
Cesarean delivery	
Postoperative infection	

https://doi.org/10.1515/9783110487817-021

21.2 Definition of obesity

At present, there is no definition of obesity specific to pregnancy; however, the most clinically relevant definition is based on the body mass index (BMI) [4]. A pregnant woman is classified as overweight when her BMI is 25 to 29.9 kg/m^2, and obese when her BMI is 30 kg/m^2 or greater. Obesity can then be categorized as Class 1 (BMI 30–34.9 kg/m^2), Class 2 (BMI 35–39.9 kg/m^2), and Class 3 (BMI ≥40 kg/m^2) with additional subgroups in this category (see Tab. 21.2). It is important to establish the BMI of pregnant women as early as possible. The American College of Obstetricians and Gynaecologists recommends checking the BMI at the first prenatal visit. This is to allow for the expected increase in body weight during pregnancy due to an increase in the size of the fetus, blood volume, placenta, and amniotic fluid. Early identification of obese women also allows for early nutritional counseling, intervention, and attempts to minimize the complications associated with obesity. BMI should be tracked throughout pregnancy and obese women with a BMI ≥ 30 kg/m^2 should be advised to gain no more than 5 to 9 kg during their pregnancy as per recent National Research Council guidelines [5]. Studies have shown that this target can prove difficult with more than 50% of obese women gaining weight during pregnancy in excess of current recommendations [6].

Tab. 21.2: Obesity classification.

Classification	BMI (kg/m^2)
Normal	18.5–24.9
Overweight	25–29.9
Obese	
Class 1	30–34.9
Class 2	35–39.9
Class 3	≥40
– Morbid obese	40–49.9
– Superobese	≥50

21.3 Physiological changes of pregnancy and their anesthetic implications in the obese parturient

Several physiological changes occur during pregnancy with obesity often resulting in further limitation of the already stretched physiological reserve (Tab. 21.3). These changes can have a significant effect on the conduct of anesthesia in the obese parturient.

Tab. 21.3: Physiological changes of pregnancy and anesthetic implications in obese parturients.

Physiological changes of the obese parturient	Anesthetic implications
Respiratory	
Reduced chest wall compliance	Increased ventilation requirements
Increased O_2 consumption	Increased O_2 requirements
Increased V/Q mismatch	Decreased time to desaturation
Cardiovascular	
Left ventricular hypertrophy	Increased incidence of hypertension, peripartum cardiomyopathy, and arrhythmias
Intra-abdominal hypertension causing aortocaval compression	Exaggerated bradycardia and hypotension on supine position
Gastrointestinal	
Higher incidence of gastric reflux, hiatus hernia, and delayed gastric emptying	Increased risk of pulmonary aspiration on induction of anesthesia
Coagulation system	
Procoagulopathic state	Timing of neuraxial techniques difficult if on antithrombotic agents
Endocrine system	
Increased incidence of diabetes and gestational diabetes	Difficult peripartum glucose control Fetal macrosomia

21.3.1 Respiratory system

I. Increased work of breathing: Significant energy is required during ventilation to move the increased weight of the chest and abdominal wall in obesity. Chest wall compliance can be reduced by up to one-third of normal in obesity [7]. In contrast to women who increase their minute ventilation during pregnancy by increasing their tidal volume, obese individuals with reduced chest wall compliance increase their minute ventilation by increasing their respiratory rate, thus avoiding diaphragmatic fatigue.

II. Poor oxygenation: Obese parturients use a significantly higher percentage of total oxygen consumption when compared with nonobese controls during respiration even during quiet breathing [8]. Any weight gain during pregnancy further exacerbates this. Furthermore, an increased ventilation-perfusion (V/Q) mismatch is seen in obesity with ventilation occurring in the more compliant nondependent portion of the lung and perfusion occurring in the dependent portion of the lung. Oxygenation further deteriorates when the patient is in the supine or Trendelenburg position.

III. Changes in lung volumes: Both pregnancy and obesity are independently associated with significant changes in lung volumes. Both result in a reduction in the expiratory reserve volume, residual volume, and functional residual capacity (FRC). Intuition would lead us to believe that these changes are exacerbated in the obese parturient; however, this has been shown not to be the case. In obese pregnant women with reduced FRC in the prepregnancy state, further reduction in FRC during pregnancy is generally not significant [9]. As pregnancy progresses, the gravid uterus pushes the diaphragm in the cephalad direction and this may result in the closing volume becoming greater than the FRC with resultant alveolar collapse and thus significant V/Q mismatch. This phenomenon is unique to the obese pregnant women and can be further exacerbated by lying in the supine or Trendelenburg position [10].

Consequences of the respiratory physiological changes of obese parturients include:

- Decreased time to desaturation during periods of apnea [11].
- Increased O_2 requirements [12].
- Greater ventilator pressures required during positive pressure ventilation.
- Increased incidence of postoperative atelectasis.

21.3.2 Cardiovascular system

I. Both obesity and pregnancy independently result in an increase in blood volume and cardiac output (CO). The increase in CO is a result of both an increase in stroke volume and heart rate. In obese patients, there is an increase in preload as well as afterload, which results in left ventricular hypertrophy [13]. This is in contrast to nonobese patients who have an increased preload but decreased afterload and an increase in left ventricular diameter but not wall thickness.

II. Obese parturients are also more prone to hypertensive disorders, the risk being three times more in those over BMI of 30 kg/m^2 as compared to normal weight women [14].

III. Upon lying in the supine position, obese women are more prone to aortocaval compression syndrome due to the extra abdominal weight on the inferior vena cava impeding venous return.

Consequences of the cardiovascular physiological changes include:

- Increased incidence of peripartum cardiomyopathy as a result of an increase in CO around the time of delivery. This occurs when patients with limited reserve cannot tolerate this increase in cardiac demand [15].
- Increased incidence of serious arrhythmias, especially around the time of delivery [16]. This is a result of a hypertrophied myocardium and also increased levels of catecholamines during labor.
- Increased incidence of hypotension and bradycardia upon lying in the supine position due to aortocaval compression.

21.3.3 Gastrointestinal system

In both the obese and nonobese population, there is a delay in gastric emptying during labor, thus putting these patients at risk of Mendelson's syndrome (aspiration pneumonitis) if they were to proceed to general anesthesia. Obesity carries with it additional risk factors, which include an increased incidence of hiatus hernia [17], gastroesophageal reflux [17], gastroparesis from diabetes mellitus [18], difficult bag mask ventilation [19], and difficult intubation [20].

Consequences of the gastrointestinal physiological changes include:

- An increased risk of aspiration pneumonitis during induction or extubation of general anesthesia due to the associated risk factors, in addition to a higher rate of both operative delivery and failure of neuraxial techniques in the obese population.

21.3.4 Coagulation system

Venous thromboembolism is the leading cause of direct maternal mortality [1]. Obesity potentiates all aspects of Virchow's triad putting this cohort of patients at particular risk for thromboembolic events in the peripartum period.

Consequences of the coagulation changes include:

- Obese patients are more likely to be commenced on low-molecular weight heparin or similar medications in the later stages of pregnancy to reduce the incidence of thromboembolic events [21]. These medications may interfere with the placement or removal of an epidural catheter or spinal insertion if the interval between the administration of anticoagulants and neuraxial procedure is short.
- There is also a risk of postpartum hemorrhage if anticoagulants are not stopped prior to delivery.

21.3.5 Endocrine system

Patients with a BMI ≥40 kg/m^2 are about seven times more likely to have diabetes mellitus than those with a normal BMI [22]. The incidence of gestational diabetes mellitus is also increased in the obese parturients.

Consequences of the endocrine changes include:

- Difficult blood glucose control in the peripartum period.
- Increased incidence of fetal macrosomia [23] leading to a higher rate of assisted and operative delivery requiring anesthetic intervention.

21.4 Obstructive sleep apnea and the obese parturient

Obstructive sleep apnea (OSA) is characterized by recurrent partial or complete episodes of upper airway obstruction during sleep leading to hypoxemia, hypercarbia, and a poor sleep pattern. Obesity and OSA are closely related, with obesity being a significant risk factor for the development of OSA [24]. There should be a high index of suspicion for undiagnosed OSA in all obese parturients.

The exact prevalence of OSA among the pregnant population has yet to be fully ascertained; however, results of a recent small prospective cohort study suggested the prevalence to be approximately 8.4% in the first trimester and up to 19.7% in the third trimester for all BMI groups [25]. This number is very concerning as it is greater than the incidence in the general population. Often, OSA is underdiagnosed in pregnancy leading to undertreatment and related complications.

The repeated episodes of hypoxemia seen in OSA can lead to both endocrine and metabolic disturbances, which may result in both maternal and fetal side effects. Potential maternal side effects of OSA include an increased risk of severe maternal morbidity [26], preeclampsia and gestational hypertension [27], gestational diabetes [28], and preterm delivery [29]. The effects of OSA on the fetus are as of yet unclear with studies having conflicting results. Some studies attribute OSA to fetal heart decelerations [30]; however, other studies have failed to repeat these results and found no correlation between OSA and fetal heart rate changes [31].

Screening tools such as the STOP-BANG [32] and Berlin questionnaires [33], which are used to detect the presence of OSA in the general population, are poorly predictive in pregnancy [31]. The low sensitivity and specificity yield of these questionnaires almost makes them obsolete, although they seem to improve as the pregnancy progresses. The development of OSA questionnaires specific to pregnancy is an evolving area of current research. Facco et al. [34] have demonstrated greater sensitivity and specificity using a four-variable prediction rule, which incorporates the presence of frequent snoring and chronic hypertension as well as age and BMI. Larger validation studies are required to identify the exact maternal characteristics associated with OSA and incorporate them into a questionnaire that will reliably detect OSA in the obstetric population. If there is a suspicion of OSA, formal testing in the form of an overnight polysomnogram should be undertaken to detect and categorize the severity of OSA.

With regard to treatment modalities for OSA, there are currently no pregnancy-specific guidelines and the approach to treatment of OSA in pregnancy is similar to that in the general population. Indeed, there is no evidence at present that the treatment has any effect on maternal or neonatal morbidity; however, it is suggested that all women with moderate to severe OSA should be treated. The mainstay of treatment is nocturnal continuous positive airway pressure (CPAP), which is generally effective and well tolerated but often compliance rates fall to less than 50% [35]. Other measures that can be taken include avoiding excessive weight gain during pregnancy and sleeping in the lateral recumbent or head elevated position.

Extra care during the intrapartum and postpartum period should be undertaken for patients with documented or suspected OSA. Neuraxial techniques are favored for these patients who require a cesarean delivery and indeed siting an early epidural for labor should be considered. Avoiding concomitant administration of systemic opioids and sedatives, which may cause respiratory depression, is of paramount importance. Adequate monitoring of all patients including those who received neuraxial opioids should be undertaken due to the possibility of delayed respiratory depression. CPAP devices should be continued and supplemental oxygen given if hypoxemia is observed. The latest American Society of Anesthesiologists' (ASA) guideline suggests at least 24 hours of monitoring in high-risk patients who receive neuraxial opioids [36].

21.5 Anesthesia and perioperative care of the obese parturient

The most important component of caring for the obese parturient during labor or operative delivery is good communication between the various healthcare providers, including midwives, obstetricians, and anesthesiologists. Ideally, the patient should have been seen in a preanesthesia consultation clinic and an anesthetic plan be formulated to best suit the anticipated mode of delivery. Potential difficulties such as those with palpating intervertebral spaces, accessing airway or veins, monitoring with regular-sized blood pressure (BP) cuff, and the presence of OSA, should be flagged early. Ultrasound-guided intravenous (IV) access and invasive BP monitoring may be required. On arrival to the labor ward, early involvement of anesthesia should be undertaken.

21.6 Labor and vaginal delivery

Neuraxial analgesia is considered the best option for labor analgesia in the obese patient. Given that there is a higher incidence of fetal macrosomia [23] in this population, it is imperative that adequate analgesia is provided to facilitate vaginal delivery. Also, the incidence of conversion to operative delivery is up to 33% in obese parturients [37]; hence, having a functional epidural in-situ allows the cesarean delivery to be done with epidural top-up, thus avoiding a general anesthetic and the inherent risks associated with it.

Early establishment of epidural analgesia is highly recommended in the obese population due to the increased incidence of difficult insertion, epidural failure, and the need to re-site epidural catheters. The incidence of failed labor analgesia requiring a repeat neuraxial procedure in obese parturients is reported to be up to 42% [38] and multiple attempts at catheter insertion or manipulation are not uncommon.

21.6.1 Ultrasound use for epidural placement

Technically, siting the epidural is more difficult in the obese parturient and adequate measures should be undertaken to optimize conditions and improve success rate. The sitting position is preferred and time should be spent to optimize the position with possibly the aid of a positioning device, which is commercially available (see Fig. 21.1). Prepuncture neuraxial ultrasound (see Fig. 21.2) may be beneficial in this group of patients to improve success. Studies have shown that the use of prepuncture ultrasound in obese parturients facilitated the identification of the correct lumbar interspace more accurately than palpation [39], accurately predicted the depth to the epidural space, and resulted in increased success and ease of performance [19]. Poor visualization and underestimation of the depth to the epidural space are possible due to the deep location of the ligamentum flavum and a greater degree of subcutaneous tissue compression by the ultrasound transducer, respectively. However, it should be noted that the visibility in the paramedian sagittal plane is likely to be superior to that in the transverse median plane. The estimates of ultrasound-determined distance to the epidural space in both these planes are comparable to each other and can be used interchangeably [40]. For accurate measurement of the depth and avoidance of underestimation from tissue compression, it may be advisable to release the pressure on the transducer after obtaining an optimized image. If the ultrasound-predicted depth to the epidural space is longer than 8 cm, a longer needle should be considered [41].

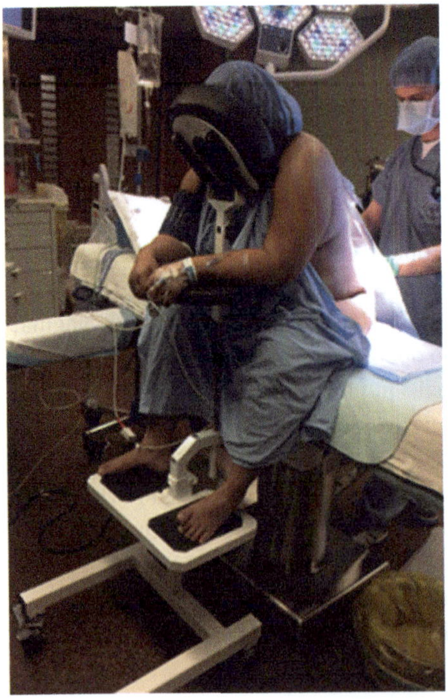

Fig. 21.1: Patient positioned for combined spinal epidural in the operating room using epidural positioning device. Written consent from patient obtained for this image.

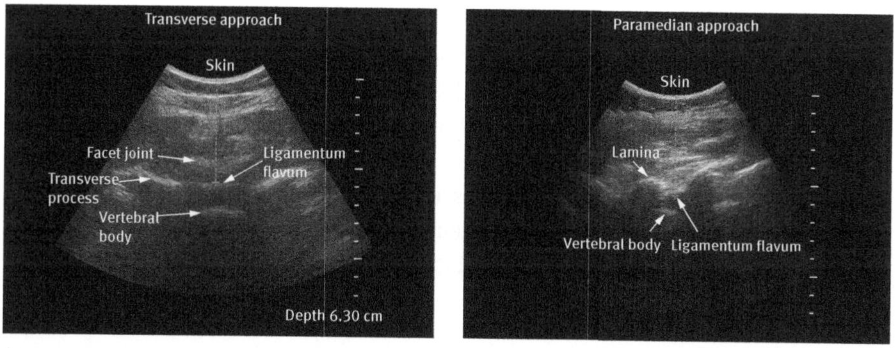

Fig. 21.2: Spinal ultrasound image in obese parturient. (**A**) Scanning in transverse approach; (**B**) scanning in paramedian longitudinal approach. Vertical dotted line represents the depth to the epidural space.

Once the epidural space has been identified, the catheter should be threaded to leave at least 5 to 7 cm length in the epidural space. This will help reduce the likelihood of epidural catheter migration. Confirmation of correct epidural catheter is again essential and we would advocate the use of either the Tsui test [42] (epidural electrical stimulation test) or a local anesthetic test dose to confirm correct placement prior to administrating a loading dose through the catheter. During the labor process, the adequacy of analgesia should be constantly evaluated and there should be a low threshold to re-site the epidural catheter if analgesia is suboptimal.

21.6.2 Choice of interspace

With regards to what is the ideal interspace for the placement of epidural catheter in the obese population, we feel siting at a higher interspace than the traditional L3/L4 level is more advantageous. Technically, in this population, the higher lumbar interspaces are easier to puncture and the depth to the epidural space is shorter, thus allowing the operator to use normal length needles. Also, at this level, there is less catheter movement thus reducing the incidence of epidural catheter dislodgement. Having an epidural sited in the upper lumbar region also provides an adequate coverage of the dermatomal levels and superior anesthesia if the patient was to proceed to an operative delivery. This is because the obstetricians most often use either a higher Pfannenstiel incision than traditional or perform a classical uterine incision.

21.6.3 Dural puncture

The incidence of inadvertent dural puncture with epidural needle is higher in the obese population [43]; approximately four times that of the nonobese population.

However, the progression to postdural puncture headache seems to be less [44]. This is thought to be because obese parturients have an increased intra-abdominal pressure, thus reducing the leakage of cerebrospinal fluid through the dural puncture site. If the dura is accidently punctured, the operator can consider threading the catheter into the subarachnoid space and use a continuous spinal for analgesia. We do not routinely opt for this during labor because of the possibility of excessive motor block, unpredictability, lack of experience, and poor evidence to support its use, but instead elect to re-site the epidural, unless the epidural placement was technically very challenging.

21.7 Cesarean delivery

Central neuraxial blockade is the anesthetic technique of choice in obese parturients, as long as there are no contraindications. Despite an increase in the rate of cesarean deliveries over the last three decades, there has been a decline in overall maternal mortality [45]; this has largely been attributed to the increased use and safety of regional anesthesia. Here, we will discuss general considerations for both regional and general anesthesia and also the specific considerations for each technique for obese parturients (see Tab. 21.4).

Tab. 21.4: Anesthetic considerations for obese parturients.

Neuraxial anesthesia	General anesthesia
– Early placement of epidural	– Consider aspiration prophylaxis
– Use positioning device for optimal patient positioning	– Position on TROOP pillow
– Site epidural catheter in high lumbar interspace	– Optiflow for pre- and apneic oxygenation
– Use ultrasound guidance	– Prepare for difficult airway, consider awake fiber-optic intubation if difficulty anticipated
– Test epidural catheter location with Tsui test or local anesthetic test dose	– Consider multimodal analgesia including regional blocks
– Review regularly for adequacy of analgesia, replace as soon as deemed inadequate	– Extubate awake, sitting upright, and when adequate tidal volumes achieved
– Consider a combined spinal epidural anesthesia for cesarean delivery	– Monitor for postoperative respiratory depression

Note: General considerations for both regional and general anesthesia.

21.7.1 Positioning

Regardless of the mode of anesthesia used, all obese parturients should be positioned on a bariatric table in a ramped up position with left uterine displacement.

The ramped position can be achieved with either the use of a commercially available positioning device such as the TROOP pillow (see Fig. 21.3) or by the use of blankets. Either way, the aim is to achieve horizontal alignment of the external auditory meatus and the sternal notch. This position has been shown to improve laryngoscopic view in morbidly obese patients [45] while also conferring benefit in terms of improving hemodynamic and respiratory parameters during the cesarean delivery. Another consideration is to carefully retract the often large panniculus in such a way so as not to cause any hemodynamic or respiratory compromise. We suggest to perform vertical and cephalad retraction, which has been shown to reduce the risk of hypotension and hypoxemia. An additional advantage of the ramped up position is the prevention of gastroesophageal reflux.

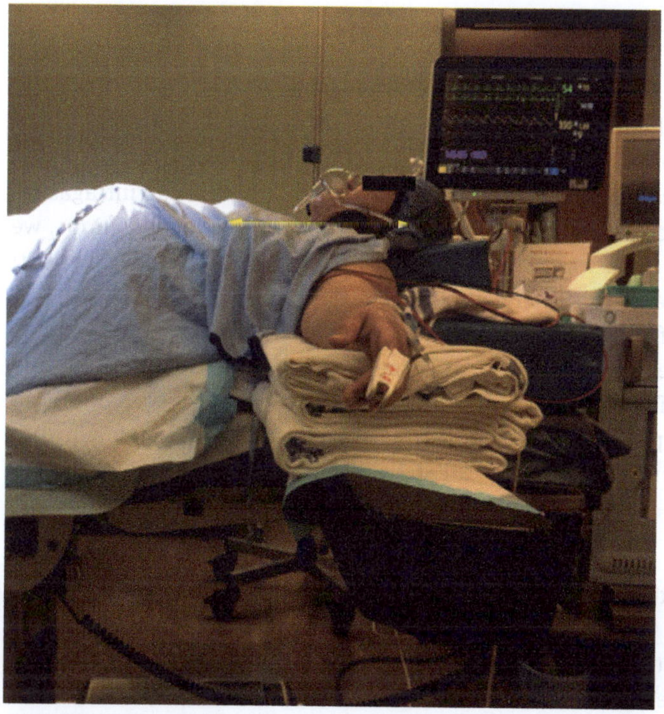

Fig. 21.3: Patient positioned on TROOP pillow showing optimal intubating conditions with horizontal alignment of the external auditory meatus with the sternal notch. Written consent from patient obtained for this image.

21.7.2 Monitoring

Adequate monitoring of the obese parturient during cesarean delivery is essential but often challenging. Appropriately sized cuffs must be used for accurate noninvasive

BP measurements. A forearm cuff may be used, which has shown to have a good correlation with upper arm readings [46]. In certain instances, where there are any comorbidities such as cardiac disease or there is a potential risk for bleeding, invasive monitoring in the form of an arterial line may be indicated.

21.7.3 Intravenous access

Secure IV access is essential for the safe delivery of anesthesia. The advent of ultrasound has made this easier in those patients who have poor venous access. At least two large-bore IVs should be secured prior to the commencement of anesthesia.

21.7.4 Aspiration prophylaxis

Pulmonary aspiration prophylaxis should be considered in all obese patients regardless of the mode of delivery. The routine use of sodium citrate, H_2 antagonists, and proton pump inhibitors is well established and studies have shown that administration of these medications significantly reduces the risk of having an intragastric pH < 2.5 [47]. In our center, in addition to the above-mentioned medications, we routinely administer metoclopramide, which we feel confers an added benefit; however, the evidence for this intervention is limited [47]. The use of gastric ultrasound to rule out a full stomach may also be considered in this population as standard fasting times may not necessarily mean an empty stomach, especially in laboring women. This is a very current and ongoing area of research, and in our experience, has proven very useful in identifying those with stomach contents despite complying with current Canadian Anesthesiologists' Society fasting guidelines [48].

21.7.5 Regional anesthesia

Various regional anesthetic techniques may be used for cesarean deliveries in obese women. These include, spinal (single shot or continuous), combined spinal epidural (CSE), or epidural. In general, if the patient has a good functioning labor epidural catheter, this can be topped up to achieve surgical anesthesia; otherwise, a technique that involves a spinal component is preferred.

21.7.6 Single shot spinal

Spinal anesthesia is an excellent choice for cesarean delivery as it delivers a fast, reliable, and dense block with superior operating conditions. It also facilitates the administration of intrathecal opioids for sustained postoperative analgesia. However, in morbidly obese populations, the surgery is often prolonged, and inability to extend the duration of the block with a single shot technique limits its use. Exaggerated cephalad spread of local anesthetic in the intrathecal space of obese patients, resulting in a high block with conventional doses, is a highly debated subject in the literature. Studies using magnetic resonance imaging have shown reduced lumbar cerebrospinal fluid volume due to increased abdominal pressure in obese nonpregnant subjects possibly from the inward movement of soft tissue in the intervertebral foramen, resulting in diminished dilution of anesthetic and a high block [49]. However, these effects do not seem to be apparent in clinical practice. Lee et al. [50] have shown that the effective dose (ED95) of bupivacaine for cesarean deliveries in obese parturients is the same as in nonobese parturients. Thus, reducing the spinal dose of local anesthetic in obese patients is not warranted and may even increase the risk of inadequate anesthesia.

21.7.7 Continuous spinal anesthesia

This technique offers all the advantages of a single shot spinal with the added benefit of being able to titrate the dose for greater hemodynamic stability and prolong the duration of the block by repeated top-ups. Despite these advantages, its use is limited by the high incidence of postdural puncture headache, as well as the risk of failure and need for supplemental analgesia in 9% to 24% of patients [51]. Another reported complication associated with continuous spinal anesthesia is cauda equina syndrome. Rigler et al. [52] reported four cases of cauda equine syndrome after continuous spinal anesthesia. It was initially suggested that the microcatheters themselves could be the cause due to maldistribution of anesthetic agent; however, subsequent studies implicated the slow flow rate of very hyperbaric solutions and subsequent pooling in the sacral area as the cause. At present, there are no commercially available continuous spinal kits in Canada; however, in other countries, the available kits (Wiley Spinal®) consist of a 23G catheter over a 27G atraumatic pencil tip needle, thus reducing but not eliminating the incidence of postdural puncture headache. To date, studies are limited on the use of this technique in routine obstetric practice and further studies are needed to see what role, if any, this technique has. In emergent situations, some authors may even consider the use of deliberate dural puncture with a Tuohy needle followed by intrathecal catheter placement, as it is often easier to identify the intrathecal space with a large-bore Tuohy needle and thus induce anesthesia quickly in morbidly obese women [53]. In our institution, we do not advocate the routine use of continuous spinal catheters; however, if there is an inadvertent dural puncture with a Touhy needle, we opt to thread the catheter approximately 3 to 5 cm into the intrathecal space and use this for anesthetic coverage.

21.7.8 Epidural

An epidural catheter that has been functioning well during labor can be topped up to achieve surgical anesthesia for cesarean delivery; however, the use of an epidural as a sole technique is not routine for elective cesarean deliveries. In the event of an emergency, we prefer topping up the epidural catheter with 5 to 10 mL local anesthetic in the labor room, so that adequate block can be quickly achieved with additional 5 to 10 mL local anesthetic top-up in the operating room and general anesthesia can be avoided. An epidural does allow for a slow gradual top-up, thus limiting the hemodynamic effects, which may be desirable in certain patients such as those with cardiac disease. An advantage of epidural catheter is that it allows for prolonged postoperative analgesia, which is beneficial for early recovery in these patients.

21.7.9 Combined spinal epidural

A CSE, in our view, is the best way to manage the obese parturient for a cesarean delivery. A CSE confers the benefit of a spinal while also having the ability to extend the duration of surgical anesthesia if the procedure is prolonged. There is also the ability to provide excellent postoperative analgesia with the epidural catheter, which can reduce the incidence of respiratory complications in this high-risk group. If there is a concern of the possibility of a high block or excessive sympathetic block with a spinal, the intrathecal dose of local anesthetic can be reduced and anesthesia titrated up slowly through epidural top-up. One concern with a CSE approach is the potential failure of the epidural component when the effect of the spinal wears off. However, the incidence of epidural failure when a needle-through-needle technique is used is much less than when an epidural is placed alone [54]. Some institutions suggest a double-segment technique with placement of spinal in the L3/4 interspace and a high lumbar or low thoracic epidural. This technique may be useful if a very high supraumbilical or midline incision is used by the operator. To date, there is no evidence to support one method over another and the technique used is often based on local experience. In our institution, we have very good communication with the surgeons and a detailed plan is formulated for each patient. With the aid of devices such as the self-retaining elastic abdominal retractor (MOBIUS™), high supraumbilical or midline incisions are generally not required and we find we can provide adequate anesthesia with a lumbar needle-through-needle CSE technique.

21.7.10 General anesthesia

Every effort should be made to avoid general anesthesia for cesarean delivery in the obese parturient as it is associated with significant morbidity and potential mortality [55].

However, if deemed necessary, certain principles must be adhered to in order to provide a safe anesthetic.

21.7.11 Airway

All obese pregnant patients should be regarded as having difficult airways. The incidence of difficult intubation in the obstetric population is between 1.3% and 16.3% [56], and the incidence of failed intubation up to 1 in 390 [57]. The incidence of difficult or failed intubation is likely to be even higher in the case of obese parturients. In addition, these patients are often difficult to bag mask ventilate and can easily end up into a "can't intubate, can't ventilate" scenario. A properly sized laryngeal mask airway could be life-saving in these situations. If a neuraxial technique is deemed to be contraindicated, then steps to maximize the success of tracheal intubation should be undertaken. It is important to properly position the patient in the ramped position with left uterine displacement as discussed before. Consideration for awake fiber-optic or video laryngoscope-assisted intubation should be undertaken. A difficult airway cart, appropriate size supraglottic device and skilled assistance should be readily available. Two anesthesiologists with experience in difficult airway management should be present. In case of failure, the anesthetist should be familiar with algorithms for managing difficult airways in the obstetric patient such as those set out by the Difficult Airway Society (DAS) [58].

21.7.12 Preoxygenation and apneic oxygenation

Good preoxygenation in this population is essential to try and prolong safe apnea time after the administration of muscle relaxant. Desaturation in the obese parturient can occur very precipitously, often occurring in less than 40 seconds of apnea even after adequate preoxygenation. Various methods of preoxygenation can be used such as tidal volume ventilation with 100% oxygen for 3 minutes or eight maximal inspiratory breaths. Another concept that is becoming popular is apneic oxygenation using high-flow nasal oxygenation with a device such as Optiflow™ system (Fisher and Paykel Healthcare Ltd., Panmure, Auckland, New Zealand). Devices such as this deliver O_2 at flow rates of up to 70 L/min and can significantly prolong the safe apneic period by maintaining oxygenation. In a recent study, the safe apnea time in a patient with a BMI of 54 kg/m^2 was prolonged to 5 minutes [59]. This extended safe apnea time may be life-saving in a difficult airway scenario. In our practice, we have started considering the use of an Optiflow device in morbidly obese patients undergoing a cesarean delivery, particularly for general anesthesia. DAS guidelines also advocate the use of gentle bag and mask ventilation (maximum inflation pressure <20 cm H_2O) before tracheal intubation after the administration of induction drugs to minimize desaturation and to allow an estimation of the likelihood of successful ventilation should a situation of difficult or failed intubation arise [58].

21.7.13 Induction and maintenance of anesthesia

Induction of general anesthesia should be achieved with drugs that suit the hemodynamic profile of the patient. Doses should be calculated using lean body weight as opposed to total body weight or ideal body weight, which are likely to overdose and underdose the obese parturient, respectively. Equations to calculate lean body weight such as the Boer formula [60] have limitations at extremes of obesity; however, more accurate equations from Janmahasatian et al. [61] have recently been developed, which are more suited to the obese parturient. In any case, a rapid sequence induction will be required unless there is a plan for awake fiber-optic intubation. Propofol and succinylcholine are the most common agents used to induce anesthesia. In our practice, we routinely use fentanyl as part of our induction, as we believe it confers a better hemodynamic profile during induction with minimal effects on the fetus [62]. Remifentanil could alternatively be considered to obtund pressor response [63]. Rocuronium can be used for neuromuscular blockade if there is a contraindication to succinylcholine. In this incidence, it is imperative that the neuromuscular reversal agent sugammadex be available in case immediate reversal is required in the event of difficult intubation/ventilation. Nerve stimulators should be used to monitor neuromuscular blockade. Maintenance of anesthesia is generally done with a mixture of volatile anesthetic mixed with nitrous oxide. Another option is to use total IV anesthesia with propofol and remifentanil. Use of bispectral index monitor can help ensure adequate depth of anesthesia. Long-acting hydrophilic opioids such as morphine or hydromorphone could be administered for postoperative analgesia. To minimize the use of systemic opioids, nonsteroidal anti-inflammatory drugs, acetaminophen, intraperitoneal instillation of local anesthetic, or transversus abdominis plane block should be considered for postoperative analgesia.

21.7.14 Intraoperative ventilation

Intraoperative ventilation and oxygenation can prove difficult in the obese parturients. High FiO_2 requirements are not uncommon and this is often accompanied by high driving pressures to overcome the reduced compliance of the chest wall. This puts these patients at an increased risk of lung trauma and postoperative pulmonary complications. The optimal way to ventilate obese patients is currently unknown; however, this is currently under investigation in a large international multicenter clinical trial [64]. In general, a lung-protective mode of ventilation should be used with low tidal volumes based on ideal body weight and starting with low positive end-expiratory pressure levels, which can be titrated upward to improve oxygenation if required.

21.7.15 Extubation

Extubating an obese parturient at the end of surgery is a critical stage and also a time when major complications can occur. In a recent report [65], it was noted that maternal mortality most often occurred during emergence and recovery, highlighting how crucial this particular period of anesthesia is. Extubation in the obese parturient should only take place when the patient is fully awake, alert, and obeying commands with adequate minute ventilation. If there are any doubts about the adequacy of ventilation prior to extubation, either from inadequate reversal of muscle relaxation or excessive narcotization, then the patient should remain intubated with a secure airway until it is safe to do so.

21.7.16 Postoperative analgesia and respiratory monitoring

Adequate analgesia is of the upmost importance so as to ensure early mobilization and reduce the incidence of pulmonary and thromboembolic complications. Postoperative analgesia will almost always take the form of opioid medications through neuraxial or systemic routes. Given that the incidence of diagnosed and occult OSA is high in this patient group, extended monitoring of respiratory parameters should be undertaken. Patients known to have OSA that use nocturnal CPAP should continue to use this in the postoperative period. If systemic opioids are to be used, they should be used in conjunction with a multimodal analgesic regimen and the dose of opioid be reduced as sensitivity to systemic opioids is common in this population group.

Regional analgesia techniques should be used whenever possible so as to reduce the use of systemic opioids [66] and to minimize the likelihood of adverse outcomes in patients at increased perioperative risk from OSA. Our recommended analgesic regimen consists of the use of either intrathecal fentanyl 10 μg and epimorph 100 μg, or epidural fentanyl 50 to 100 μg and epimorph 2.5 mg. Often, an epidural catheter is left in place postoperatively for 12 hours and an infusion of bupivacaine 0.0625% to 0.125% with fentanyl 2 μg/mL is administered at the rate of 5 to 10 mL/h. We also use nonopioid analgesic adjuncts such as acetaminophen and diclofenac. If general anesthesia is administered, patient-controlled analgesia with either morphine or hydromorphone at standard doses should be considered.

Morbidly obese patients or those with associated OSA should be monitored in high-acuity care units. As per ASA standards [36], patients should undergo monitoring for adequacy of ventilation (e.g., respiratory rate, depth of respiration), oxygenation (e.g., pulse oximetry when appropriate), and level of consciousness for a minimum of 24 hours after neuraxial morphine administration. The monitoring should be performed at least once per hour for the first 12 hours, followed by at least once every 2 hours for the next 12 hours. After 24 hours, frequency of monitoring should be dictated by the patient's overall clinical condition and concurrent medications. CPAP use should be considered and supplemental oxygen administered as needed to maintain acceptable arterial oxygen saturation.

21.8 Postoperative complications

Postoperative complications are common in obese parturients and hence their care should not end directly postpartum but should extend into the days after delivery. Some of the commonly encountered complications are listed below.

21.8.1 Postpartum hemorrhage

There is a high incidence of postpartum hemorrhage in the Class III obese population [67, 68]. This increased risk is seen in spontaneous vaginal deliveries, instrumental deliveries, and cesarean deliveries. In addition to an increased challenge to the operator to control hemorrhage, this group also poses a significant challenge to the anesthesiologist who may need to convert to a general anesthetic in an emergent situation to secure the airway and achieve a better hemodynamic control.

21.8.2 Thromboprophylaxis

Thromboembolic events are one of the leading causes of direct maternal mortality [2]. Adequate prophylaxis should be undertaken in the form of low-molecular weight heparin and the dose used should be weight-adjusted to ensure adequate dosing in this group. Timing of dosing should be discussed between the surgical and anesthesia teams to factor in the timing of neuraxial technique and catheter removal. According to the latest guidelines of the American Society of Regional Anesthesia and Pain Medicine, neuraxial anesthesia should be avoided for at least 10 h to 12 h after prophylactic and 24 h after therapeutic dosing of low-molecular weight heparin. Subsequent administration of low-molecular weight heparin should commence after at least 2 h of epidural catheter removal or 6–8 h postoperatively [69].

21.8.3 Infection

The incidence of postpartum infection is significantly high in the obese parturient. The risk of postoperative endometriosis is almost three times higher in obese than in normal weight parturient [70]. Postcesarean wound infection is almost doubled with every five-unit increment in BMI [71]. Both surgeons and anesthesiologists need to be vigilant to ensure adequately timed and dosed antibiotic administration. In our practice, we ensure preincision antibiotic dosing and adjust according to the patient's weight. We routinely dose 3 g of Cefazolin for morbid obese parturients to ensure adequate serum and tissue levels of antibiotic.

21.9 Summary

- The incidence of maternal obesity and its associated complications is increasing at an alarming rate and poses a significant challenge to the obstetric anesthesiologist and allied health staff.
- A multidisciplinary team approach and careful antepartum anesthetic planning is required to formulate the optimal conduct of anesthesia for the chosen mode of delivery.
- When possible, a neuraxial technique should be considered for both labor analgesia and surgical anesthesia for cesarean delivery.
- If a general anesthetic is required for the obese parturient, specific considerations and principles must be adhered to in order to deliver a safe anesthetic.
- The risk of OSA must be evaluated and suspected in all obese parturients and steps taken to minimize complications associated with it especially in the postoperative period.
- Postoperative complications are more common in the obese parturient and adequate analgesia, antibiotic prophylaxis and thromboprophylaxis are required to minimize complications.

Bibliography

[1] Balki M, Liu S, León JA, Baghirzada L. Epidemiology of cardiac arrest during hospitalization for delivery in Canada: a nationwide study. Anesth Analg 2017;124:890–7.
[2] Knight M, Nair M, Tuffnell D, Kenyon S, Shakespeare J, Brocklehurst P, Kurinczuk JJ (Eds.) on behalf of MBRRACE-UK. Saving Lives, Improving Mothers' Care—Surveillance of maternal deaths in the UK 2012–14 and lessons learned to inform maternity care from the UK and Ireland Confidential Enquiries into Maternal Deaths and Morbidity 2009–14. Oxford: National Perinatal Epidemiology Unit, University of Oxford 2016.
[3] Branum A, Kirmeyer SE, Gregory ECW. Prepregnancy body mass index by maternal characteristics and state: data from the birth certificate, 2014. Natl Vital Stat Rep 2016;65:1–11.
[4] National Institutes of Health. National Heart, Lung, and Blood Institute. Clinical guidelines on the identification, evaluation, and treatment of overweight and obesity in adults: the evidence report. Obes Res 1998;6 Suppl 2:51S-209S.
[5] IOM (Institute of Medicine) and NRC (National Research Council). Weight gain during pregnancy: reexamining the guidelines. Washington, DC: The National Academies Press, 2009.
[6] Lowell H, Miller DC. Weight gain during pregnancy: adherence to Health Canada's guidelines. Health Rep 2010;21:31–6.

[7] Sharp JT, Henry JP, Sweany SK, Meadows WR, Pietras RJ. The total work of breathing in normal and obese men. J Clin Invest 1964;43:728–39.
[8] Littleton SW. Impact of obesity on respiratory function. Respirology 2012;17:43–9.
[9] Eng M, Butler J, Bonica JJ. Respiratory function in pregnant obese women. Am J Obstet Gynecol 1975;123:241–5.
[10] Yap JC, Watson RA, Gilbey S, Pride NB. Effects of posture on respiratory mechanics in obesity. J Appl Physiol 1995;79:1199–205.
[11] Jense HG, Dubin SA, Silverstein PI, O'Leary-Escolas U. Effect of obesity on safe duration of apnea in anesthetized humans. Anesth Analg 1991;72:89–93.
[12] Kabon B, Nagele A, Reddy D, et al. Obesity decreases perioperative tissue oxygenation. Anesthesiology 2004;100:274–80.
[13] Veille JC, Hanson R. Obesity, pregnancy, and left ventricular functioning during the third trimester. Am J Obstet Gynecol 1994;171:980–3.
[14] Weiss JL, Malone FD, Emig D, et al. FASTER research consortium. Obesity, obstetric complications and cesarean delivery rate-a population-based screening study. Am J Obstet Gynecol 2004;190:1091–7.
[15] Shnaider R, Ezri T, Szmuk P, et al. Combined spinal-epidural anesthesia for Cesarean section in a patient with peripartum dilated cardiomyopathy. Can J Anaesth 2001;48:681–3.
[16] Drenick EJ, Fisler JS. Sudden cardiac arrest in morbidly obese surgical patients unexplained after autopsy. Am J Surg 1988;155:720–6.
[17] Eslick GD. Gastrointestinal symptoms and obesity: a meta-analysis. Obes Rev 2012;13:469–79.
[18] Landon MB, Gabbe SG. Diabetes mellitus and pregnancy. Obstet Gynecol Clin North Am 1992;19:633–54.
[19] Kheterpal S, Han R, Tremper KK, et al. Incidence and predictors of difficult and impossible mask ventilation. Anesthesiology 2006;105:885–91.
[20] Juvin P, Lavaut E, Dupont H, et al. Difficult tracheal intubation is more common in obese than in lean patients. Anesth Analg 2003;97:595–600.
[21] Bates SM, Greer IA, Middeldorp S, et al. VTE, thrombophilia, antithrombotic therapy, and pregnancy: antithrombotic therapy and prevention of thrombosis, 9th ed: American College of Chest Physicians Evidence-Based Clinical Practice Guidelines. Chest 2012;141:e691S-736S.
[22] Chu SY, Callaghan WM, Kim SY, et al. Maternal obesity and risk of gestational diabetes mellitus. Diabetes Care 2007;30:2070–6.
[23] Ehrenberg H, Mercer B, Catalano P. The influence of obesity and diabetes on the prevalence of macrosomia. Am J Obstet Gynecol 2004;191:964–8.
[24] Edwards N, Middleton PG, Blyton DM, Sullivan CE. Sleep disordered breathing and pregnancy. Thorax 2002;57:555–8.
[25] Pien GW, Pack AI, Jackson N, et al. Risk factors for sleep-disordered breathing in pregnancy. Thorax 2014;69:371–7.
[26] Louis JM, Mogos MF, Salemi JL, et al. Obstructive sleep apnea and severe maternal-infant morbidity/mortality in the United States, 1998–2009. Sleep 2014;37:843–9.
[27] Louis JM, Auckley D, Sokol RJ, Mercer BM. Maternal and neonatal morbidities associated with obstructive sleep apnea complicating pregnancy. Am J Obstet Gynecol 2011;202:261.e1–5.
[28] Reutrakul S, Zaidi N, Wroblewski K, et al. Sleep disturbances and their relationship to glucose tolerance in pregnancy. Diabetes Care 2011;34:2454–7.
[29] Chen YH, Kang JH, Lin CC, et al. Obstructive sleep apnea and the risk of adverse pregnancy outcomes. Am J Obstet Gynecol 2012;206:136.e1–6.e5.
[30] Sahin FK, Koken G, Cosar E, et al. Obstructive sleep apnea in pregnancy and fetal outcome. Int J Gynaecol Obstet 2008;100:141–6.
[31] Olivarez SA, Maheshwari B, McCarthy M, et al. Prospective trial on obstructive sleep apnea in pregnancy and fetal heart rate monitoring. Am J Obstet Gynecol 2010;202:552.e1–7.

[32] Chung F, Yegneswaran B, Liao P, et al. STOP questionnaire: a tool to screen patients for obstructive sleep apnea. Anesthesiology 2008;108:812–21.
[33] Netzer NC, Stoohs RA, Netzer CM, et al. Using the Berlin Questionnaire to identify patients at risk for the sleep apnea syndrome. Ann Intern Med 1999;131:485–91.
[34] Facco FL, Ouyang DW, Zee PC, Grobman WA. Development of a pregnancy-specific screening tool for sleep apnea. J Clin Sleep Med 2012;8:389–94.
[35] Flemons WW. Clinical practice. Obstructive sleep apnea. N Engl J Med 2002;347:498–504.
[36] The American Society of Anesthesiologists Committee on Standards and Practice Parameters, the American Society of Anesthesiologists Task Force on Neuraxial Opioids and the American Society of Regional Anesthesia and Pain Medicine. Practice guidelines for the prevention, detection and management of respiratory depression associated with neuraxial opioid administration: an updated report. Anesthesiology 2016;124:535–52.
[37] Weiss JL, Malone FD, Emig D, Ball RH, Nyberg DA, Comstock CH, et al. FASTER Research Consortium. Obesity, obstetric complications and cesarean delivery rate–a population based screening study. Am J Obstet Gynecol 2004;190:1091–7.
[38] Dresner M, Brocklesby J, Bamber J. Audit of the influence of body mass index on the performance of epidural analgesia in labour and the subsequent mode of delivery. BJOG 2006;113:1178–81.
[39] Balki M, Lee Y, Halpern S, Carvalho JC. Ultrasound imaging of the lumbar spine in the transverse plane: the correlation between estimated and actual depth to the epidural space in obese parturients. Anesth Analg 2009;108:1876–81.
[40] Sahota JS, Carvalho JC, Balki M, Fanning N, Arzola C. Ultrasound estimates for midline epidural punctures in the obese parturient: paramedian sagittal oblique is comparable to transverse median plane. Anesth Analg 2013;116:829–35.
[41] Balki M. Locating the epidural space in obstetric patients — ultrasound a useful tool: continuing professional development. Can J Anaesth 2010;57:1111–26.
[42] Tsui B, Gupta S, Finucane B. Confirmation of epidural catheter placement using nerve stimulation. Can J Anaesth. 1998;45:640–4.
[43] Faure E, Moreno R, Thisted R. Incidence of postdural puncture headache in morbidly obese parturients. Reg Anesth 1994;19:361–3.
[44] Peralta F, Higgins N, Lange E, Wong CA, McCarthy RJ. The relationship of body mass index with the incidence of postdural puncture headache in parturients. Anesth Analg 2015;121:451–6.
[45] Collins JS, Lemmens HJ, Brodsky JB, Brock-Utne JG, Levitan RM. Laryngoscopy and morbid obesity: a comparison of the “sniff” and “ramped” positions. Obes Surg 2004;14:1171–5.
[46] Pierin AM, Alavarce DC, Gusmão JL, Halpern A, Mion D Jr. Blood pressure measurement in obese patients: comparison between upper arm and forearm measurements. Blood Press Monit 2004;9:101–5.
[47] Paranjothy S, Griffiths JD, Broughton HK, Gyte GM, Brown HC, Thomas J. Interventions at caesarean section for reducing the risk of aspiration pneumonitis. Cochrane Database Syst Rev 2014;2:Cd004943.
[48] Barboni E, Mancinelli P, Bitossi U, DE Gaudio AR, Micaglio M, Sorbi F, DI Filippo A. Ultrasound evaluation of the stomach and gastric emptying in pregnant women at term: a case-control study. Minerva Anestesiol 2016;82:543–9.
[49] Hogan QH, Prost R, Kulier A, Taylor ML, Liu S, Mark L. Magnetic resonance imaging of cerebrospinal fluid volume and the influence of body habitus and abdominal pressure. Anesthesiology 1996;84:1341–9.
[50] Lee Y, Balki M, Parkes R, Carvalho JC. Dose requirement of intrathecal bupivacaine for cesarean delivery is similar in obese and normal weight women. Rev Bras Anestesiol 2009;59:674–83.
[51] Alonso E, Gilsanz F, Gredilla E, Martinez B, Canser E, Alsina E. Observational study of continuous spinal anesthesia with the catheter-over-needle technique for cesarean delivery. Int J Obstet Anesth 2009;18:137–41.

[52] Rigler ML, Drasner K, Krejcie TC, Yelich SJ, Scholnick FT, DeFontes J, Bohner D. Cauda equina syndrome after continuous spinal anesthesia. Anesth Analg 1991;72:275–81.
[53] Soens MA, Birnbach DJ, Ranasinghe JS, Van Zundert A. Obstetric anesthesia for the obese and morbidly obese patient: an ounce of prevention is worth more than a pound of treatment. Acta Anaesthesiol Scand 2008;52:6–19.
[54] Pan PH, Bogard TD, Owen MD. Incidence and characteristics of failures in obstetric neuraxial analgesia and anesthesia: a retrospective analysis of 19,259 deliveries. Int J Obstet Anesth 2004;13:227–33.
[55] Hawkins JL, Chang J, Palmer SK, Gibbs CP, Callaghan WM. Anesthesia-related maternal mortality in the United States: 1979–2002. Obstet Gynecol 2011;117:69–74.
[56] Mcdonnell NJ, Paech MJ, Clavisi OM, Scott KL. ANZCA trials group. Difficult and failed intubation in obstetric anaesthesia: an observational study of airway management and complications associated with general anaesthesia for caesarean section. Int J Obstet Anesth 2008;17:292–7.
[57] Kinsella SM, Winton AL, Mushambi MC, Ramaswamy K, Swales H, Quinn AC, Popat M. Failed tracheal intubation during obstetric general anaesthesia: a literature review. Int J Obstet Anesth 2015;24:356–74.
[58] Mushambi MC, Kinsella SM, Popat M, Swales H, Ramaswamy KK, Winton AL, & Quinn AC. Obstetric Anaesthetists' Association and Difficult Airway Society guidelines for the management of difficult and failed tracheal intubation in obstetrics. Anaesthesia 2015;70:1286–306.
[59] Patel A, Nouraei SA. Transnasal Humidified Rapid-Insufflation Ventilatory Exchange (THRIVE): a physiological method of increasing apnoea time in patients with difficult airways. Anaesthesia 2015;70:323–9.
[60] Boer P. Estimated lean body mass as an index for normalization of body fluid volumes in man. Am J Physiol 1984;247:F632–6.
[61] Janmahasatian S, Duffull SB, Ash S, et al. Quantification of lean body weight. Clin Pharmacokinet 2005;44:1051–65.
[62] Portella AAV, Reis GFF, Silva GAM, Cyreno NU. General anesthesia for cesarean section with fentanyl: maternal and fetal plasma concentrations. Rev Bras Anestesiol 1991;41:377–80.
[63] Heesen M, Klöhr S, Hofmann T, Rossaint R, Devroe S, Straube S, Van de Velde M. Maternal and foetal effects of remifentanil for general anaesthesia in parturients undergoing caesarean section: a systematic review and meta-analysis. Acta Anaesthesiol Scand 2013;57:29–36.
[64] de Abreu MG, Bluth T. Protective ventilation with higher versus lower PEEP during general anesthesia for surgery in obese patients (PROBESE). ClinicalTrials.gov Identifier: NCT02148692.
[65] Mhyre JM, Riesner MN, Polley LS, et al. A series of anesthesia-related maternal deaths in Michigan, 1985–2003. Anesthesiology 2007;106:1096–104.
[66] Chin KJ, McDonnell JG, Carvalho B, Sharkey A, Pawa A, Gadsden J. Essentials of our current understanding: abdominal wall blocks. Reg Anesth Pain Med 2017;42:133–83.
[67] Tran G, Kanczuk M, Balki M. The association between the time of oxytocin cessation during labor until cesarean delivery and postpartum blood loss: a retrospective cohort study. Can J Anesth 2017;64:820–827.
[68] Blomberg M. Maternal obesity and risk of postpartum hemorrhage. Obstet Gynecol 2011;118:561–8.
[69] Horlocker TT, Wedel DJ, Rowlingsonet JC, et al. Regional anesthesia in the patient receiving antithrombotic or thrombolytic therapy: American Society of Regional Anesthesia and Pain Medicine Evidence-Based Guidelines. Reg Anest Pain Med 2010;35:64–101.
[70] Perlow JH, Morgan MA. Massive maternal obesity and perioperative cesarean morbidity. Am J Obstet Gynecol 1994;170:560–5.
[71] Myles TD, Gooch J, Santolaya J. Obesity as an independent risk factor for infectious morbidity in patients who undergo cesarean delivery. Obstet Gynecol 2002;100:959–64.

Susan Guest, Merihan Abdel Malek and Cynthia Maxwell

22 Obstetric nursing and team organization in planning for obese parturient

22.1 Introduction

The care of pregnant women with increased body mass index (BMI) is increasingly pertinent as a subject of discussion and planning for all healthcare services, as obesity is a growing health problem globally. Nursing care of the bariatric pregnant, laboring, or postpartum patient requires consideration of a number of factors related not just to the medical issues of the patient but also to the psychological concerns as well as the facility resources, accessibility issues, and preparedness of the interprofessional team—nurses, obstetrics/midwifery, anesthesia, lactation specialists, and learners. This chapter is intended to give a general overview of these considerations in the context of this population.

As with all our patients, underlying the experience of the pregnant bariatric patient are the many experiences that she has already had in her life or in relation to her healthcare. It is well documented that this population have experienced stigmatization related to their habitus and health [1]. Weight bias in healthcare contributes to feelings of humiliation, neglect, and can have an enormous effect on the patient's experience. Paradoxically, this may negatively affect a woman's physical and psychological health during the healthcare encounter. Some examples of care elements that would understandably contribute to these sensitivities might be the use of inappropriate or unsuitable equipment (unsteady scales for those with high BMI; blood pressure cuffs or hospital gowns that are not sized appropriately), healthcare spaces that are unaccommodating (chairs/doorways lacking adequate width) and importantly staff, visitor, and/or family language and demeanor that creates an unwelcoming and discriminatory environment. The healthcare team must develop an awareness of this to provide a helpful and healing environment. Having a skilled and knowledgeable team with easy access to appropriate equipment and standardized approaches to care can facilitate a seamless experience and will normalize the patient's care in a way that inspires confidence and minimizes conflict and complication [2].

22.2 Antenatal considerations

Assessing risk is a key factor in planning. Thus, identification of medical conditions such as chronic hypertension, type 2 diabetes, obstructive sleep apnea, depression, and cardiac or respiratory conditions is crucial as all can be exacerbated by the additional demands of the pregnancy and postpartum periods. The requirement

https://doi.org/10.1515/9783110487817-022

for access to specialized, skilled personnel who can manage these conditions in the context of a pregnancy or postpartum mother is a key element to providing safe and effective care. Consulting services, in addition to anesthesiology, may include dieticians and bariatric medicine specialists, obstetrical medicine, hematology, endocrinology, cardiology, diagnostic imaging, psychiatry, neonatology, and wound care specialists. In our tertiary level institution, we have access to these providers who have specific expertise in these areas as they relate to pregnancy.

Antenatal assessment may generate the need for testing such as polysomnography (sleep studies), pulmonary function, and cardiac and renal testing to ensure optimal pregnancy and in-hospital care. Occasionally, an unexpected health event in labor or during pregnancy may prompt the need for urgent assessment, for example, a cardiac event in a young woman with elevated BMI.

On the other hand, the automatic categorization of the pregnant patient as medically complex solely due to her high BMI carries with it the risk of increased medical surveillance and intervention that might not be medically indicated, and possibly decreased options for birth that might be available with alternative types of surveillance. The team is obliged to consider all indications for intervention and offer all opportunities for elements of a normal birth experience. Having quick access to an interdisciplinary team with expertise, as well as access to specialized equipment and adequate spaces, allows for a more seamless and simpler transition to an emergent situation. In all cases, the awareness of potential for need will underlie the quick initiation of a higher level of care, if the need arises.

In our institution, we offer a specialized antenatal clinic for the bariatric population, which focuses on comprehensive screening and care planning for both mother and fetus. A "BMI checklist" (Fig. 22.1) can serve as a prompt and may facilitate communication of important results, such as pregestational diabetes parameters, ECG and echocardiogram reports, and serial fetal growth readings.

Standardization of the patient record in the flow sheet may trigger appropriate specialist referrals and can record ongoing information such as the use of continuous positive-airway pressure, initiation of prophylactic anticoagulation, notes regarding challenging peripheral intravenous access and the resulting plan, as well as appropriate blood pressure cuff size (thigh cuff, for example) and location for optimal and consistent assessment of blood pressure recordings (in some cases, radial rather than upper arm blood pressure readings may be the only realistic option available on an ambulatory basis). This information can direct the team in their effort to address each issue early in the pregnancy. It will also support consistency across caregivers and across the continuum of care, thereby optimizing safety and the patient experience.

Our specialized antenatal clinic is directed by maternal fetal medicine and supported by bariatric medicine. The bariatric medicine physician works simultaneously with the maternal fetal medicine team in the same physical setting with the support of a pregnancy dietician. The aim of this weekly collaboration is to continuously support

Checklist for High BMI Obstetric Patient Care Planning:

Patient Name______________________________

MRN______________________________

MOUNT SINAI HOSPITAL
Joseph and Wolf Lebovic Health Complex

ANTENATAL:		
Blood Pressure monitoring Arm/forearm/leg Cuff size		
Cardiac testing O ECG O ECHO	RESULTS	
O Pulmonary Function tests	RESULT	
O Sleep Apnea Testing Need for CPAP	RESULT	
GCT O Early O 26w GTT Hgb A1c	RESULTS	
Consults: O OB Medicine O Anesthesia O Dietician O Bariatric Medicine O Haematology O Endocrine O Cardiology O Neonatology O Clinical Nurse Specialist	DATES:	PLAN:

Fig. 22.1: The BMI checklist.

optimal nutrition and weight management throughout pregnancy and into postpartum care. This post discharge opportunity can be a wonderful addition to the holistic care planning that occurred in the pregnancy and offers a follow-up solution that may have a big effect on the long-term maternal and neonatal health.

The role of the advanced practice nurse in caring for the complex pregnant patient is multifaceted. Care-planning with the patient and her family is one aspect of the role, and can ensure that all elements of care are communicated. The benefits of having an advanced practice nurse who follows a patient along the continuum of her care, and communicates her interactions with the patient, can clearly support not only the healthcare team but also the patient by offering some anticipatory guidance and allowing for full patient involvement in the care planning process. Frontline nursing will use the plan to anticipate the individual and equipment needs of the patient to create an experience of well-coordinated, thoughtful, and empathetic care. Frontline nursing can also use the plan to communicate to the intrapartum and postpartum interdisciplinary team, the specific planning that the antepartum team and the patient have already negotiated.

Even when that plan of care cannot be fulfilled completely, out of medical or safety necessity, the opportunity to have these discussions and create something that speaks for the patient and family secures the role of the patient as a part of the team and as an active contributor to her own care. A written plan of care, that a patient can carry, and which also is incorporated into the legal health record of the patient, promotes transparency of the team communications, as well as self-efficacy for the patient. Along with a medical and obstetric history, the plan will consider all the medical and psychosocial issues that have been discussed with the patient over the course of her pregnancy. Each issue and the related decision-making is recorded to create a level of understanding for the patient's choices and provider counseling for the entire team. The discussions with the patient support her understanding of the position the team might take under certain circumstances. In the case of unplanned events, the patient will have some background knowledge regarding her management and potential risks, and the team will know to circle back with the patient and family at the earliest opportunity so that debriefing on some level can occur.

22.3 Accessibility

Additionally, the care planning for the bariatric population requires that the institution be committed to being an accessible facility. Such a commitment requires that the facility accommodate the bariatric patient in terms of equipment capacity needs as well as spaces that allow for wider equipment to maneuver. Antenatal clinics must have appropriate scales, wider and appropriate weight-bearing seating, examining tables with stepping stools as well as accessible spaces that will accommodate the patient who must mobilize with a walker or bariatric wheelchair (see Fig. 22.2) due to the added pregnancy challenges. The hospital may need to consider acquisition of designated bariatric equipment such as wider stretchers, hospital beds and operating tables (with extenders, see Fig. 22.3) that not only support the added weight but also offer the added comfort and safety of a wider surface. In some cases, the additional risk of skin breakdown related to increased weight or vulnerable tissues in the setting of edema or diabetes, specialized therapeutic surfaces are recommended. An accessible, barrier-free washroom in the women's and infants' units will include additional hand rails for patients with mobility challenges. Showers are ideally single-level entry and toilets have the added support underneath (see Fig. 22.4) rather than being wall mounted. In addition, hospital gowns that can accommodate the fuller figure of the gravid bariatric patient will be available and blood pressure cuffs that are in larger sizes will be in all rooms.

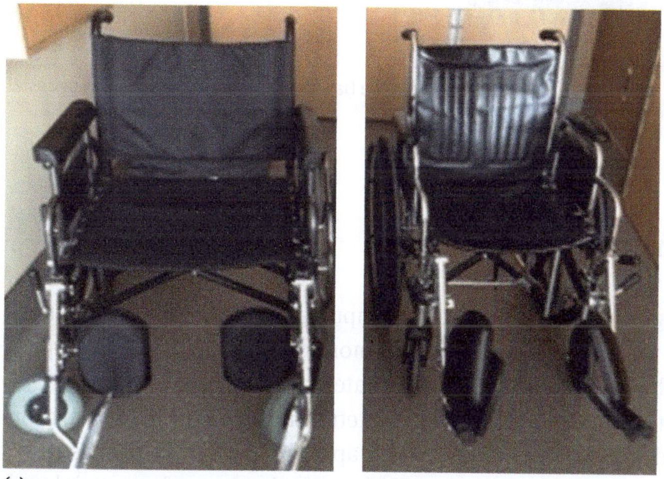

(a) (b)

Fig. 22.2: The bariatric wheelchair (**a**) and standard wheelchair (**b**) for comparison.

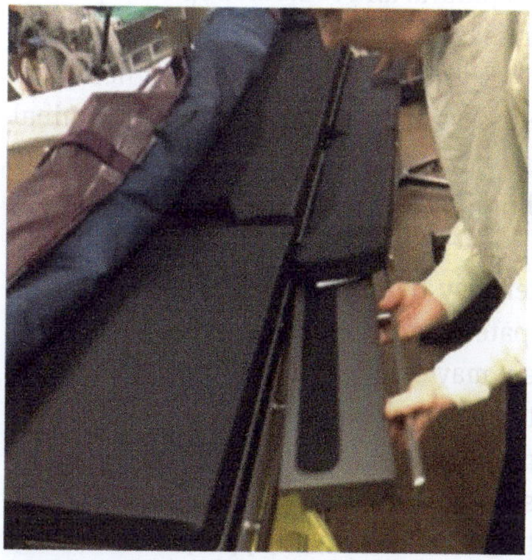

Fig. 22.3: Operating room bed extenders.

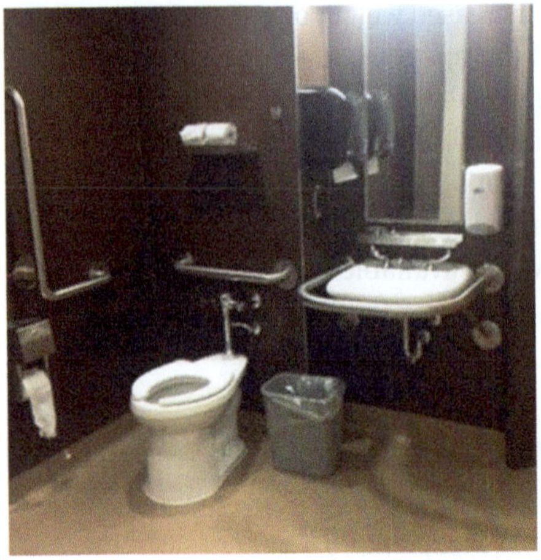

Fig. 22.4: Bariatric inpatient bathroom with pedestal toilet.

22.4 Intrapartum care planning

Planning for the obese gravida in the labor ward prompts several points of consideration:

A. Labor monitoring will include fetal heart rate monitoring and may require longer belts or other methods to attach them to the maternal abdomen.

B. Ideally, the patient will have consulted with obstetric anesthesia prior to admission to the labor ward and consideration to the approach of regional anesthesia would have been discussed (reviewed in Chapter 21). In cases where peripheral intravenous access will be challenging or impossible, we will arrange for the patient to have a peripherally inserted central catheter line placed to ensure safe accessibility. Ensuring that longer spinal, epidural and combined spinal/epidural kits are available may save time in urgent situations. Our labor unit is equipped with several portable ultrasound machines to facilitate placement of neuraxial anesthesia (as well as the preoperative assessment of the maternal abdominal pannus to gauge level of abdominal entry for cesarean entry). Difficult airway trays as well as the Troop Elevation™ pillow [3] are easily located in the operating room suite.

C. Use of the intrauterine pressure catheter may be indicated more frequently as uterine activity may not be easily palpated through the maternal abdominal wall. As it is often the case that the patient may be undergoing induction of labor for medical reasons or having augmentation for slow progress in labor, both of which are more common in the obese gravida, we have noted greater utilization of intrauterine pressure catheter devices in our unit.

D. In the operating room, having an operating room table with appropriate capacity should be predetermined. Our labor and delivery operating room tables are equipped with an inflatable patient transfer device (Hovermatt™) [4] under the linens will avoid any last minute delays in the surgery. This device offers an air-assisted lateral transfer that supports the patient safely and comfortably and protects the caregivers in the transfer process.

E. Our institution has assembled a specialized bariatric cesarean section tray with specially sized instruments (see Fig. 22.5) and utilizes a disposable retractor device (the Mobius™, for example) [5] for complex cases. Devices such as the Traxi™ retractor [6] can be used to elevate the pannus during cesarean section.

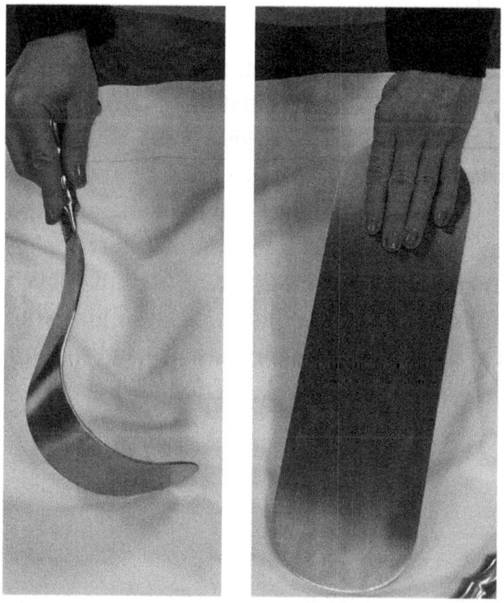

(a) (b)

Fig. 22.5: Surgical instruments from the BMI C-section kit: extra-large Dever retractor (**a**); extra-large Malleable retractor (**b**).

Following skin closure, we use a negative pressure wound therapy system (one example is the PICO™ system) [7] that can be applied after the surgical site is closed to facilitate wound closure and healing potential.

Awareness of availability and use of equipment will be a great comfort to the nurses and other team members who are providing care. This, in turn, will minimize the patient's discomfort, anxiety, and sensitivity to her situation and will increase her confidence in the care she is receiving. Attention to this level of detail is necessary in the provision of safe care as well as care that is patient-focused and nonjudgmental.

F. Nursing time management requires thought as the laboring patient with increased BMI may require additional surveillance related to fetal monitoring (i.e., hands-on placement of the Doppler to ensure adequate detection in light of maternal pannus) and uterine activity monitoring (frequently slow labors are identified and it can be difficult to palpate contractions manually). Mobility in labor may be compromised or may be a safety concern with the high-BMI patient. Labor dystocia is a common occurrence and coupled with the monitoring challenges and potential for shoulder dystocia in second stage can result in a lower threshold for decision-making around cesarean birth. Additional nursing support would be welcomed in the care of this laboring mother, to assist with mobility, surveillance, and positioning of the patient in the case of shoulder dystocia or transfer to the operating room for surgical intervention.

If anesthesia is not initiated until arrival in the operating room, significant time may be needed for this procedure. The technical challenges in initiating neuraxial anesthesia are often chosen over a general anesthetic procedure, given the potential for airway and ventilation problems. Anesthesia itself can take up to an hour or more of the operating room time. Positioning for the surgery and final assessment of the patient, with determination of approach, including decisions regarding skin incision can also take some time, especially if the obstetric team is different from the physician who counseled the patient in pregnancy. The surgery itself is slower given the additional tissue and the added technical challenges. Nursing presence and support throughout these steps is central to the care of the patient and functioning of the labor and delivery team.

22.5 Postpartum care

After the birth, the patient may require closer monitoring with one-to-one nursing care, and anesthesia availability. This is especially true of the bariatric patient with a history of obstructive sleep apnea. Postoperative pain management can require extra attention. Although not always the case, the additional need for pain medication in the postoperative period, if not well addressed, can have implications for the patient's ability to take on infant care as well as her mobility. Disposition of the patient as well as pain management challenges increase the length of stay of the patient and contribute to general delays in the flow of patients through the labor and delivery setting.

Breastfeeding presents specific challenges in women with increased BMI [8, 9]. During the postpartum period, medical comorbidities and the associated care needs can delay discharge as can the added nursing care challenges associated with breastfeeding support. Polycystic ovarian syndrome, a condition that is common in the bariatric population, can have implications for the experience of breastfeeding. Often, positioning of the infant at the breast can present a difficult task. Encouragement and support for skin to skin care, frequent feeding, and frequent breast stimulation and emptying will optimize breastfeeding. Lactation consultant support while in hospital and after discharge can sustain breastfeeding efforts. Given the associations between breastfeeding and the lowered incidence of diabetes and obesity in childhood [10], the additional time and effort in establishing and sustaining breastfeeding in this population is a public health priority.

Lastly, women with a high BMI are known to have a higher incidence of postpartum depression. Risk assessment and referral early in pregnancy can offer reassurance. The role of nursing and perinatal social work is important in assisting in the identification of women at risk as well as ensuring appropriate follow-up with a psychiatric provider, counselor, or family physician.

22.6 Summary

Care of the pregnant, laboring, or postpartum bariatric patient can present many challenges to the resources of an institution. This chapter has attempted to outline some of the general considerations and special challenges with the bariatric population that can benefit from a specialized process for care, with specific reference to the role of nursing as a part of the interdisciplinary team. This outline is summarized in Tab. 22.1. The role of the advanced practice nurse in care coordination is also addressed as a possible solution to the communication issues that are especially prevalent when many team members are involved in a patient's and family's care.

Tab. 22.1: BMI pregnancy care coordination summary.

1. General concerns in caring for the high BMI population
   a. Access to
      i. Personnel with training—ultrasonography anesthesia, surgeon, endocrine, OB medicine, hematology, maternal and fetal cardiac assessment, interventional radiology, wound care
      ii. Facilities and equipment—space requirements, mobility requirements, special equipment needs
      iii. Respectful care—the sensitivities we express in our care
   b. Added risks with increased BMI
      i. Comorbidities—CHTN, type 2 diabetes, OSA, cardiac/respiratory challenges, PCOS, mobility challenges, depression
      ii. Fall risk
      iii. Peripheral IV access
      iv. Fetal health surveillance—U/S and FHR monitoring in labor
      v. Risk of wound dehiscence and infection
      vi. Intrapartum and postpartum pain issues
      vii. Breastfeeding—PCOS and specialty care r/t habitus
      viii. Stigma and psychosocial concerns
         1. Depression risk
   c. Time issues
      i. Anticipated length of time
         1. Intrapartum for anesthesia, surgery, labor
         2. LOS r/t wound, breastfeeding challenges, sleep apnea

Tab. 22.1 (continued)

2. Preconception planning
   a. Infertility
   b. Counseling
   c. Weight optimization
   d. Fetal risks
      i. Folic acid supplementation
3. Prenatal care and planning
   a. Consults
   b. Ultrasound scanning
   c. Cardiac assessment
   d. Sleep apnea assessment
   e. Pulmonary function testing
   f. Early gestational diabetes testing
      i. GCT in first trimester
      ii. HgA1c
4. Intrapartum care
   a. Obstetrical challenges
      i. Birth options
         1. Accommodation of birth planning requests for mobility, hydrotherapy, room (intra- and postpartum)
      ii. Intrauterine pressure monitoring and FHR monitoring in labor
      iii. Labor dystocia
   b. Nursing
      i. Monitoring challenges, mobility challenges
      ii. Team notification/communication
      iii. Needs for gown, BP cuff, monitoring belts
      iv. OR table and Hovermatt
      v. PICO negative pressure system
   c. Anesthesia
      i. GERD prophylaxis
      ii. Intravenous access
      iii. Neuraxial vs. GA
         1. Epidural needles, portable U/S for imaging of back
         2. Troop pillow
         3. Difficult airway tray and Glidescope
      iv. Pain management
   d. Cesarean births
      i. Incision planning—location and closure, negative pressure system
      ii. Other equipment needs—special BMI tray C/S instruments including Mobius
5. Postpartum care
   a. LOS in L&D considerations with anesthesia
   b. Mobility
   c. Infection risk and pain management
   d. VTE prophylaxis for in-hospital
   e. Endocrine management

Tab. 22.1 (continued)

f. HTN follow-up
g. Breastfeeding support
h. Wound care
i. Psychosocial
j. Fetal—macrosomia, hypoglycemia

6. Discharge planning
   a. Medical—depending on comorbidities
      i. Wound—delayed removal of staples/negative pressure system
   b. Breastfeeding—ongoing support
   c. Psychosocial support

Bibliography

[1] Mulherin K, Miller Y, Barlow F, Diedrich P, Thompson R. Weight stigma in maternity care: women's experiences and care providers attitudes. BMC Pregnancy Childbirth 2013;13(19).
[2] Centre for Maternal and Child Enquiries/Royal College of Obstetricians and Gynaecologists. Management of women with obesity in pregnancy. 1–29, March 2010.
[3] Troop Elevation Pillow (Accessed April 7, 2017 at http://www.mercurymed.com/product-category/troop-elevation-pillows-and-accessories/).
[4] Mobius (Accessed April 7, 2017 at http://www.coopersurgical.com/Products/Detail/ob-mobius-self-retaining-c-section-retractor).
[5] Hovermatt (Accessed April 7, 2017 at http://www.hovermatt.com/).
[6] Traxi (Accessed April 7, 2017 at http://clinicalinnovations.com/portfolio-items/traxi-panniculus-retractor/).
[7] PICO (Accessed April 7, 2017 at http://www.smith-nephew.com/key-products/advanced-wound-management/pico/).
[8] Garner C, Ratcliff S, Devine C, Thornburg L, Rasmussen K. Health professionals experiences providing breastfeeding related care for obese women. Breastfeed Med 2014;9(10):503–9.
[9] Amir L, Donath S. A systematic review of maternal obesity and breastfeeding intention, initiation and duration. BMC Pregnancy Childbirth 2007;7:9.
[10] Yan J. Liu L, Zhu Y, Huong G, Wang P. The association between breastfeeding and childhood obesity: a meta-analysis. BMC Public Health 2014;14:1267.

Yair Sagi and Cindy Maxwell

23 Cesarean delivery in women with obesity

23.1 Introduction

Cesarean delivery (CD) is one of the most common surgical procedures in the United States [1]. Pregnant women with obesity have unique risks that may affect their need for and outcome from CD. Obesity places pregnant women at increased risk for CD and complications such as hypertensive disorders, diabetes, macrosomia, and stillbirth [2–6].

A review of 11 cohort studies reported that the risk of CD increased by 50% in women with a body mass index (BMI) of 30 to 35 kg/m^2 and more than doubled in women with a BMI >35 kg/m^2 as compared with women with a normal BMI [7]. The frequency of wound complications following CD ranges from 3% to 17% [8–13]; however, in women with morbid obesity, it is as high as 30% [14]. Finally, wound complications are a burden for the patient, her family, and the health care system; one study estimated that a post discharge wound complications costs on average an additional $3,000 US dollars [15].

As is true for any abdominal surgery, CD presents unique challenges in obese women. There is the question of how urgent the procedure is and how a delay might affect the fetal outcome, for example. The steps taken during the surgical planning may have a direct effect on the rates of intraoperative and postoperative complications such as endometritis, wound complications (infection, separation, hematoma, seroma, and fascial dehiscence), and bladder and bowel injury.

23.2 Prophylactic antibiotics

CD increases the risk of infection compared with vaginal birth by fivefold to 20-fold. Surgical site infection (SSI) rates after CD are estimated to be as high as 7% to 20% [16]. These can be attributed mainly to two major factors: unscheduled CD and maternal obesity. Obesity alone may increase the likelihood of the development of an SSI after CD by threefold to fivefold, whereas obese parturients are up to three times more likely to require a CD than no obese control subjects.

There are many reasons why obese parturients experience these increased risks. Increased rates of medical comorbidities (e.g., diabetes mellitus, hypertension, preoperative skin breakdown, intertriginous infection) can directly affect the healing process. Obesity is associated with longer operative times and higher blood loss. Due to greater depth of subcutaneous adipose tissue, tissue perfusion can be compromised, inhibiting proper tissue oxygenation, delivery of immune cells and

https://doi.org/10.1515/9783110487817-023

subsequently reduced ability to prevent and respond to infection. Furthermore, prophylactic antibiotics have lower tissue concentrations in obese patients [9, 17, 18].

The prophylactic use of antibiotics in women undergoing CS[Q1] has been shown in randomized controlled trials (RCTs) to reduce the incidence of wound infection (RR 0.39; 95% CI 0.32–0.48), puerperal endometritis (RR 0.38; 95% CI 0.34–0.42), and serious maternal infectious complications (RR 0.31; 95% CI 0.19–0.48) [19]. When administered before skin incision, as opposed to intraoperatively following umbilical cord clamping, it has been shown to decrease puerperal endometritis (RR 0.59; 95% CI 0.37–0.94) [20], with a nonsignificant trend toward a reduction in wound infection. The appropriate dosing of prophylactic antibiotics, specifically for the obese obstetric population, has been studied recently. The most common antibiotics used are the first generation cephalosporins, especially cefazolin 1 or 2 g intravenously (IV) given 30 to 60 minutes prior to skin incision [16].

Few data exist regarding the optimal dose specific to obesity in pregnancy. Most studies suggest the administration of at least 2 g of cefazolin 60 minutes before the operation, although this dosage may be insufficient in women with increased BMI [21]. A recent prospective cohort study evaluating the effects of obesity on tissue concentrations after a prophylactic 3 g of IV cefazolin doses at the time of CD. The tissue concentration was compared with that of historic control subjects who had received a 2 g dose. Higher adipose tissue concentrations of cefazolin were observed after the administration of the 3 g prophylactic dose. On the other hand, a multicenter retrospective cohort study in 2015 showed that administration of the higher 3 g dose of cefazolin did not reduce SSIs in obese pregnant women undergoing CD [22].

The pharmacokinetics of antibiotic metabolism is important and may differ in adiposity and therefore more studies are needed to determine the optimal antibiotic dosing.

23.3 Skin incision

Lower abdominal transverse skin entry (Pfannenstiel) is generally favored for the normal weight woman undergoing a nonemergent CD. However, the optimal skin incision type for the obese woman is unknown.

There are no randomized clinical trials comparing the risks and benefits of skin incision type (vertical or transverse) for CD in obese women. The choice of skin incision for CS in obese patients is still a matter of controversy, as mixed findings have been reported in observational studies. Current practice is largely based on surgeon or institutional preference [23].

In pelvic surgery, low transverse or Pfannenstiel skin incisions give adequate exposure while providing a good cosmetic result, but this may not be the case when the abdominal pannus is significant in size. Furthermore, the incision will be covered over by the large pannus postoperative, which interferes with wound healing and physical integrity of the incision. It is a common practice to apply pressure dressings to lessen postoperative bleeding below the skin incision, yet this may impair wound healing by compromising tissue circulation and perfection and may cause fat necrosis below the incision. Alternatively, a vertical incision could be used. There are healing concerns with this approach as well, as these incisions typically need to be long to have adequate exposure and may result in greater tension in keeping the wound edges together. To avoid the dissection of thickened layers of adipose tissue below the umbilicus, a supraumbilical vertical incision could be an alternative approach. However, this type of incision requires careful anesthetic planning given the higher level of entry and dermatomes affected.

Another option is the transverse supra-pannus incision and can be considered appropriate if the pannus displaced the umbilicus downward to the level of the pubic symphysis when standing. To choose the best level of incision, using an ultrasound can be helpful to assess adipose thickness. A transverse cutaneous incision is followed by standard entry into peritoneal cavity, and generally a transverse lower uterine incision. The subcutaneous fat layer tended to be less thick than the pannus, and surgical exposure and access to the lower uterine segment is not compromised by the alternative skin approach [23, 24].

In a US hospital cohort of 239 patients with BMI >35 kg/m^2 undergoing their first CD, a vertical skin incision was associated with higher risk of wound complications requiring reopening of the incision (OR 12.4; 95% CI 3.9–39.3) when compared with a transverse incision [8]. A similar study of 623 women with BMI >35 kg/m^2 undergoing primary CD showed that vertical skin incisions were associated with a fourfold risk of infection and wound separation [25]. On the other hand, a large US retrospective cohort of 3,200 women with BMI >40 kg/m^2 undergoing primary CD reported a significantly lower rate of wound complication with vertical skin incision, including infection, seroma, hematoma, evisceration, and fascial dehiscence (OR 0.32; 95% CI 0.17–0.62) [6, 26]. In conclusion, there is conflicting evidence on the benefits of vertical versus transverse skin incisions for CD in obese women and therefore an RCT is necessary to clarify this clinical dilemma.

23.4 Uterine incision

Uterine entry may pose challenges depending on the surgical approach and fetal position. Making the traditional lower uterine transverse incision can pose a risk if there are inadvertent lateral extensions of the incision downward, particularly in the setting of the macrosomic fetus or late second stage CD. Repair of such extensions is complicated by inadequate exposure with the maternal pannus and the depth of pelvic cavity and place the mother at risk for hemorrhage, blood transfusion, bladder and ureter injuries, and even cesarean hysterectomy. Our approach has been to use a sharp, crescentic opening that stays well above the uterovesical peritoneal reflection to minimize the chance of downward extension.

To enhance the surgical exposure, self-retaining retractors (both reusable and disposable such as the Mobius™ retractor) can facilitate the retraction process and delivery of the baby. Additionally, specialized extra-large retractors organized for such cases may be of benefit to the surgical team (see Fig. 22.5 in Chapter 22).

23.5 Closure of peritoneum

A Cochrane review in 2014 concluded that there was no difference in terms of postoperative adhesion formation, but a significant reduction in the operative time in cases where the peritoneum was not closed, as compared with closure of both peritoneal layers. In addition to the reduction in operative time, hospital stay and wound infection rates were also decreased [27]. That being said, our practice has been to routinely close this layer to minimize the intra-abdominal contents from being extruded and complicating the subsequent closure of the peritoneum, keeping in mind that the patients are generally awake for surgery, there is tremendous intra-abdominal pressure and the reduction in the uterine size just after delivery contribute to the bowel obscuring the operative field.

23.6 Closure of the subcutaneous tissue layer and drain placement

There is robust evidence that in the general CD population, if the subcutaneous tissue layer exceeds 2 cm, closure of the subcutaneous layer is recommended. A meta analysis of six studies has shown that this measure decreases wound complications by 34%, particularly seroma formation [28]. Our practice is to re-approximate the tissue with multiple layers of interrupted rapidly absorbable sutures to close the dead space.

RCTs evaluating CD performed in the general population have found no difference in the incidence of wound complications or any other maternal morbidity when subcutaneous drains are left in place [29, 30].

In a prospective case control study conducted in Egypt evaluating 118 women with a BMI >32 kg/m^2 undergoing CD with a Pfannenstiel incision, no difference in wound dehiscence or hematoma formation was found with the placement of subcutaneous drains [31]. However, in a retrospective US cohort of 194 patients with a BMI >50 kg/m^2 undergoing CD, the use of subcutaneous drains was associated with an increased risk of wound complication (OR 2.3; 95% CI 1.23–4.38) [14]. A multicenter RCT in the US, including 280 women with >4 cm of subcutaneous thickness undergoing CD, were randomized to subcutaneous layer closure alone or in combination with subcutaneous suction drainage. The incidence of composite wound morbidity (subcutaneous or fascial dehiscence, seroma, hematoma, and abscess) was similar in both groups [32].

In summary, current evidence does not support the use of subcutaneous drainage to reduce the incidence of wound complication.

23.7 Closure of the skin

Choice of closure continues to vary among clinicians, with the most common choices being absorbable subcuticular suturing and nonabsorbable metal staples. The literature available on skin closure methods is inconclusive.

A systematic review identified eight RCTs evaluating these two options, and found similar incidences of wound complication, pain, and cosmetic results [33]. This study investigated a general population and was not able to observe the effect of BMI. [Q2] In contrast, two RCTs among women with BMI >30 kg/m^2 showed that subcuticular closure reduced the risk of postoperative wound complication. However, when wound complications were analyzed for the effect on disruption as compared with infection, infection was not affected by method of closure.

More recently, a meta-analysis from 2015 by Mackeen et al. [34] compared skin closure with absorbable subcuticular suture versus metal staples and found that sutures decreased wound morbidity. Wound complications occurred 51% less frequently in patients closed with sutures as compared with those closed with staples. This benefit persisted even when data were stratified into obese and nonobese BMI categories.

In conclusion, recent literature shows that suture closure of transverse skin incisions significantly decreases wound morbidity, specifically wound separation, without significant differences in pain, patient satisfaction, or cosmesis.

23.8 Wound dressing

Maintenance of wound closure is a challenge as excessive suture tension, infection, diabetes mellitus, peripheral vascular disease, use of steroid or immunosuppressive drugs, and smoking may delay proper closure [35].

Conventional dressing consisting of sterile dry gauzes, topical antimicrobial dressing, and more recently, negative pressure wound therapy (NPWT) may be used to enhance healing.

Although it is not part of the current guidelines, NPWT has emerged as an accepted technique in contemporary wound management [36] and has become increasingly popular over the last two decades, particularly for the treatment of pressure and post-traumatic wounds, diabetic leg ulcers, and skin grafts [36–42].

The NPWT is comprised of two units: a therapy unit, which delivers a constant negative pressure by means of a pump, and a dressing, which is a self-adhesive system. It requires sealed edges to achieve its effect, and reduces lateral tension and tissue edema. This results in increased blood circulation, decreased edema, enhanced granulation tissue formation, and reduced bacterial colonization. Moreover, NPWT acts by stimulating cell-mediated immune response and fibroblast viability, migration, and proliferation within 48 hours after its application. Two commonly used systems are the PICO™ and Prevena™ dressings. Patients can be safely discharged with these dressings in place [43, 44].

Two RCTs and two observational studies demonstrated faster wound closure and a higher percentage of treatment success with NPWT [45]. Meta-analysis also favored NPWT regarding decrease in wound size [42].

The use of NPWT for wound dehiscence and infection in CD patients requires further study. A case series of three patients with superficial wound dehiscence after CD showed full wound healing after 25 to 41 days of treatment, with no reported complications [16].

23.9 Anesthesia for the obese woman undergoing CD

This topic is covered in detail in Chapter 21.

23.10 Venous thromboembolism prophylaxis

This topic is covered in detail in Chapter 17.

23.11 Conclusion

Careful predelivery assessment in addition to planning with other relevant caregivers is essential for the management of the obese pregnant woman. Both the American College of Obstetricians and Gynecologists and the Society of Obstetricians and Gynaecologists of Canada recommend a multidisciplinary approach.

Key things to remember:

A. Additional time for patient positioning and surgical setup
B. Additional time allocation for anesthesia placement
C. Perioperative antibiotics
D. Thoughtful approach to skin entry, specialized instruments for retraction and wound dressing
E. Postpartum venous thromboembolism prophylaxis, which must be coordinated with the anesthesia team
F. Consider early wound assessment (i.e., in 2–4 weeks postdelivery) to monitor for complications

Bibliography

[1] Osterman MJ, Martin JA. Changes in cesarean delivery rates by gestational age: United States, 1996–2011. NCHS Data Brief 2013(124):1–8.

[2] ACOG Committee Opinion number 315, September 2005. Obesity in pregnancy. Obstet Gynecol 2005;106(3):671–5.

[3] Cnattingius S, Bergstrom R, Lipworth L, Kramer MS. Prepregnancy weight and the risk of adverse pregnancy outcomes. N Engl J Med 1998;338(3):147–52.

[4] Cedergren MI. Maternal morbid obesity and the risk of adverse pregnancy outcome. Obstet Gynecol 2004;103(2):219–24.

[5] Nohr EA, Bech BH, Davies MJ, Frydenberg M, Henriksen TB, Olsen J. Prepregnancy obesity and fetal death: a study within the Danish National Birth Cohort. Obstet Gynecol 2005;106(2):250–9.

[6] Brocato BE, Thorpe EM, Jr., Gomez LM, Wan JY, Mari G. The effect of cesarean delivery skin incision approach in morbidly obese women on the rate of classical hysterotomy. J Pregnancy 2013;2013:890296.

[7] Poobalan AS, Aucott LS, Gurung T, Smith WC, Bhattacharya S. Obesity as an independent risk factor for elective and emergency caesarean delivery in nulliparous women—systematic review and meta-analysis of cohort studies. Obes Rev 2009;10(1):28–35.

[8] Wall PD, Deucy EE, Glantz JC, Pressman EK. Vertical skin incisions and wound complications in the obese parturient. Obstet Gynecol 2003;102(5 Pt 1):952–6.

[9] Schneid-Kofman N, Sheiner E, Levy A, Holcberg G. Risk factors for wound infection following cesarean deliveries. Int J Gynaecol Obstet 2005;90(1):10–5.

[10] Tran TS, Jamulitrat S, Chongsuvivatwong V, Geater A. Risk factors for postcesarean surgical site infection. Obstet Gynecol 2000;95(3):367–71.

[11] Myles TD, Gooch J, Santolaya J. Obesity as an independent risk factor for infectious morbidity in patients who undergo cesarean delivery. Obstet Gynecol 2002;100(5 Pt 1):959–64.

[12] Caesarean section surgical techniques: a randomised factorial trial (CAESAR). BJOG 2010;117(11):1366–76.

[13] Vermillion ST, Lamoutte C, Soper DE, Verdeja A. Wound infection after cesarean: effect of subcutaneous tissue thickness. Obstet Gynecol 2000;95(6 Pt 1):923–6.

[14] Alanis MC, Villers MS, Law TL, Steadman EM, Robinson CJ. Complications of cesarean delivery in the massively obese parturient. Am J Obstet Gynecol 2010;203(3):271.e1–7.

[15] Perencevich EN, Sands KE, Cosgrove SE, Guadagnoli E, Meara E, Platt R. Health and economic impact of surgical site infections diagnosed after hospital discharge. Emerg Infect Dis 2003;9(2):196–203.

[16] Ayres-de-Campos D. Obesity and the challenges of caesarean delivery: prevention and management of wound complications. Best Pract Res Clin Obstet Gynaecol 2015;29(3):406–14.

[17] Witter FR, Lawson P, Ferrell J. Decreasing cesarean section surgical site infection: an ongoing comprehensive quality improvement program. Am J Infect Control 2014;42(4):429–31.

[18] Corcoran S, Jackson V, Coulter-Smith S, Loughrey J, McKenna P, Cafferkey M. Surgical site infection after cesarean section: implementing 3 changes to improve the quality of patient care. Am J Infect Control 2013;41(12):1258–63.

[19] Smaill FM, Grivell RM. Antibiotic prophylaxis versus no prophylaxis for preventing infection after cesarean section. Cochrane Database Syst Rev 2014(10):Cd007482.

[20] Baaqeel H, Baaqeel R. Timing of administration of prophylactic antibiotics for caesarean section: a systematic review and meta-analysis. BJOG 2013;120(6):661–9.

[21] Pevzner L, Swank M, Krepel C, Wing DA, Chan K, Edmiston CE, Jr. Effects of maternal obesity on tissue concentrations of prophylactic cefazolin during cesarean delivery. Obstet Gynecol 2011;117(4):877–82.

[22] Swank ML, Wing DA, Nicolau DP, McNulty JA. Increased 3-gram cefazolin dosing for cesarean delivery prophylaxis in obese women. Am J Obstet Gynecol 2015;213(3):415.e1–8.
[23] Marrs CC, Moussa HN, Sibai BM, Blackwell SC. The relationship between primary cesarean delivery skin incision type and wound complications in women with morbid obesity. Am J Obstet Gynecol 2014;210(4):319.e1–4.
[24] Stirrat LI, Milne A, Paul A, Denison FC. Suprapannus transverse caesarean section incision in morbidly obese women. Eur J Obstet Gynecol Reprod Biol 2015;186:110–1.
[25] Thornburg LL, Linder MA, Durie DE, Walker B, Pressman EK, Glantz JC. Risk factors for wound complications in morbidly obese women undergoing primary cesarean delivery. J Matern Fetal Neonatal Med 2012;25(9):1544–8.
[26] McLean M, Hines R, Polinkovsky M, Stuebe A, Thorp J, Strauss R. Type of skin incision and wound complications in the obese parturient. Am J Perinatol 2012;29(4):301–6.
[27] Bamigboye AA, Hofmeyr GJ. Closure versus non-closure of the peritoneum at caesarean section: short- and long-term outcomes. Cochrane Database Syst Rev 2014(8):Cd000163.
[28] Chelmow D, Rodriguez EJ, Sabatini MM. Suture closure of subcutaneous fat and wound disruption after cesarean delivery: a meta-analysis. Obstet Gynecol 2004;103(5 Pt 1):974–80.
[29] Gates S, Anderson ER. Wound drainage for caesarean section. Cochrane Database Syst Rev 2013(12):Cd004549.
[30] Hellums EK, Lin MG, Ramsey PS. Prophylactic subcutaneous drainage for prevention of wound complications after cesarean delivery—a metaanalysis. Am J Obstet Gynecol 2007;197(3):229–35.
[31] Al-Inany H, Youssef G, Abd ElMaguid A, Abdel Hamid M, Naguib A. Value of subcutaneous drainage system in obese females undergoing cesarean section using Pfannenstiel incision. Gynecol Obstet Invest 2002;53(2):75–8.
[32] Ramsey PS, White AM, Guinn DA, Lu GC, Ramin SM, Davies JK, et al. Subcutaneous tissue reapproximation, alone or in combination with drain, in obese women undergoing cesarean delivery. Obstet Gynecol 2005;105(5 Pt 1):967–73.
[33] Ibrahim MI, Moustafa GF, Al-Hamid AS, Hussein MR. Superficial incisional surgical site infection rate after cesarean section in obese women: a randomized controlled trial of subcuticular versus interrupted skin suturing. Arch Gynecol Obstet 2014;289(5):981–6.
[34] Mackeen AD, Schuster M, Berghella V. Suture versus staples for skin closure after cesarean: a metaanalysis. Am J Obstet Gynecol 2015;212(5):621.e1–10.
[35] Beattie PG, Rings TR, Hunter MF, Lake Y. Risk factors for wound infection following caesarean section. Aust N Z J Obstet Gynaecol 1994;34(4):398–402.
[36] Webster J, Scuffham P, Sherriff KL, Stankiewicz M, Chaboyer WP. Negative pressure wound therapy for skin grafts and surgical wounds healing by primary intention. Cochrane Database Syst Rev 2012(4):Cd009261.
[37] Pauli EM, Krpata DM, Novitsky YW, Rosen MJ. Negative pressure therapy for high-risk abdominal wall reconstruction incisions. Surg Inf 2013;14(3):270–4.
[38] Karlakki S, Brem M, Giannini S, Khanduja V, Stannard J, Martin R. Negative pressure wound therapy for management of the surgical incision in orthopaedic surgery: a review of evidence and mechanisms for an emerging indication. Bone Joint Res 2013;2(12):276–84.
[39] Allen G. Evidence appraisal of Blackham AU, Farrah JP, McCoy TP, Schmidt BS, Shen P. Prevention of surgical site infections in high-risk patients with laparotomy incisions using negative-pressure therapy. Am J Surg 2013;205(6):647–54. AORN J 2013;98(3):320–4.[Q3]
[40] Stevens P. Vacuum-assisted closure of laparostomy wounds: a critical review of the literature. Int Wound J 2009;6(4):259–66.
[41] Stannard JP, Volgas DA, Stewart R, McGwin G, Jr., Alonso JE. Negative pressure wound therapy after severe open fractures: a prospective randomized study. J Orthop Trauma 2009;23(8):552–7.

[42] Ubbink DT, Westerbos SJ, Nelson EA, Vermeulen H. A systematic review of topical negative pressure therapy for acute and chronic wounds. Br J Surg 2008;95(6):685–92.
[43] Anglim B, O'Connor H, Daly S. Prevena, negative pressure wound therapy applied to closed Pfannenstiel incisions at time of caesarean section in patients deemed at high risk for wound infection. J Obstet Gynaecol 2015;35(3):255–8.
[44] Payne C, Edwards D. Application of the single use negative pressure wound therapy device (PICO) on a heterogeneous group of surgical and traumatic wounds. Eplasty 2014;14:e20.
[45] Gregor S, Maegele M, Sauerland S, Krahn JF, Peinemann F, Lange S. Negative pressure wound therapy: a vacuum of evidence? Arch Surg 2008;143(2):189–96.

Christina M. Nowik and Gregory A. Davies

24 Vaginal delivery in the obese patient

24.1 Introduction

Maternal obesity presents several specific challenges to the labor and delivery process, including compromised myometrial contractility, prolonged labor, and challenges in monitoring. While acknowledging the unique risks faced by obese parturients, health care providers should take an evidence-based approach, wherever possible, to the intrapartum care of this population. Interventions without demonstrated benefit may, in fact, subject patients to harm. This is especially true as obese women undergoing cesarean delivery are at increased risk for anesthetic, infectious, and thromboembolic complications [1].

24.2 Altered uterine contractility

Biochemical and clinical studies both point to derangements of uterine contractility in obese pregnant women. This principle underlies many of the obstetrical complications that occur more frequently among obese patients [2].

In one study, female rats that were fed a high-fat, high-cholesterol diet demonstrated altered expression of several myometrial contractile-associated proteins. Myometrial strips from these rats also produced asynchronous contractions of variable amplitude during ex vivo studies, whereas rats that were fed a control diet exhibited stronger and more consistent contractions [3].

Myometrial biopsies from women undergoing elective cesarean delivery show a decline in myometrial activity, measured in vitro, with increasing body mass index (BMI). Human adipocytokines, a term representing a group of secretory products from adipose tissue, are also thought to affect myometrial contraction. Leptin and apelin concentration are both found to be elevated in obese patients. In vitro studies of myometrial strips exposed to each of these adipocytokines demonstrate a strong inhibitory effect on myometrial contractility [4, 5].

Furthermore, in the human uterus, ether-a-go-go potassium channels suppress contraction amplitude and duration. Beta inhibitory protein normally reduces this suppressive activity to achieve longer duration of uterine action potentials and contractions. However, increasing BMI has been associated with decreased beta inhibitory peptide, lending further support to the notion of impaired uterine contractility in obese women [6].

These findings are corroborated by clinical outcomes, as obesity is associated with prolonged labors and increased rates of cesarean delivery [7].

https://doi.org/10.1515/9783110487817-024

24.3 Management of the first stage of labor

Obesity seems to have a more marked effect on the first stage of labor than the second. It has been noted in multiple observational trials that obese women are more likely to have a prolonged first stage of labor [9, 10]. In particular, progress between 4 cm and 6 cm dilatation is significantly slower among pregnant women with BMI higher than 30 [10, 11]. The Consortium on Safe Labor examined detailed labor and delivery information from more than 118,000 eligible live, term singleton, cephalic deliveries in the United States [11]. Figures 24.1 and 24.2 depict the labor curves for nulliparas and multiparas, respectively, according to BMI. Overall, both nulliparous and multiparous women demonstrated prolongation of the first stage of labor with increasing BMI. Women with BMI higher than 40 required an average of 7.7 hours to achieve full dilatation, compared with 5.4 hours for women with BMI less than 25 [11].

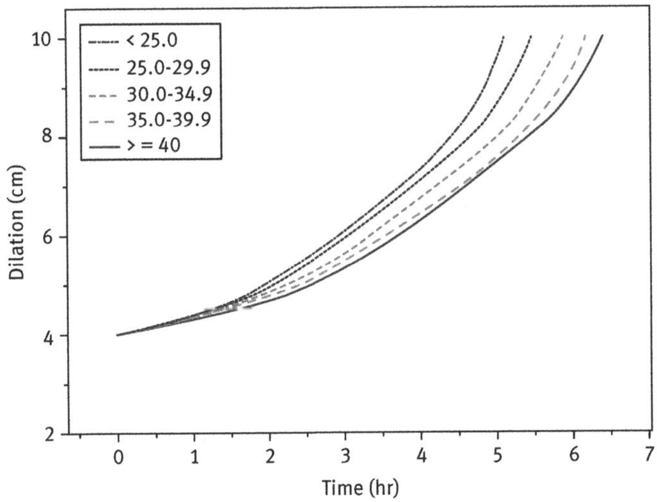

Fig. 24.1: Labor curves in nulliparas by BMI [11].

Obesity is associated with a significantly increased risk for cesarean delivery in the first stage of labor [12], primarily due to a higher incidence of labor dystocia/failure to progress [13]. Soni et al. [14] found that, in comparison to women with a BMI of <25, women with BMI greater than 35 were significantly more likely to require cesarean delivery after oxytocin augmentation for arrest of dilatation (69.6% vs. 11.4%).

In one large Swedish observational study, the odds ratios for cesarean delivery for ineffective uterine contractility were 2.14, 2.72, and 3.98 for class I, II, and III obesity, respectively (see Tab. 24.1) [13].

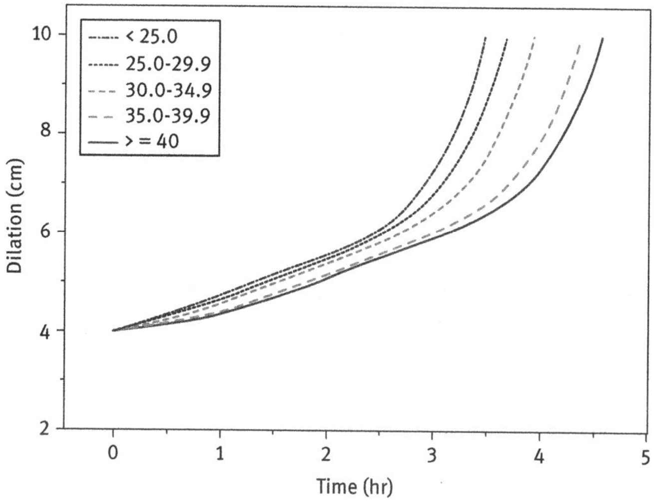

Fig. 24.2: Labor curves in multiparas by BMI [11].

Tab. 24.1: Definition of classes of obesity.

Category	**BMI (kg/m²)**
Underweight	<18.5
Normal weight	18.5–24.9
Overweight	25.0–29.9
Class I obesity	30.0–34.9
Class II obesity	35.0–39.9
Class III obesity*	≥40.0

*, Morbid obesity is usually defined as BMI ≥40.0 or BMI ≥35.0 with severe, obesity-related morbidity. Adapted from Erlanger & Henson, 2008; "Gastrointestinal surgery for severe obesity: National Institutes of Health Consensus Development Conference Statement," 1992) [75].

These findings have led many to question whether the standard management of labor should be altered to accommodate labor patterns that are expected to differ from those characterized by Friedman [15]. Given the proposed inhibitory effects of leptin on myometrial contractility, Wuntakal et al. [16] advocates for the early use of oxytocin augmentation to achieve five contractions in 10 minutes.

The Society of Obstetricians and Gynaecologists of Canada (SOGC) updated its clinical practice guideline for the management of spontaneous labor at term in healthy women in 2016 [17]. This guideline recommends that in a low-risk, nulliparous woman, cervical dilation after 4 cm as slow as 0.5 cm/h should be considered normal [17]. When oxytocin augmentation is required, the SOGC states that "a minimum of 4 to 6 hours of adequate uterine activity may be required to have the desired response" [17].

When oxytocin is used in response to arrested dilatation, women with BMI greater than 35 require significantly more oxytocin [14]. The American College of Obstetricians and Gynecologists recommends that, as long as there is reassuring maternal and fetal status, cesarean delivery should only be performed for active phase arrest if (a) there is at least 6 cm cervical dilatation and (b) there is no progress despite membrane rupture and either 4 hours of adequate contractions (i.e., >200 Montevideo units) or 6 hours of inadequate contractions [18].

It should be noted that obese women have an increased incidence of difficult vaginal examinations (OR 8.9) [19]. Under ideal circumstances, determination of cervical dilatation and effacement is subjective. In the case of a difficult vaginal examination, it may be necessary to place the patient in lithotomy position [19]. Furthermore, it may be advisable to minimize the number of different examiners to optimize the reliability of the assessment.

24.4 Management of the second stage of labor

In contrast to the dysfunctional patterns seen in the first stage of labor, obesity does not seem to be associated with an increased risk for dystocia in the second stage of labor. In fact, Carlhall et al. [9] noted the duration of the second stage of labor to be significantly shorter among obese nulliparous singletons in spontaneous labor, relative to normal weight women. One must take into account, however, that significantly more obese women had nonelective cesarean deliveries already in the first stage. It does seem, however, that based on large observational studies, obese women are not at increased risk of second stage cesarean delivery [20, 21].

24.5 Intrapartum monitoring

The SOGC recommends intermittent auscultation for "fetal surveillance during labor for healthy women without risk factors for adverse perinatal outcome" [22]. In women who are morbidly obese, the SOGC further suggests that "intrapartum electronic fetal surveillance may be beneficial" [22]. Although intermittent auscultation is a reasonable option in overweight and nonmorbidly obese women, an observational study in a Canadian academic health sciences center noted that women with increasing BMI were significantly less likely to receive intermittent auscultation at any point during labor (75.0% for BMI 18.5 to 24.9 vs. 64.4% for BMI 25.0 to 29.9 vs. 40.0% for BMI ≥30.0) [23]. It could not be determined in this study as to what extent the decreased use of intermittent auscultation in patients of higher BMI might be related to technical challenges of transducing the fetal heart rate through a thicker abdominal wall or maternal pannus, or to perceived risk for adverse perinatal outcome. The authors similarly could not glean whether the decreased use of intermittent auscultation might be independently associated with increased interventions in overweight and obese patients [23].

As obesity presents technical challenges for intermittent auscultation, continuous external fetal monitoring also has decreasing reliability with increasing BMI, especially when BMI is greater than 40 [24]. Similarly, morbidly obese patients are more likely to receive internal fetal monitoring during labor [19]. Abdominal-fetal electrocardiography is an emerging technology not commonly available at the time of this publication. Unlike continuous external monitoring, it does not seem to show a decline in reliability with increasing maternal BMI [24, 25], and this may evolve as an improved method of noninvasive fetal monitoring for obese patients.

Contractions are usually monitored with external tocodynamometry and manual palpation of the maternal abdomen. These techniques may not provide adequate monitoring of uterine contractions in obese patients where there is increased subcutaneous fat, thicker abdominal wall, and, possibly, a pannus [19, 26]. Therefore, an intrauterine pressure catheter, although not recommended for routine use, may be beneficial where a patient's contraction pattern cannot otherwise be reliably assessed. In particular, where there are concerns about labor progress, intrauterine pressure catheters accurately measure uterine contractility, which can inform the health care provider whether the patient has an adequate contraction pattern (i.e., 200 Montevideo units) [17].

Electrohysterography, which measures uterine electrical activity from the surface of the maternal abdomen, correlates well with readings from intrauterine pressure catheters [27, 24]. This represents a promising new technology for noninvasive monitoring of uterine contractions in the obese.

24.6 Fetal overgrowth and shoulder dystocia

Fetal overgrowth is typically characterized by the terms "large for gestational age" (≥90th percentile) or "macrosomia," which is usually defined as birth weight greater than 4,000 g [28]. A systematic review and meta-analysis including more than 214,000 deliveries of large-for-gestational age infants and more than 13,000 macrosomic infants solidified the association between obesity and fetal overgrowth. Specifically, BMI ≥30.0 was associated with a statistically significantly increased risk of large for gestational age (OR 2.423), birth weight greater than 4,000 g (OR 2.014), and birth weight greater than 4,500 g (OR 3.009) [28]. However, it was not possible to control for maternal diabetes in this meta-analysis. In a large retrospective analysis of more than 287,000 births, women with BMI ≥30 had a significantly increased risk of having a large-for-gestational age infant (OR 2.36), even after controlling for maternal diabetes [29]. Another observational study also noted an increased risk for birth weight greater than 4,000 g and 4,500 g (OR 1.58 and 1.87, respectively) among patients with BMI ≥50.0 compared with lean controls. This relationship was independent of gestational diabetes [30].

Several studies have noted an increased incidence of shoulder dystocia in obese patients. One Swedish population-based cohort study including 3,840 women with BMI >40 noted a significantly increased risk of shoulder dystocia when compared with lean controls (OR 2.14) [31]. However, this was not adjusted for birth weight or gestational diabetes, both known to contribute to shoulder dystocia [32]. A Canadian population-based cohort study noted that women with BMI ≥50.0 were at significantly higher risk of shoulder dystocia compared with normal weight patients (OR 1.51), even after controlling for gestational diabetes or macrosomia [30]. Conversely, a retrospective observational study that sought to identify the independent effects of obesity, gestational weight gain, and gestational diabetes, did not find a significant association between shoulder dystocia and obesity [33]. In general, it is not clear that obesity presents an independent risk factor for shoulder dystocia [8, 34]. Regardless, whether or not obesity is independently associated with shoulder dystocia, health care providers must be prepared for a greater incidence in the obese population.

Clinicians have sought to estimate the risk of shoulder dystocia by estimating fetal size. Fetal growth, however, is also more difficult to assess in obese patients. The accuracy of symphysis fundal height measurement declines with increasing maternal obesity [35]. Although it was thought that routine fetal growth assessment by ultrasound might be helpful, it has not been shown to confer significant benefit.

Despite improved ultrasound technology, the images obtained in obese patients are of generally lower quality because adipose tissue negatively affects the propagation of sound waves [37]. A prospective study comparing estimated fetal weight within 48 hours of delivery with birth weight demonstrated significantly increased absolute error with increasing BMI. Normal weight patients had an average absolute error of 106.97 g, compared with 248.82 g, 308.31 g, and 446.00 g for class I, class II, and class III obesity, respectively [37]. Another study examined third trimester estimated fetal weight with use of the gestation-adjusted projection method to estimate birth weight in obese women with singleton pregnancies [38]. Overall, ultrasound measurement tended to overestimate the birth weight of smaller infants and to underestimate the birth weight of larger infants. Ultrasound generally had low sensitivity and positive predictive value for birth weight of more than 4,000 g, although the specificity was high (see Tab. 24.2) [38]. Furthermore, the accuracy of ultrasound estimated fetal weight declines with advancing gestational age, particularly in patients with BMI >25, and with increasing fetal weight [39].

Tab. 24.2: Diagnostic accuracy of GAP method to predict birth weight at more than 4,000 g. Patients with BMI 35.1 to 39.9 were not included in the study [38].

Test characteristic	BMI (kg/m²)		
	30–35	40–50	>50
Sensitivity (%)	40.0	72.2	25.0
Specificity (%)	93.4	96.1	95.5
Positive predictive value (%)	45.5	76.5	42.9
Negative predictive value (%)	91.9	95.2	90.4

There is concern that false positive ultrasound findings of macrosomia may put patients at risk for unnecessary obstetrical interventions. In a retrospective cohort study, patients who had an estimated fetal weight of more than 4,000 g, but had birth weight between 3,500 and 4,000 g, were significantly more likely to have a cesarean delivery than patients with birth weights between 3,500 and 4,000 g but without the prenatal diagnosis of macrosomia [41].

It is unclear that obstetrical interventions for presumed macrosomia will prevent shoulder dystocia. Approximately 25% to 50% of deliveries complicated by shoulder dystocia occur in patients with birth weight less than 4,000 g, and most macrosomic fetuses will not have shoulder dystocia [42, 43]. Most cases of shoulder dystocia will not be associated with long-term injury. Brachial plexus injury complicates between 4% and 16% of deliveries with shoulder dystocia [44, 40]; however, the majority will resolve without permanent dysfunction [44].

A randomized controlled trial demonstrated that induction of labor between 37 and 38 + 6 weeks gestation for estimated fetal weight greater than the 95th percentile significantly decreased the incidence of shoulder dystocia without increasing the rate of cesarean delivery [45]. However, there is no evidence that such a policy would have a significant effect on fetal morbidity.

Despite the limitations of antenatal assessment of fetal weight, the risk of shoulder dystocia does increase significantly with increasing macrosomia; 13% of deliveries of infants greater than 5,000 g will be complicated by shoulder dystocia [43]. Although they have identified the level of evidence supporting their recommendation is of low quality, the American College of Obstetricians and Gynecologists recommends primary cesarean delivery when estimated fetal weight exceeds 4,500 g in diabetic patients or 5,000 g in nondiabetic patients, but does not recommend routine fetal biometry [18]. The Royal College of Obstetricians and Gynaecologists supports consideration of primary cesarean delivery in diabetic patients only with estimated fetal weight greater than 4,500 g, citing the large numbers needed to treat to prevent one brachial plexus injury in nondiabetic patients [46].

24.7 Operative vaginal delivery

There is no clear association between obesity and operative vaginal delivery. An analysis from the prospective Norwegian Mother and Child Cohort Study revealed a small but significantly increased incidence of vacuum-assisted vaginal delivery among women with prepregnancy BMI greater than 40 (OR 1.5) [47]. Another prospective observational study of more than 16,000 patients revealed a significant association between BMI ≥35, but not BMI 30 to 34.9, and operative vaginal delivery, although the OR was only 1.7 [48]. Neither Sebire et al.'s [29] large Swedish cohort study nor the Canadian All Our Babies Cohort study [49] demonstrated any significant difference in the rate of operative vaginal delivery among obese patients. It is not possible to determine to what extent provider bias or comfort with operative vaginal delivery in obese patients may explain these variable results [49].

24.8 Obstetrical trauma

Higher birth weight and operative vaginal delivery are both independent risk factors for perineal tears, particularly obstetrical anal sphincter injuries (OASIS) [50]. However, obesity is not clearly associated with increased perineal lacerations, and may be protective against OASIS. In a retrospective cohort study of 5,569 term vaginal deliveries, obesity was not associated with having any perineal laceration versus no laceration, and there was no association between BMI and OASIS [50]. In another retrospective analysis of more than 210,000 primiparous deliveries in Sweden, obesity was associated with a small but significant increased risk of first- and second-degree perineal tears (OR 1.32 when BMI ≥35). Conversely, obesity was protective against OASIS in a dose-dependent fashion. In multivariate analysis, the odds ratios for OASIS were 0.84 for BMI 30.0 to 34.9 and 0.70 for BMI ≥35 [51]. A case control study including 605 OASIS cases noted a significantly decreased incidence of OASIS in women with BMI ≥30 (OR 0.75). The risk of OASIS was further reduced in patients with BMI ≥40.0 (OR 0.52) [52]. Crane et al. [30] found no association between BMI ≥50 and OASIS.

24.9 Post-dates pregnancy

Obese women are more likely to have post-dates pregnancy, with odds ratios between 1.26 and 1.69 in large observational studies [53–55]. The risk of prolonged pregnancy is even further increased with morbid obesity (OR 2.27 compared with normal BMI) [56]. This may be a product of the inhibitory effect of adipocytokines on myometrial contractility [57]. Furthermore, proinflammatory cytokines are thought to play an important role in triggering local prostaglandin synthesis [10], and obese women demonstrate inflammatory upregulation, including elevated C-reactive protein [58].

Most obese women with post-dates pregnancy will still deliver vaginally. Arrowsmith et al. [56] noted in a large observational study that 61.3% of obese nulliparas and 90.1% of obese multiparas delivered vaginally after induction of labor for post-dates pregnancy.

24.10 Induction of labor

Obese women undergo induction of labor more often than lean controls [29, 49, 59]. In the latter Canadian cohort study by Vinturache et al. [49], 49% of obese patients were induced, compared with 28.8% of their normal weight population. Crane et al. [30] noted that 39% of women with BMI ≥50 were induced versus 30% of lean controls. This can be explained, at least in part, by increased incidence of post-dates pregnancy [54], hypertension, and diabetes [60].

Patients with an unfavorable cervix typically receive some form of cervical ripening to reduce the chance of cesarean delivery [61]. Obese patients may be less likely to achieve a favorable cervix. An observational study by Gauthier et al. [62] noted that obese women with a Bishop score of ≤3 undergoing cervical ripening with PGE2 vaginal inserts or gel were significantly less likely to achieve a Bishop score of 6 after one dose compared with normal weight, parity-matched controls. Obese women also received significantly more PGE2 (mean number of PGE2 administrations 1.4 vs. 1.2), but the clinical significance of such a difference is unclear. Moreover, a secondary analysis of the Misoprostol Vaginal Insert Trial (a randomized trial of misoprostol and dinoprostone) demonstrated that, after adjusting for race, parity, and treatment allocation, women with BMI 30 to 39.9 and ≥40 were significantly less likely than women with BMI less than 30 to deliver within 24 hours (OR 0.75 and 0.52, respectively) [63].

In keeping with the increased incidence of failure to progress in the first stage of labor, inductions are more likely to fail in obese patients [63]. The risk of failed induction increases with increasing BMI. Gunatilake et al. [60] noted that 39.7% of nulliparous women with BMI 40 to 50 who were induced beyond 34 weeks with a singleton pregnancy eventually had cesarean delivery. This increased to 65% for BMI 50 to 60 and 77.8% for BMI >60. Arrest of labor and failed induction of labor accounted for 64% of the cesarean deliveries in that study [60]. Among multiparas, obesity was not an independent predictor of cesarean delivery [60]. This study was somewhat limited in sample size. As there were only 19 subjects with BMI >60, the authors cautioned that their findings required validation [60]. Pevzner et al. [63] similarly found that the incidence of cesarean delivery after cervical ripening and induction of labor was 21.3% for women with BMI less than 30, but increased to 29.8% for BMI 30 to 39.9 and to 39.9% for BMI 40 or higher.

Having highlighted these concerns, contemporary large population-based cohort studies suggest that induction of labor does not increase risk for cesarean delivery relative to expectant management [64]. A large, retrospective cohort study compared induction of labor of patients with BMI ≥30 at 37, 38, and 39 weeks gestational age with expectant management. Elective induction of labor at 37 and 39 weeks (compared with expectant management) was associated with a significantly decreased risk of cesarean delivery among nulliparous women (OR 0.55 and 0.77, respectively) [66]. Multiparous women who had elective induction of labor at 38, 39, and 40 weeks similarly had a decreased risk of cesarean delivery. It was not possible to control for cervical status in that study [66]. Elective induction of labor at 37 to 39 weeks was also associated with a significantly decreased risk of macrosomia, without a significant change in shoulder dystocia or brachial plexus injury [66]. This study is limited by its retrospective nature, and major societies have not endorsed such a policy of elective induction, but this provides interesting direction for future research.

24.11 Vaginal birth after cesarean

Trial of labor after a previous cesarean delivery is associated with a small increase in perinatal mortality and major maternal complications (i.e., uterine rupture, hysterectomy, operative injury), although the absolute risks are small [67, 68]. Patients who have a failed trial of labor are subject to the greatest risk of major complications [67], and obese patients attempting vaginal birth after cesarean (VBAC) are at increased risk for failed trial of labor compared with normal weight patients. In a retrospective analysis of 510 eligible patients attempting VBAC, only 54.6% of obese patients had a successful VBAC compared with 70.3% of patients with normal BMI [69].

The risks associated with VBAC seem to increase with increasing obesity. In another prospective observational study of term singletons attempting VBAC, 15.2% of normal weight women had failed trial of labor, compared with 29.9% of patients with BMI 30.0 to 39.9 and 39.3% of patients with BMI ≥40.0 [70]. Chauhan et al. [71] performed a prospective observational study of 30 women weighing greater than 300 lb. who attempted VBAC; only four patients (13%) had a successful VBAC. Another observational study of patients with BMI ≥50.0 noted a 35% (9/26) rate of successful VBAC [72].

Obese patients attempting VBAC are at increased risk for emergency cesarean delivery; in addition, the interval from decision to delivery is generally longer in obese patients [26]. A retrospective study of 826 emergency cesarean deliveries at a Canadian tertiary level hospital showed that the decision-to-incision and decision-to-delivery intervals were both increased by an average of 4.5 minutes among obese versus nonobese patients. The majority were nonetheless delivered in less than 30 minutes in both groups [73]. Because the mean difference for the two intervals was equivalent, this suggests that the increased time required to carry out a cesarean delivery in obese patients is related to patient transportation and anesthetic preparation rather than surgical time [73]. However, another observational study noted that increasing BMI was associated with significantly increased time from skin incision to infant delivery [74].

When counseling an obese patient about VBAC options, health care providers should communicate the increased risks of failed VBAC, particularly in the morbidly obese, and the associated risks for complications. This counseling should also take into account the capabilities of an individual center to provide emergency cesarean delivery to obese patients who may require extra time and resources for transportation, anesthesia, and surgery. It would be reasonable for such considerations to sway some patients and health care providers toward elective repeat cesarean delivery, particularly in the morbidly obese patient.

24.12 Planned cesarean delivery

Given the increased risk for failure to progress and other complications faced by obese patients, in addition to the added morbidity of an emergency (versus elective) cesarean delivery, some have suggested planned primary cesarean delivery for some obese patients. Crane et al. [30] noted a 31.7% primary cesarean delivery rate in an observational study of patients with BMI ≥50.0. In another observational study comparing outcomes of women with BMI ≥50.0 planning vaginal versus cesarean delivery, 30.5% of those who had planned a vaginal delivery required cesarean delivery [72]. There was a trend towards decreased major maternal morbidity (a composite of haemorrhage, thromboembolism, septicaemia, septic shock, and/or admission to an intensive care unit) amongst the planned vaginal delivery group, although there were no differences in anesthetic complications, wound complications, or neonatal morbidity [72]. These findings should be interpreted with caution, as the groups were not randomized.

In the absence of evidence supporting planned cesarean delivery for obesity, such a broad policy should not be recommended, even for extreme BMI. However, the relationship between obesity, labor, and delivery is especially complex when one takes into account other complicating factors that are associated with obesity (e.g., preeclampsia, gestational diabetes, macrosomia). The effect of obesity and related conditions should be discussed with the obese patient seeking vaginal delivery well before the onset of labor. The clinical approach should be individualized, respecting the autonomy of the patient who may be faced with difficult decisions.

Bibliography

[1] Machado LSM. Cesarean section in morbidly obese parturients: practical implications and complications. N Am J Med Sci 2012;4(1):13–8. doi:10.4103/1947-2714.92895.

[2] Lowe NK, Corwin EJ. Proposed biological linkages between obesity, stress, and inefficient uterine contractility during labor in humans. Med Hypotheses 2011;76(5):755–60. doi:10.1016/j.mehy.2011.02.018.

[3] Muir R, Ballan J, Clifford B, McMullen S, Khan R, Shmygol A, Elmes M. Modelling maternal obesity: the effects of a chronic high-fat, high-cholesterol diet on uterine expression of contractile-associated proteins and ex vivo contractile activity during labour in the rat. Clin Sci (Lond) 2016;130(3):183–92. doi:10.1042/cs20150539.

[4] Moynihan AT, Hehir MP, Glavey SV, Smith TJ, Morrison JJ. Inhibitory effect of leptin on human uterine contractility in vitro. Am J Obstet Gynecol 2006;195(2):504–9. doi:10.1016/j.ajog.2006.01.106.

[5] Hehir MP, Morrison JJ. The adipokine apelin and human uterine contractility. Am J Obstet Gynecol 2012;206(4):359.e351–5. doi:10.1016/j.ajog.2012.01.032.

[6] Parkington HC, Stevenson J, Tonta MA, Paul J, Butler T, Maiti K, Smith R. Diminished hERG K+ channel activity facilitates strong human labour contractions but is dysregulated in obese women. Nat Commun 2014;5:4108. doi:10.1038/ncomms5108.

[7] Norman SM, Tuuli MG, Odibo AO, Caughey AB, Roehl KA, Cahill AG. The effects of obesity on the first stage of labor. Obstet Gynecol 2012;120(1):130–5. doi:10.1097/AOG.0b013e318259589c.

[8] Sheiner E, Levy A, Menes TS, Silverberg D, Katz M, Mazor M. Maternal obesity as an independent risk factor for caesarean delivery. Paediatr Perinat Epidemiol 2004;18(3):196–201. doi:10.1111/j.1365-3016.2004.00557.x.

[9] Carlhall S, Kallen K, Blomberg M. Maternal body mass index and duration of labor. Eur J Obstet Gynecol Reprod Biol 2013;171(1):49–53. doi:10.1016/j.ejogrb.2013.08.021.
[10] Bogaerts A, Witters I, Van den Bergh BR, Jans G, Devlieger R. Obesity in pregnancy: altered onset and progression of labour. Midwifery 2013;29(12):1303–13. doi:10.1016/j.midw.2012.12.013.
[11] Kominiarek MA, Zhang J, Vanveldhuisen, P, Troendle J, Beaver J, Hibbard JU. Contemporary labor patterns: the impact of maternal body mass index. Am J Obstet Gynecol 2011;205(3):244.e241–8. doi:10.1016/j.ajog.2011.06.014.
[12] Zhang J, Bricker L, Wray S, Quenby S. Poor uterine contractility in obese women. BJOG 2007;114(3):343–8. doi:10.1111/j.1471-0528.2006.01233.x.
[13] Cedergren MI. Non-elective caesarean delivery due to ineffective uterine contractility or due to obstructed labour in relation to maternal body mass index. Eur J Obstet Gynecol Reprod Biol 2009;145(2):163–6. doi:10.1016/j.ejogrb.2009.05.022.
[14] Soni S, Chivan N, Cohen WR. Effect of maternal body mass index on oxytocin treatment for arrest of dilatation. J Perinat Med 2013;41(5):517–21. doi:10.1515/jpm-2013-0024.
[15] Friedman EA. Primigravid labor: a graphicostatistical analysis. Obstet Gynecol 1955;6(6):567–89.
[16] Wuntakal R, Kaler M, Hollingworth T. Women with high BMI: should they be managed differently due to antagonising action of leptin in labour? Med Hypotheses 2013;80(6):767–8. doi:10.1016/j.mehy.2013.03.006.
[17] Lee L, Dy J, Azzam H. Management of spontaneous labour at term in healthy women. J Obstet Gynaecol Can 2016;38(9):843–65. doi:10.1016/j.jogc.2016.04.093.
[18] Caughey AB, Cahill AG, Guise JM, Rouse DJ. Safe prevention of the primary cesarean delivery. Am J Obstet Gynecol 2014;210(3):179–93. doi:10.1016/j.ajog.2014.01.026.
[19] Ray A, Hildreth A, Esen UI. Morbid obesity and intra-partum care. J Obstet Gynaecol 2008;28(3):301–4. doi:10.1080/01443610802042548.
[20] Fyfe EM, Anderson NH, North RA, Chan EH, Taylor RS, Dekker GA, McCowan LM. Risk of first-stage and second-stage cesarean delivery by maternal body mass index among nulliparous women in labor at term. Obstet Gynecol 2011;117(6):1315–22. doi:10.1097/AOG.0b013e318217922a.
[21] Hirshberg A, Levine LD, Srinivas S. Labor length among overweight and obese women undergoing induction of labor. J Matern Fetal Neonatal Med 2014;27(17):1771–5. doi:10.3109/14767058.2013.879705.
[22] Liston R, Sawchuck D, Young D. Fetal health surveillance: antepartum and intrapartum consensus guideline. J Obstet Gynaecol Can 2007;29(9 Suppl 4):S3–56.
[23] Sheth Thakkar S, Lammers S, Hahn PM, Waddington A. The use of intermittent auscultation in parturients of varying BMI categories: experience from a mid-sized tertiary care obstetrical unit. J Obstet Gynaecol Can 2015;37(4):310–13.
[24] Cohen WR, Hayes-Gill B. Influence of maternal body mass index on accuracy and reliability of external fetal monitoring techniques. Acta Obstet Gynecol Scand 2014;93(6):590–5. doi:10.1111/aogs.12387.
[25] Jezewski J, Matonia A, Kupka T, Roj D, Czabanski R. Determination of fetal heart rate from abdominal signals: evaluation of beat-to-beat accuracy in relation to the direct fetal electrocardiogram. Biomed Tech (Berl) 2012;57(5):383–94. doi:10.1515/bmt-2011-0130.
[26] Davies GA, Maxwell C, McLeod L, Gagnon R, Basso M, Bos H, Wilson K. SOGC clinical practice guidelines: obesity in pregnancy. No. 239, February 2010. Int J Gynaecol Obstet 2010;110(2):167–73.
[27] Euliano TY, Nguyen MT, Marossero D, Edwards RK. Monitoring contractions in obese parturients: electrohysterography compared with traditional monitoring. Obstet Gynecol 2007;109(5):1136–40. doi:10.1097/01.aog.0000258799.24496.93.
[28] Gaudet L, Ferraro ZM, Wen SW, Walker M. Maternal obesity and occurrence of fetal macrosomia: a systematic review and meta-analysis. Biomed Res Int 2014;2014:640291. doi:10.1155/2014/640291.

[29] Sebire NJ, Jolly M, Harris JP, Wadsworth J, Joffe M, Beard RW, Robinson S. Maternal obesity and pregnancy outcome: a study of 287,213 pregnancies in London. Int J Obes Relat Metab Disord 2001;25(8):1175–82. doi:10.1038/sj.ijo.0801670.
[30] Crane JM, Murphy P, Burrage L, Hutchens D. Maternal and perinatal outcomes of extreme obesity in pregnancy. J Obstet Gynaecol Can 2013;35(7):606–11.
[31] Cedergren MI. Maternal morbid obesity and the risk of adverse pregnancy outcome. Obstet Gynecol 2004;103(2):219–24. doi:10.1097/01.aog.0000107291.46159.00.
[32] Acker DB, Sachs BP, Friedman EA. Risk factors for shoulder dystocia. Obstet Gynecol 1985;66(6):762–8.
[33] Cosson E, Cussac-Pillegand C, Benbara A, Pharisien I, Nguyen MT, Chiheb S, Carbillon L. Pregnancy adverse outcomes related to pregravid body mass index and gestational weight gain, according to the presence or not of gestational diabetes mellitus: a retrospective observational study. Diabetes Metab 2016;42(1):38–46. doi:10.1016/j.diabet.2015.06.001.
[34] Deneux-Tharaux C, Delorme P. [Epidemiology of shoulder dystocia]. J Gynecol Obstet Biol Reprod (Paris) 2015;44(10):1234–47. doi:10.1016/j.jgyn.2015.09.036.
[35] Drassinower D, Timofeev J, Huang CC, Benson JE, Driggers RW, Landy HJ. Accuracy of clinically estimated fetal weight in pregnancies complicated by diabetes mellitus and obesity. Am J Perinatol 2014;31(1):31–7. doi:10.1055/s-0033-1334450.
[36] Rai L, Kurien L, Kumar P. Symphysis fundal height curve—a simple method for foetal growth assessment. J Postgrad Med 1995;41(4):93–4.
[37] Aksoy H, Aksoy U, Karadag OI, Yucel B, Aydin T, Babayigit MA. Influence of maternal body mass index on sonographic fetal weight estimation prior to scheduled delivery. J Obstet Gynaecol Res 2015;41(10):1556–61. doi:10.1111/jog.12755.
[38] Ahmadzia HK, Thomas SM, Dude AM, Grotegut CA, Boyd BK. Prediction of birthweight from third-trimester ultrasound in morbidly obese women. Am J Obstet Gynecol 2014;211(4):431.e431–7. doi:10.1016/j.ajog.2014.06.041.
[39] Paganelli S, Soncini E, Comitini G, Palomba S, La Sala GB. Sonographic fetal weight estimation in normal and overweight/obese healthy term pregnant women by gestation-adjusted projection (GAP) method. Arch Gynecol Obstet 2016;293(4):775–81. doi:10.1007/s00404-015-3910-z.
[40] Politi S, D'Emidio L, Cignini P, Giorlandino M, Giorlandino C. Shoulder dystocia: an evidence-based approach. J Prenat Med 2010;4(3):35–42.
[41] Parry S, Severs CP, Sehdev HM, Macones GA, White LM, Morgan MA. Ultrasonographic prediction of fetal macrosomia. Association with cesarean delivery. J Reprod Med 2000;45(1):17–22.
[42] Baskett TF, Allen AC. Perinatal implications of shoulder dystocia. Obstet Gynecol 1995;86(1):14–17. doi:10.1016/0029-7844(95)00099-d.
[43] Overland EA, Vatten LJ, Eskild A. Risk of shoulder dystocia: associations with parity and offspring birthweight. A population study of 1 914 544 deliveries. Acta Obstet Gynecol Scand 2012;91(4):483–88. doi:10.1111/j.1600-0412.2011.01354.x.
[44] Gherman RB, Ouzounian JG, Goodwin TM. Obstetric maneuvers for shoulder dystocia and associated fetal morbidity. Am J Obstet Gynecol 1998;178(6):1126–30.
[45] Boulvain M, Senat MV, Perrotin F, Winer N, Beucher G, Subtil D, Rozenberg P. Induction of labour versus expectant management for large-for-date fetuses: a randomised controlled trial. Lancet 2015;385(9987):2600–605. doi:10.1016/s0140-6736(14)61904-8.
[46] Royal College of Obstetricians and Gynaecologists. "Shoulder Dystocia." Green-Top Guideline No. 42. 2012. 2nd edition.
[47] Morken NH, Klungsoyr K, Magnus P, Skjaerven R. Pre-pregnant body mass index, gestational weight gain and the risk of operative delivery. Acta Obstet Gynecol Scand 2013;92(7):809–15. doi:10.1111/aogs.12115.

[48] Weiss JL, Malone FD, Emig D, Ball RH, Nyberg DA, Comstock CH, D'Alton ME. Obesity, obstetric complications and cesarean delivery rate—a population-based screening study. Am J Obstet Gynecol 2004;190(4):1091–97. doi:10.1016/j.ajog.2003.09.058.
[49] Vinturache A, Moledina N, McDonald S, Slater D, Tough S. Pre-pregnancy body mass index (BMI) and delivery outcomes in a Canadian population. BMC Pregnancy Childbirth 2014;14:422. doi:10.1186/s12884-014-0422-y.
[50] Meister MR, Cahill AG, Conner SN, Woolfolk CL, Lowder JL. Predicting obstetric anal sphincter injuries in a modern obstetric population. Am J Obstet Gynecol 2016;215(3):310.e311–17. doi:10.1016/j.ajog.2016.02.041.
[51] Lindholm ES, Altman D. Risk of obstetric anal sphincter lacerations among obese women. BJOG 2013;120(9):1110–15. doi:10.1111/1471-0528.12228.
[52] Garretto D, Lin BB, Syn HL, Judge N, Beckerman K, Atallah F, Bernstein PS. Obesity may be protective against severe perineal lacerations. J Obes 2016;2016:9376592. doi:10.1155/2016/9376592.
[53] Usha Kiran TS, Hemmadi S, Bethel J, Evans J. Outcome of pregnancy in a woman with an increased body mass index. BJOG 2005;112(6):768–72. doi:10.1111/j.1471-0528.2004.00546.x.
[54] Caughey, AB, Stotland NE, Washington AE, Escobar GJ. Who is at risk for prolonged and postterm pregnancy? Am J Obstet Gynecol 2009;200(6):683.e681–5. doi:10.1016/j.ajog.2009.02.034.
[55] Stotland NE, Washington AE, Caughey AB. Prepregnancy body mass index and the length of gestation at term. Am J Obstet Gynecol 2007;197(4):378.e371–5. doi:10.1016/j.ajog.2007.05.048.
[56] Arrowsmith S, Wray S, Quenby S. Maternal obesity and labour complications following induction of labour in prolonged pregnancy. BJOG 2011;118(5):578–88. doi:10.1111/j.1471-0528.2010.02889.x.
[57] AlSaif S, Mumtaz S, Wray S. A short review of adipokines, smooth muscle and uterine contractility. Life Sci 2015;125:2–8. doi:10.1016/j.lfs.2015.02.001.
[58] Ramsay JE, Ferrell WR, Crawford L, Wallace AM, Greer IA, Sattar N. Maternal obesity is associated with dysregulation of metabolic, vascular, and inflammatory pathways. J Clin Endocrinol Metab 2002;87(9):4231–7. doi:10.1210/jc.2002-020311.
[59] Hermann M, Le Ray C, Blondel B, Goffinet F, Zeitlin J. The risk of prelabor and intrapartum cesarean delivery among overweight and obese women: possible preventive actions. Am J Obstet Gynecol 2015;212(2):241.e241–249. doi:10.1016/j.ajog.2014.08.002.
[60] Gunatilake RP, Smrtka MP, Harris B, Kraus DM, Small MJ, Grotegut CA, Brown HL. Predictors of failed trial of labor among women with an extremely obese body mass index. Am J Obstet Gynecol 2013;209(6):562.e561–5. doi:10.1016/j.ajog.2013.07.023.
[61] Leduc D, Biringer A, Lee L, Dy J, Corbett T, Leduc D, Senikas, V. Induction of labour. J Obstet Gynaecol Can 2016;35(9):840–57. doi:10.1016/S1701-2163(15)30842-2.
[62] Gauthier T, Mazeau S, Dalmay F, Eyraud JL, Catalan C, Marin B, Aubard Y. Obesity and cervical ripening failure risk. J Matern Fetal Neonatal Med 2012;25(3):304–7. doi:10.3109/14767058.2011.575485.
[63] Pevzner L, Powers BL, Rayburn WF, Rumney P, Wing DA. Effects of maternal obesity on duration and outcomes of prostaglandin cervical ripening and labor induction. Obstet Gynecol 2009;114(6):1315–21. doi:10.1097/AOG.0b013e3181bfb39f.
[64] Darney BG, Snowden JM, Cheng YW, Jacob L, Nicholson JM. Kaimal A, Caughey AB. Elective induction of labor at term compared with expectant management: maternal and neonatal outcomes. Obstet Gynecol 2013;122(4):761–9. doi:10.1097/AOG.0b013e3182a6a4d0.
[65] Stock SJ, Ferguson E, Duffy A, Ford I, Chalmers J, Norman JE. Outcomes of elective induction of labour compared with expectant management: population based study. BMJ 2012;344:e2838. doi:10.1136/bmj.e2838.

[66] Lee VR, Darney BG, Snowden JM, Main EK, Gilbert W, Chung J, Caughey AB. Term elective induction of labour and perinatal outcomes in obese women: retrospective cohort study. BJOG 2016;123(2):271–8. doi:10.1111/1471-0528.13807.
[67] McMahon MJ, Luther ER, Bowes WAJ, Olshan AF. Comparison of a trial of labor with an elective second cesarean section. N Engl J Med 1996;335(10):689–95. doi:doi:10.1056/NEJM199609053351001.
[68] Mozurkewich EL, Hutton EK. Elective repeat cesarean delivery versus trial of labor: a meta-analysis of the literature from 1989 to 1999. Am J Obstet Gynecol 2000;183(5):1187–97. doi:10.1067/mob.2000.108890.
[69] Durnwald CP, Ehrenberg HM, Mercer BM. The impact of maternal obesity and weight gain on vaginal birth after cesarean section success. Am J Obstet Gynecol 2004;191(3):954–7. doi:10.1016/j.ajog.2004.05.051.
[70] Hibbard JU, Gilbert S, Landon MB, Hauth JC, Leveno KJ, Spong CY, Gabbe SG. Trial of labor or repeat cesarean delivery in women with morbid obesity and previous cesarean delivery. Obstet Gynecol 2006;108(1):125–33. doi:10.1097/01.aog.0000223871.69852.31.
[71] Chauhan SP, Magann EF, Carroll CS, Barrilleaux PS, Scardo JA, Martin JN, Jr. Mode of delivery for the morbidly obese with prior cesarean delivery: vaginal versus repeat cesarean section. Am J Obstet Gynecol 2001;185(2):349–54. doi:10.1067/mob.2001.116729.
[72] Homer CS, Kurinczuk JJ, Spark P, Brocklehurst P, Knight M. Planned vaginal delivery or planned caesarean delivery in women with extreme obesity. BJOG 2011;118(4):480–7. doi:10.1111/j.1471-0528.2010.02832.x.
[73] Pulman KJ, Tohidi M, Pudwell J, Davies GAL. Emergency caesarean section in obese parturients: is a 30-minute decision-to-incision interval feasible? J Obstet Gynaecol Can 2016;37(11):988–94. doi:10.1016/S1701-2163(16)30048-2.
[74] Conner SN, Tuuli MG, Longman RE, Odibo AO, Macones GA, Cahill AG. Impact of obesity on incision-to-delivery interval and neonatal outcomes at cesarean delivery. Am J Obstet Gynecol 2013;209(4):386.e381–386. doi:10.1016/j.ajog.2013.05.054.
[75] Erlanger SR, Henson EA. Classification and pharmacological management of obesity. P&T 2008;33(12):724–8.

Index

https://doi.org/10.1515/9783110487817-025

Printed and bound by CPI Group (UK) Ltd, Croydon, CR0 4YY
13/09/2026
14960858-0002